Preoperative Patient Evaluation

Editors

ZDRAVKA ZAFIROVA
RICHARD D. URMAN

ANESTHESIOLOGY CLINICS

www.anesthesiology.theclinics.com

Consulting Editor
LEE A. FLEISHER

December 2018 • Volume 36 • Number 4

ELSEVIER

1600 John F. Kennedy Boulevard • Suite 1800 • Philadelphia, Pennsylvania, 19103-2899

http://www.theclinics.com

ANESTHESIOLOGY CLINICS Volume 36, Number 4
December 2018 ISSN 1932-2275, ISBN-13: 978-0-323-64308-5

Editor: Colleen Dietzler
Developmental Editor: Kristen Helm

Anesthesiology Clinics (ISSN 1932-2275) is published quarterly by Elsevier Inc., 360 Park Avenue South, New York, NY 10010-1710. Months of issue are March, June, September, and December. Periodicals postage paid at New York, NY and at additional mailing offices. Subscription prices are $100.00 per year (US student/resident), $346.00 per year (US individuals), $437.00 per year (Canadian individuals), $657.00 per year (US institutions), $830.00 per year (Canadian institutions), $225.00 per year (Canadian and foreign student/resident), $460.00 per year (foreign individuals), and $830.00 per year (foreign institutions). To receive student and resident rate, orders must be accompanied by name of affiliated institution, date of term, and the *signature* of program/residency coordinator on institutions letterhead. Orders will be billed at individual rate until proof of status is received. Foreign air speed delivery is included in all *Clinics'* subscription prices. All prices are subject to change without notice. POSTMASTER: Send address changes to *Anesthesiology Clinics,* Elsevier Health Sciences Division, Subscription Customer Service, 3251 Riverport Lane, Maryland Heights, MO 63043. Customer Service (orders, claims, online, change of address): Elsevier Health Sciences Division, Subscription Customer Service, 3251 Riverport Lane, Maryland Heights, MO 63043. **Tel:1-800-654-2452 (U.S. and Canada); 314-447-8871 (outside U.S. and Canada). Fax: 314-447-8029. E-mail: journalscustomerservice-usa@elsevier.com (for print support); journalsonlinesupport-usa@elsevier.com (for online support).**

Reprints. For copies of 100 or more of articles in this publication, please contact the Commercial Reprints Department, Elsevier Inc., 360 Park Avenue South, New York, NY 10010-1710. Tel.: 212-633-3874; Fax: 212-633-3820; E-mail: reprints@elsevier.com.

Anesthesiology Clinics, is also published in Spanish by McGraw-Hill Inter-americana Editores S. A., P.O. Box 5-237, 06500 Mexico D. F., Mexico.

Anesthesiology Clinics, is covered in *MEDLINE/PubMed (Index Medicus), Current Contents/Clinical Medicine, Excerpta Medica, ISI/BIOMED,* and *Chemical Abstracts.*

Printed in the United States of America.

Contributors

CONSULTING EDITOR

LEE A. FLEISHER, MD
Robert D. Dripps Professor and Chair of Anesthesiology and Critical Care, Professor of Medicine, Perelman School of Medicine, University of Pennsylvania, Philadelphia, Pennsylvania, USA

EDITORS

ZDRAVKA ZAFIROVA, MD
Associate Professor, Section of Critical Care, Department of Cardiovascular Surgery, Mount Sinai Hospital System, Icahn School of Medicine at Mount Sinai, Mount Sinai Medical Center, New York, New York, USA

RICHARD D. URMAN, MD, MBA, CPE, FASA
Associate Professor, Department of Anesthesiology, Perioperative and Pain Medicine, Center for Perioperative Research, Brigham and Women's Hospital, Harvard Medical School, Boston, Massachusetts, USA

AUTHORS

ALISON M. A'COURT, MD
Assistant Clinical Professor, Department of Anesthesiology, Director, Preoperative Care Clinic, University of California, San Diego, La Jolla, California, USA

BASEM ABDELMALAK, MD, FASA
Professor of Anesthesiology, Cleveland Clinic Lerner College of Medicine of Case Western Reserve University, Director of Anesthesia for Bronchoscopic Surgery, Director, Center for Procedural Sedation, Departments of General Anesthesiology and Outcomes Research, Anesthesiology Institute, Cleveland Clinic, Cleveland, Ohio, USA

DUSICA BAJIC, MD, PhD
Assistant Professor of Anaesthesia, Department of Anesthesiology, Critical Care and Pain Medicine, Boston Children's Hospital, Department of Anaesthesia, Harvard Medical School, Boston, Massachusetts, USA

ALLISON BASEL, MD
Anesthesiology Resident, Department of Anesthesia, Critical Care, and Pain Medicine, Beth Israel Deaconess Medical Center, Department of Anesthesiology, Critical Care and Pain Medicine, Boston Children's Hospital, Boston, Massachusetts, USA

JEANNA D. BLITZ, MD
Medical Director, Preadmission Testing, NYU Langone Health, Assistant Professor, Department of Anesthesiology, Perioperative Care and Pain Medicine, NYU School of Medicine, New York, New York, USA

DELIA BORUNDA, MD
Department of Anesthesiology and Perioperative Medicine, Centro de Desarrollo de
Destrezas Medicas CEDDEM, Instituto Nacional de Ciencias Medicas y Nutrición
"Salvador Zubirán", Mexico City, Mexico

ETHAN Y. BROVMAN, MD
Fellow, Cardiothoracic Anesthesia, Department of Anesthesiology, Perioperative and
Pain Medicine, Harvard Medical School, Brigham and Women's Hospital, Boston,
Massachusetts, USA

REBECCA BUDISH, MS
Medical Student, Department of Anesthesiology, LSU Health Shreveport, Shreveport,
Louisiana, USA

BRITTANY N. BURTON, MHS
Medical Student, School of Medicine, University of California, San Diego, La Jolla,
California, USA

FRANCES CHUNG, MBBS, FRCPC
Professor, Department of Anesthesiology, Toronto Western Hospital, University Health
Network, University of Toronto, Toronto, Ontario, Canada

SHEELA PAI COLE, MD, FASE
Clinical Associate Professor, Anesthesiology, Perioperative and Pain Medicine, Stanford
University, Stanford, California, USA

ELYSE M. CORNETT, PhD
Assistant Professor, Department of Anesthesiology, LSU Health Shreveport, Shreveport,
Louisiana, USA

ALLISON DALTON, MD
Assistant Professor, Department of Anesthesia and Critical Care, The University of
Chicago, Chicago, Illinois, USA

GERMÁN ECHEVERRY, MD
Assistant Professor, Department of Anesthesiology and Critical Care Medicine, Memorial
Sloan Kettering Cancer Center, Cornell University, New York, New York, USA

ANGELA F. EDWARDS, MD, FASA
Associate Professor, Section Head of Perioperative Medicine, Department of
Anesthesiology, Wake Forest University School of Medicine, Winston-Salem, North
Carolina, USA

TREVOR FLYNN, BS
Department of Anesthesiology, LSU School of Medicine, New Orleans, Louisiana, USA

DANIEL J. FOREST, MD
Assistant Professor, Medical Director, Preoperative Assessment Clinic, Department of
Anesthesiology, Wake Forest University School of Medicine, Winston-Salem, North
Carolina, USA

RODNEY A. GABRIEL, MD, MAS
Chief, Division of Regional Anesthesia and Acute Pain, Assistant Clinical Professor,
Departments of Anesthesiology and Medicine, Division of Biomedical Informatics,
University of California, San Diego, La Jolla, California, USA

MICHAEL P.W. GROCOTT, MBBS, MD, FRCP, FRCA, FFICM
Critical Care Research Group, NIHR Biomedical Research Centre, University Hospital
Southampton NHS Foundation Trust, Southampton, United Kingdom

BRENDON HART, DO
Resident, Department of Anesthesiology, LSU Health Shreveport, Shreveport, Louisiana,
USA

ERIK M. HELANDER, MBBS
Department of Anesthesiology, LSU School of Medicine, New Orleans, Louisiana, USA

ALAN DAVID KAYE, MD, PhD
Chairman, Program Director, Professor, Departments of Anesthesiology and
Pharmacology, LSU School of Medicine, LSU Health Science Center, New Orleans,
Louisiana, USA

DUSTIN LATIMER, BS
Medical Student, Department of Anesthesiology, LSU Health Shreveport, Shreveport,
Louisiana, USA

CHRISTIAN MABRY, MD
Assistant Professor, Department of Anesthesiology, Perioperative Care and Pain
Medicine, NYU School of Medicine, New York, New York, USA

ASHLEY R. MEYN, MD
Department of Anesthesiology, Oschner Clinic, Jefferson, Louisiana, USA

TIMOTHY E. MILLER, MB ChB, FRCA
Associate Professor of Anesthesiology, Duke University School of Medicine, Duke
University Health System, Durham, North Carolina, USA

TALHA MUBASHIR, MD
Research Fellow, Department of Anesthesiology, Toronto Western Hospital, University
Health Network, University of Toronto, Toronto, Ontario, Canada

MAHESH NAGAPPA, MD
Assistant Professor, Department of Anesthesia and Perioperative Medicine, London
Health Science Centre, St. Joseph Health Care, Western University, University Hospital,
London, Ontario, Canada

TIMOTHY D. QUINN, MD
Assistant Professor, Department of Anesthesiology, Jacobs School of Medicine
and Biomedical Sciences, University at Buffalo, The State University of New York,
Assistant Professor of Oncology, Department of Anesthesiology, Critical Care,
Pain Medicine, Roswell Park Comprehensive Cancer Center, Buffalo, New York,
USA

DEBORAH C. RICHMAN, MBChB, FFA (SA)
Associate Professor, Department of Anesthesiology, Stony Brook Medicine, Stony Brook,
New York, USA

MICHAEL J. SCOTT, MD, ChB, FRCP, FRCA, FFICM
Professor, Department of Anesthesiology, Virginia Commonwealth University
Health System, Richmond, Virginia, USA; Department of Anesthesiology, Perelman
School of Medicine, University of Pennsylvania, Philadelphia, Pennsylvania,
USA

ROSHNI SREEDHARAN, MD
Program Director, Critical Care Anesthesiology Fellowship, Assistant Professor of
Anesthesiology, Cleveland Clinic Lerner College of Medicine of Case Western Reserve
University, Staff Anesthesiologist and Intensivist, Department of General Anesthesiology,
Center for Critical Care, Anesthesiology Institute, Cleveland Clinic, Cleveland, Ohio, USA

RAYMOND SROKA, PharmD, MD
Assistant Professor, Department of Anesthesiology, Jacobs School of Medicine and
Biomedical Sciences, University at Buffalo, The State University of New York, Assistant
Professor of Oncology, Department of Anesthesiology, Critical Care, Pain Medicine,
Roswell Park Comprehensive Cancer Center, Buffalo, New York, USA

YAMINI SUBRAMANI, MD
Clinical Fellow, Department of Anesthesia and Perioperative Medicine, London Health
Science Centre, St. Joseph Health Care, Western University, Centre, Victoria Hospital,
London, Ontario, Canada

VAHÉ S. TATEOSIAN, MD
Assistant Professor, Department of Anesthesiology, Stony Brook Medicine, Stony Brook,
New York, USA

RICHARD D. URMAN, MD, MBA, CPE, FASA
Associate Professor, Department of Anesthesiology, Perioperative and Pain Medicine,
Center for Perioperative Research, Brigham and Women's Hospital, Harvard Medical
School, Boston, Massachusetts, USA

KARINA G. VÁZQUEZ-NARVÁEZ, MD
Head of Perioperative Medicine, Department of Anesthesiology and Perioperative
Medicine, Instituto Nacional de Ciencias Médicas y Nutrición "Salvador Zubirán", Mexico
City, Mexico

THOMAS R. VETTER, MD, MPH
Professor, Director of Perioperative Care, Director of Comprehensive Pain Management,
Department of Surgery and Perioperative Care, Department of Population Health, Dell
Medical School, The University of Texas at Austin, Austin, Texas, USA

RUTH S. WATERMAN, MD, MSc
Chair, Associate Clinical Professor, Department of Anesthesiology, University of
California, San Diego, San Diego, California, USA

MICHAEL P. WEBB, MBChB, MSc
Department of Anesthesiology, North Shore Hospital, Auckland, New Zealand

JOHN WHITTLE, MBBS, MD, FRCA, FFICM
Assistant Professor, Anesthesiology, Duke University School of Medicine, Duke
University Health System, Durham, North Carolina, USA; Honorary Senior Lecturer,
Perioperative Medicine, University College London, London, United Kingdom

PAUL E. WISCHMEYER, MD, EDIC
Director, Nutrition Support Service, Professor of Anesthesiology and Surgery, Director of
Perioperative Research, Duke Clinical Research Institute, Duke University Hospital, Duke
University School of Medicine, Durham, North Carolina, USA

PIOTR WOLCZYNSKI, MD
Resident Physician, Department of Internal Medicine, Jacobs School of Medicine and
Biomedical Sciences, University at Buffalo, The State University of New York, Buffalo,
New York, USA

JEAN WONG, MD, FRCPC
Associate Professor, Department of Anesthesiology, Toronto Western Hospital, University Health Network, University of Toronto, Toronto, Ontario, Canada

ZDRAVKA ZAFIROVA, MD
Associate Professor, Section of Critical Care, Department of Cardiovascular Surgery, Mount Sinai Hospital System, Icahn School of Medicine at Mount Sinai, Mount Sinai Medical Center, New York, New York, USA

Contents

Value in health care has been described as quality divided by cost, where quality is the sum of patient outcomes and experience. A well-run preoperative evaluation clinic (PEC) offers many opportunities to improve the value of the care delivered to patients by reducing the associated costs and improving the quality of care. Certain patient education and medical optimization strategies initiated in the PEC clinic are linked to an improvement in patients' long-term health outcomes. When designing a PEC, it is important to address the PEC's mission and scope with all stakeholders early in the process.

Obtaining routine preoperative laboratory tests increases health care costs and has been listed, by the Choosing Wisely Campaign, as one of the top 5 practices anesthesiologists should avoid. Routine testing without clinical indication is not cost-effective and could cause harm and unnecessary delays. Abnormal findings are more likely to be false positive and costly to pursue, introduce new risks, and increase anxiety for the patient. Preoperative testing need to be performed only following a targeted history and physical examination, factoring severity of surgery, and comorbidities such that the benefit of the test outweighs risk.

Cardiac risk stratification before surgery informs consent, may advise optimization interventions, and guides intraoperative and postoperative management and monitoring. Published guidelines provide an outline for risk stratification but are only updated every 5 to 10 years; hence, cardiology expert opinion is often needed. Preoperative cardiovascular evaluation starts with an excellent history and physical examination. Accurate assessment of exercise tolerance is paramount in defining risk and determining the need for further testing. Risk/benefit ratio needs to be assessed and reviewed with all stakeholders, which pertains to deciding on cardiac

One in 4 deaths occurring within a week of surgery are related to pulmonary complications, making it the second most common serious morbidity after cardiovascular events. The most significant predictors of the postoperative pulmonary complications (PPCs) are American Society of Anesthesiologists physical status, advanced age, dependent functional status, surgical site, and duration of surgery. The overall risk of PPCs can be predicted using scores that incorporate readily available clinical data.

Perioperative acute kidney injury is associated with morbidity and mortality. Several definitions have been proposed, incorporating small changes of serum creatinine and urinary output reduction as diagnostic criteria. In the surgical patient, comorbidities, type and timing of surgery, and nephrotoxins are important. Patient comorbidities remain a significant risk factor. Urgent or emergent surgery and cardiac or transplantation procedures are associated with a higher risk of acute kidney injury. Nephrotoxic drugs, contrast dye, and diuretics worsen preexisting kidney dysfunction or act as an adjunctive insult to perioperative injury. This review includes preoperative, intraoperative, and postoperative issues that can be mitigated.

The hematologic system is responsible for several of the body's most critical functions, including delivery of oxygen and nutrients to tissues, clearance of toxic metabolic byproducts, defense against offending pathogens, and maintenance of hemostasis in the setting of trauma. Its exquisite complexity is difficult to overstate and poses a great challenge to review in short form. This article provides highlights and clinical pearls in managing patients suffering from some of the most common hematologic afflictions encountered in the perioperative setting.

Complications after major surgery account for a disproportionate amount of in-hospital morbidity and mortality. Recent efforts have focused on preoperative optimization in an attempt to modify the risk associated with major surgery. Underaddressed, but important, modifiable risk factors are physical fitness and nutritional status. Surgical patients are particularly at risk of 3 related, but distinct, conditions: frailty, sarcopenia, and reduced physical fitness. Exercise-based prehabilitation strategies have shown promise in terms of improving aerobic fitness, although their impact on key clinical perioperative outcome measures have not been fully determined. Preoperative nutritional status also has a strong bearing on perioperative outcome.

Diabetes is an important cause of morbidity in the adult population resulting in blindness, renal dysfunction, cardiovascular events, and amputation. Such morbidities may have an impact on perioperative anesthetic care and outcomes. In this review, the authors discuss the preoperative considerations in managing patients with diabetes as well as those without diabetes albeit hyperglycemic. They propose a plan for managing preoperative diabetes pharmacotherapy, including the use of a subcutaneous insulin pump to avoid both hypoglycemia and hyperglycemia. The authors also discuss the decision whether to proceed or cancel surgery for a given hemoglobin A1c percentage or blood glucose concentration.

As the population ages, more geriatric patients will be presenting for surgical procedures. Preoperative evaluation seeks to assess patients for geriatric syndromes: frailty, sarcopenia, functional dependence, and malnutrition. Age-related changes in physiology increase risk for central nervous system, cardiovascular, pulmonary, renal, hepatic, and endocrine morbidity and mortality. Identification of various comorbidities allows for preoperative optimization and for opportunities for intervention including nutritional supplementation and prehabilitation, which may improve postoperative outcomes.

Drug abuse and addiction are persistent problems in the United States and around the world. This is an ongoing issue for health care providers, as substance abuse is seen in 25% to 40% of patients admitted to hospitals for general treatment. Many patients with substance use disorders have a higher risk for adverse events; however, only a small percentage will volunteer information regarding prior substance use. This article discusses the present opioid crisis, mechanisms behind chronic pain and substance abuse, current clinical findings, treatment therapies, and abuse deterrents.

The anesthetic management of pregnant patients can present a variety of challenges and a thorough preoperative assessment is necessary before initiating any anesthetic services. Both the mother and the fetus need to be considered when formulating an anesthetic plan and discussing informed consent. The overall aims in assessing a pregnant patient are to identity potential issues that can lead to catastrophic complications, provide adequate information allowing the mother to make informed decisions, and to obtain knowledge for tailoring an anesthetic that maintains maternal and fetal homeostasis.

Pharmacogenomics (PGx) is the study of how individuals' personal genotypes may affect their responses to various pharmacologic agents. The application of PGx principles in perioperative medicine is fairly novel. Challenges in executing PGx programs into health care systems include physician buy-in and integration into usual clinical workflow, including the electronic health record. This article discusses the current evidence highlighting the potential of PGx with various drug categories (including opioids, nonopioid analgesics, sedatives, β-blockers, antiemetics, and anticoagulants) used in the perioperative process and the challenges of integrating PGx into a health care system and relevant workflows.

Shared decision-making (SDM) is essential for high-quality surgical care. Barriers to SDM exist in clinical practice but there is evidence these obstacles can be overcome. SDM requires clinician and patient engagement. Though patients may indicate understanding, deficits in decision making may persist based on language, age, or educational barriers. Multidisciplinary decision-making before surgery is an opportunity for anesthesiologists and other perioperative professionals to improve surgical care. The authors present an example of a successfully implemented pathway for high-risk surgical patients at a tertiary care center, leveraging the preoperative anesthesia evaluation.

Increasingly complex medication regimens for many comorbidities in patients for planned surgical and procedural interventions necessitate detailed preoperative evaluation of the pharmacologic therapy, including the indications, the specific drugs, and dosing amount and interval. The implications of continuing or withholding these agents in the perioperative period need to be elucidated, as well as the risks of interactions and side effects. A comprehensive plan of the management of the therapeutic agents should be devised during the preoperative visit, with input from all relevant specialists, and clearly communicated to the patients in a format that ensures their comprehension and consistent compliance.

The rising prominence of value-based health care and population health management supports evolving perioperative surgical home (PSH) models that rely on continuously evolving evidence-based best practice and telemedicine and telehealth, including mobile technologies and connectivity. To successfully deliver greater perioperative valued-based care and to effectively contribute to sustained and meaningful perioperative population health management, the scope of existing perioperative management and its associated services and care provider skills must be expanded. This article focuses on the PSH model as continued opportunity and mechanism for delivering greater value-based, comprehensive perioperative assessment and global optimization of surgical patients.

The article reviews frequently encountered preoperative concerns with a goal of minimizing complications during administration of pediatric anesthesia. It is written with general anesthesiologists in mind and provides a helpful overview of concerns for pediatric patient preparation for routine and nonemergent procedures or interventions. It covers unique topics for the pediatric population, including gestational age, respiratory and cardiovascular concerns, fasting guidelines, and management of preoperative anxiety, as well as the current hot topic of the potential neurotoxic effects of anesthetics on the developing brain.

Anemia is a decrease in red blood cell mass, which hinders oxygen delivery to tissues. Preoperative anemia has been shown to be associated with mortality and morbidity following major surgery. The preoperative care clinic is an ideal place to start screening for anemia and discussing potential interventions in order to optimize patients for surgery. This article (1) reviews the relevant literature and highlights consequences of preoperative anemia in the surgical setting, and (2) suggests strategies for screening and optimizing anemia in the preoperative setting.

ANESTHESIOLOGY CLINICS

FORTHCOMING ISSUES

March 2019
Cutting-Edge Trauma and Emergency Care
Maureen McCunn, Mohammed Iqbal
Ahmed, and Catherine M. Kuza, *Editors*

June 2019
Ambulatory Anesthesia
Michael T. Walsh, *Editor*

September 2019
Geriatric Anesthesia
Elizabeth Whitlock and
Robert A. Whittington, *Editors*

RECENT ISSUES

September 2018
Regional Anesthesia
Nabil Elkassabany and
Edward Mariano, *Editors*

June 2018
**Practice Management: Successfully Guiding
Your Group into the Future**
Amr E. Abouleish and Stanley W. Stead,
Editors

March 2018
**Quality Improvement and Implementation
Science**
Meghan B. Lane-Fall and Lee A. Fleisher,
Editors

RELATED INTEREST

Medical Clinics of North America, September 2016 (Vol. 100, No. 5)
Quality Patient Care: Making Evidence-Based, High Value Choices
Marc Shalaby and Edward R. Bollard, *Editors*
Available at: http://www.medical.theclinics.com/

THE CLINICS ARE AVAILABLE ONLINE!
Access your subscription at:
www.theclinics.com

Foreword

Preoperative Evaluation: Is It Time to View It as a Component of Perioperative Optimization?

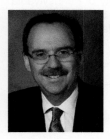

Lee A. Fleisher, MD
Consulting Editor

The preoperative evaluation of the patient undergoing surgery has been the hallmark of the role of the anesthesiologists. Traditionally, the information was used to (1) discuss the risk of surgery as part of the decision to proceed and (2) provide a database upon which to make intraoperative decisions. With the development of the perioperative medicine movement, including Enhanced Recovery After Surgery (ERAS) and the Perioperative Surgical Home, there is an increasing number of strategies to "optimize" patients prior to surgery, including anemia clinics. While the evidence to support many of these strategies is limited, it makes physiologic sense. The issue includes articles outlining the development of a preoperative evaluation clinic and the implications of several comorbidities, such as cardiac disease, kidney disease, and diabetes. They have also included important new issues such as the assessment of frailty and cognitive function. In addition, the potential utility of genomics in the preoperative evaluation is discussed. It is, therefore, exciting that the two editors have created an issue that includes both the "traditional" approach and optimization strategies.

In identifying editors for this issue, I approached leaders of the Society for Perioperative Assessment and Quality Improvement (SPAQI). Zdravka Zafirova, MD is Associate Professor of Anesthesiology and Critical Care in the Department of Cardiovascular Surgery at Icahn School of Medicine and Mount Sinai Hospital system. She is the Director of Anesthesia Pre-operative Evaluation and Testing Center at Mount Sinai Hospital. She is a member of the Board of Directors of SPAQI and has expertise in the perioperative management of medically complicated patients. Richard D. Urman, MD, MBA, CPE, FASA is an anesthesiologist at the Brigham and Women's Hospital (BWH) in Boston, Massachusetts and Associate Professor of Anesthesia at Harvard Medical School. He serves as Director of Anesthesia Services at the BWH Care Center

Anesthesiology Clin 36 (2018) xv–xvi
https://doi.org/10.1016/j.anclin.2018.08.002
1932-2275/18/© 2018 Published by Elsevier Inc.

at Chestnut Hill and Director (Anesthesia) of the interdepartmental Center for Perioperative Research at BWH and directs the newly established Perioperative Medicine Fellowship. Dr Urman is also treasurer of SPAQI. His research areas encompass patient outcomes, informatics, patient safety, novel anesthetic drugs, simulation, and operating room management. Together, they have created an important and informative issue.

Lee A. Fleisher, MD
Perelman School of Medicine at
University of Pennsylvania
3400 Spruce Street, Dulles 680
Philadelphia, PA 19104, USA

E-mail address:
Lee.Fleisher@uphs.upenn.edu

Preface

Preoperative Patient Evaluation: Practicing Evidence-Based, Cost-Effective Medicine

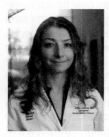
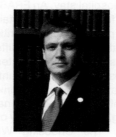

Zdravka Zafirova, MD   Richard D. Urman, MD, MBA, CPE, FASA

Editors

The idea of preoperative optimization of the surgical patient was put forth early in the twentieth century; the concept has evolved over time and has expanded into a comprehensive multidisciplinary platform in the past decades. As research about contributing factors to perioperative patient outcomes continues to accumulate, we will be able to rely on constantly evolving evidence-based principles to guide our decisions about patient care. The preoperative assessment process involves making decisions about patient and procedure selection, laboratory testing, optimization of comorbid conditions, efficient and cost-effective management of health care resources, communication among health care providers and with the patients and their social support system, and utilization of modern technological developments. The dedicated multispecialty teams play an essential role in the development and application of specialized perioperative guidelines as well as in the design and the implementation of clinical pathways for the perioperative management of medical conditions such as diabetes, chronic pain and opioid use, coagulopathy, obstructive sleep apnea, and anemia. An increasing number of facilities are now screening for cognitive impairment and frailty and introducing multidisciplinary co-management pathways involving geriatricians and other specialists. Furthermore, the mission of the perioperative teams continues through the entire perioperative period, including interventions and follow-up during the anesthesia and surgery and into the postoperative setting and postadmission health maintenance and rehabilitation venues. Emerging topics in preoperative patient optimization include personalized medicine and genetic profiling to predict response to medications and specific patient outcomes. We must think of perioperative evaluation and optimization as part of a bigger picture of population health management, including interventions such as smoking cessation counseling, nutrition, prehabilitation and postoperative rehabilitation. Many of these interventions take place

Anesthesiology Clin 36 (2018) xvii–xviii
https://doi.org/10.1016/j.anclin.2018.08.001
1932-2275/18/© 2018 Published by Elsevier Inc.
    anesthesiology.theclinics.com

in the setting of a national push for value-based care and resource optimization, which takes into consideration health care costs, quality of care, outcomes, and patient experience and satisfaction. The preoperative optimization plays an important role in the Perioperative Surgical Home model of patient-centric, team-based model of care advocated by the American Society of Anesthesiologists. Preoperative encounters also offer an opportunity for shared decision making where the needs and care goals of the patient can be assessed in a systematic way to ensure that patients are active participants in their care. Also, over the last decade, Enhanced Recovery After Surgery (ERAS) clinical pathways have been demonstrated to improve patient outcomes and reduce length of hospital stay. An ERAS program can only be successful if patients are first optimized for surgery and certain necessary interventions take place, such as exercise-based prehabilitation, nutritional supplementation, anemia management, and patient education. Nationwide, different business models exist to accomplish the preoperative assessment as it relates to billing, staffing, and other resource management strategies. It varies significantly by facility and may include an in-person visit to the preoperative assessment clinic, patient chart reviews, phone screens, or a combination thereof. There has been a national emphasis on decreasing unnecessary preoperative testing, such as frequently overused cardiac and laboratory blood testing, among others. The Choosing Wisely Campaign (http://www.choosingwisely.org) has assembled a multitude of evidence-based resources intended for both health care providers and patients to help educate them about appropriate medical testing. Also, the preoperative encounter provides an opportunity to review the pharmacotherapeutic regimen of the patient, to determine the indication for perioperative continuation or withdrawal of specific medications, such as antihypertensive agents, antiplatelet and anticoagulant agents, opioid agonists-antagonists, and immunomodulators, as well as to reduce the polypharmacy risk. Altogether, the preoperative patient's assessment should be viewed as a multidisciplinary effort involving anesthesia providers, surgeons, medical specialists, midlevel practitioners, nurses, administrative staff, and the patient and their social supports. In order to achieve the best possible patient outcomes, we must take into consideration existing evidence and practice guidelines, although we should always leave room for clinical judgment and our desire to do what is best for the patient.

Zdravka Zafirova, MD
Department of Cardiovascular Surgery
The Mount Sinai Hospital
Icahn School of Medicine
321 West 37 Street, 5A
New York, NY 10018, USA

Richard D. Urman, MD, MBA, CPE, FASA
Department of Anesthesiology
Perioperative and Pain Medicine
Brigham and Women's Hospital
Harvard Medical School
75 Francis Street
Boston, MA 02115, USA

E-mail addresses:
zzafirova@free.fr (Z. Zafirova)
rurman@bwh.harvard.edu (R.D. Urman)

Designing and Running a Preoperative Clinic

Jeanna D. Blitz, MD[a],*, Christian Mabry, MD[b]

KEYWORDS

- Preoperative evaluation • Value in health care • Quality improvement
- Triple-aim framework • Advanced practice providers • Resident education

KEY POINTS

- A preoperative evaluation clinic (PEC) may improve the value of perioperative care by reducing cost and improving quality.
- Achieving the Triple Aim in health care requires an integrator, such as a well-designed PEC, that accepts responsibility for all 3 aims for the chosen population.
- When designing a PEC, it is important to address the mission of the PEC and scope with all stakeholders early in the process.
- Advanced practice providers at a PEC have the ability to positively affect all 6 dimensions of quality in their defined roles.
- Residents at a PEC benefit from applying systems-based practice concepts, practicing patient engagement strategies, and participating in quality improvement initiatives.

IMPROVING THE VALUE OF HEALTH CARE DELIVERY: A NECESSITY AND AN OPPORTUNITY

The implementation of value-based health care initiatives is imperative to improving the health care system. Although the concept of anesthesiologists as perioperative leaders is not new, opportunities now exist for anesthesiologists to lead collaborative perioperative care teams in the redesign of the perioperative process to maximize the impact on patient outcomes. Many preoperative medicine initiatives focus on the Triple-Aim framework: improve the experience of care, improve the health of populations, and reduce per capita costs. However, achieving this Triple Aim requires an integrator who accepts responsibility for all 3 aims for the chosen population.[1] In many systems, the integrator role may be best fulfilled by a well-designed, anesthesiologist-led preoperative evaluation clinic (PEC).

Disclosure Statement: This work was funded by the department of Anesthesiology, Perioperative Care and Pain Medicine, New York University School of Medicine.
[a] Preadmission Testing, Department of Anesthesiology, Perioperative Care and Pain Medicine, NYU School of Medicine, 550 1st Avenue, TH 552, New York, NY 10016, USA; [b] Department of Anesthesiology, Perioperative Care and Pain Medicine, NYU School of Medicine, 550 1st Avenue, TH 552, New York, NY 10016, USA
* Corresponding author.
E-mail address: jeanna.viola@nyulangone.org

As directors of PECs, anesthesiologists may demonstrate their expertise in perioperative patient care and systems design. PECs have been shown to be associated with fewer cancelations, shorter length of stay, improved operating room (OR) efficiency, and a reduction in in-hospital mortality.[2–4] Furthermore, many key elements of a successful perioperative surgical home can be initiated in an anesthesiologist-directed PEC. Examples of these elements include earlier access to patients; improved adherence to standardized, evidence-based clinical pathways; increased preoperative education and counseling by anesthesiologists; more coordinated, facile communications among providers and the patient; and coordination of postoperative care.[5]

REDESIGNING THE PREOPERATIVE EVALUATION CLINIC TO ADD VALUE

$$Value = \frac{Quality}{Cost}$$

Value in health care has been described as quality divided by cost, where quality is the sum of patient outcomes and the patient experience.[6] A well-run, anesthesiologist-led PEC presents many opportunities to improve the value of the care delivered to the patients served by the health care system. This is accomplished through reducing the cost associated with the care delivered and improving the quality of the care provided to patients. With regard to the third pillar of the triple-aim framework, to improve the health of the population, patient education and medical optimization strategies initiated in PECs also have the potential to affect patient's long-term health outcomes.

Adding Value by Reducing Cost

Because many PECs are do not generate revenue, the most readily available opportunities to affect the cost of the preoperative period are to decrease the amount of unnecessary preoperative testing[7] and to ensure accurate, detailed documentation of each patient's preexisting comorbidities in the electronic health record (EHR) to facilitate the proper assignment of case mix index and Medicare Severity Diagnosis Related Groups.[8]

PECs can contribute to cost savings to the institution by improving efficiency. Day-of-surgery case cancellations are extremely costly. The lost OR time and revenue, wasted staff time, and revenue loss related to a canceled surgical case that the patient never reschedules all contribute to this. As such, the system should be designed to avoid last-minute cancellations related to circumstances that can be controlled. Unanticipated, prolonged patient admissions to the intensive care unit are also costly to the institution. PECs may further contribute to overall cost savings by contributing to the adequate assessment and optimization of medically complex, high-risk patients, selection of appropriate surgical candidates, and through shared decision-making. This will ensure that high-risk patients are well-informed about their perioperative risk and expected postoperative course.[7]

Another way that PECs contribute to a cost savings is through the use of evidence-based standards and policies for preoperative testing. PECs can reduce, if not eliminate, the costs to the hospital that are associated with unindicated tests. Prior studies have demonstrated that advanced practice providers (APPs) working in a PEC were able to incorporate standardized preoperative testing protocols, such as the Institute of Medicine (IOM) Choosing Wisely campaign, to reduce rates of unnecessary testing from 23% to 4%.[9] Reduction in the amount of routine preoperative tests in the absence of a specific clinical indication is in line with the recommendations in the

IOM Choosing Wisely campaign.[10] Initiatives to streamline preoperative testing will have financial implications for the hospital and patient given that Centers for Medicare & Medicaid Service will no longer reimburse the tests as part of a routine preoperative testing without a clinical indication.[11]

By contrast, detailed coding of a patient's preexisting medical conditions is critical for accurate reimbursement to the hospital for each episode of care. This is best accomplished by a thorough medical history-taking and detailed documentation in the medical record, and is an important function that a PEC may provide. A report may be generated from the EHR system to track how often clinically relevant medical comorbidities are captured and documented by PEC staff, such that improved reimbursement from an improvement in documentation in the EHR will be attributed to the PEC.[12]

Adding Value by Improving Quality

Although PECs may add value by improving cost, the focus of a PEC's contribution to the delivery of higher value perioperative care will be its ability to add value by improving quality. Quality, according to the IOM, has 6 domains: safety, efficiency, patient-centeredness, efficacy, equity, and timeliness of care (**Box 1**).[13] Although the specifics of which particular functions are value-added may vary greatly between institutions, PECs and the clinicians who staff them are capable of performing many valuable roles that contribute to quality improvement.

Safety

A preoperative evaluation by a physician not specifically trained in perioperative medicine has been associated with an increased length of stay and increased postoperative mortality.[14] By contrast, a PEC run by hospitalists was associated with lower mortality rates at 1 institution, and attendance at an anesthesiologist-run PEC was associated with a lower incidence of postoperative mortality at others.[2,15,16] The difference in results between the studies on preoperative assessments by internists and those of anesthesiologist or hospitalist-directed assessments in a PEC may be due to the perioperative practitioner's ability to improve coordination of care along the entire perioperative continuum, as well as the anesthesiologist's in-depth knowledge of the proposed surgery and anesthetic.

Inadequate preoperative assessment and preparation has also been linked to other critical adverse postoperative events, including major physiologic derangements, unanticipated admission to the intensive care unit, and prolonged hospital stays.[17]

Box 1
Quality health care

1. Safe: minimize risks and harm

2. Efficient: maximize resource use and avoid waste

3. Patient-centered: patient's individual preferences and culture

4. Effective: based on evidence and results in improved outcomes

5. Equitable: race, gender, ethnicity, and socioeconomic status should not be barriers to highest quality care

6. Timely: delivery of well-coordinated, accessible care

Adapted from Institute of Medicine (US) Committee on Quality of Health Care in America. Improving the 21st-century health care system. In: Richardson WC, editor. Crossing the quality chasm: a new health system for the 21st Century. Washington, DC: National Academy Press; 2003. p. 39; with permission.

Medication reconciliation and medication management are important aspects of a PEC visit, yet these may pose a challenge due to a lack of standardized recommendations and limitations in patients' health literacy. Whenever possible, a defined set of medication management protocols should be created and agreed on by the multidisciplinary teams involved in perioperative patient care. A standardized preoperative patient medication instruction sheet, in addition to verbal instructions, is associated with improved patient compliance with medication instructions on the day of surgery.[18]

Efficiency

PECs can significantly affect OR efficiency by contributing to a reduction in day-of-surgery cancelations and delays.[3] Registered nurses and APPs working in a PEC also contribute to the delivery of more efficient preoperative care. For example, an assessment during the PEC visit may contribute to the reduction in requests for additional medical or specialty consultations before surgery, and a reduction in the amount of preoperative laboratory testing ordered.[19,20] All PEC staff members should also be encouraged to participate in unit-based quality initiatives to decrease the length of the PEC appointment to improve efficiency and the patient's experience.

Patient-centered

Patient education should be the focus of the PEC visit. Topics should include preoperative preparation information (eg, bowel preparation, medication management), expectations about pain management, techniques for anxiety reduction, and risk assessment and preoperative optimization strategies (eg, smoking cessation, alcohol misuse counseling, anemia management) as appropriate. The patient should also be asked about preferred pronouns and preferred name. Their preferences related to acceptance of blood products should also be explored and documented in the medical record. Use of the pain catastrophizing scale may help to identify patients at high risk for poor pain control in the acute postoperative setting.[21] Preoperative pain management consultations may be offered on-site in the PEC for these high-risk patients. Whenever possible, colocating and/or attending to the smooth coordination of necessary preoperative services at the PEC will allow for 1-stop shopping, which will improve the patient experience.

Efficacy

Value in health care is also defined as the health outcomes achieved per dollar spent.[22] Outcomes are directly related to the time spent recovering from surgery and the return to best-attainable function.[22] The initiation of standardized, enhanced recovery pathways in the PEC may contribute to improved patient outcomes, including a reduction in length of stay and a reduction in postoperative complications.[7] Enhanced recovery pathways should incorporate elements of the surgical procedure and anesthetic, as well as the patient's preexisting medical conditions. Examples include pathways related to the medical condition regarding the perioperative management of antiplatelet agents in patients with cardiac stents, internal cardiac defibrillators and pacemakers, glycemic control, mixed opioid agonist-antagonist use, cognitive dysfunction, and obstructive sleep apnea.

Equity

Race, gender, ethnicity, and socioeconomic status should not present barriers to delivery of the highest quality care. It is important to understand the demographics of the patient population that the PEC and health care system serve. This will allow identification of areas of opportunity to improve the equity of care. A PEC visit that is free from any additional fees to the patient will improve access for patients of less financial means. Training the midlevel providers who staff the surgeon's office to provide the core services provided in PEC (ie, patient education and expectation management, care coordination) may also expand the number of patients who benefit from the quality of care that the PEC provides by increasing access to the PEC's standard evaluation process without an additional visit.

Timeliness
PECs offer the opportunity to facilitate the entire preoperative workup or assessment of the patient, thus allowing them to avoid an additional trip to their medical doctor for a preoperative evaluation. This may allow the patient to proceed with the surgery in a more timely fashion.

DELIVERING ON THE TRIPLE AIM: IMPROVING THE HEALTH OF THE POPULATION

For many patients, the preoperative period represents a window of time when they are more receptive to making lifestyle and behavioral modifications than they had been at other times in their lives. Capitalizing on this opportunity to enact preoperative optimization strategies may improve their health long beyond the postoperative period. Prehabilitation is a multimodal approach to enhance an individual's capacity to withstand the stress of surgery (see John Whittle and colleagues article, "Surgical Prehabilitation: Nutrition and Exercise", in this issue).[23] Certain components of this approach have impacts on the patient's health outcomes that extend beyond the postoperative period, such as smoking cessation counseling, screening for cognitive dysfunction, screening for sleep apnea, and correction of anemia.

Interventions in the PEC result in significantly higher rates of short-term smoking cessation (ie, within 3–6 months after surgery). Long-term smoking cessation of 12 months after surgery have also been demonstrated when smoking cessation counseling is combined with pharmacotherapy, an education pamphlet, and a referral to a smoker's quit line.[24]

Assessment of cognitive function may assist in the identification of patients who are high risk for postoperative delirium. Postoperative delirium is associated with an increased risk of postoperative morbidity and mortality, long-term cognitive decline, and an increased risk of 5-year mortality.[25,26] Counseling the patient and their loved ones about this risk and providing strategies to reduce or prevent postoperative delirium is recommended. Referral for a geriatric consultation, when possible, is also beneficial.

Anemia is among the most common diagnoses encountered during the preoperative visit and is an independent risk factor for perioperative morbidity and mortality, regardless of transfusion.[27–29] Anemia is also associated with increased long-term mortality even in the absence of surgery.[30] Preoperative iron infusions in patients with iron deficiency anemia can have a significant impact on hemoglobin levels and lower the transfusion rates in the perioperative period.[31,32] Implementation of a preoperative anemia management clinic may affect perioperative morbidity and long-term health outcomes. An anesthesia-directed preoperative anemia management clinic allows for expeditious treatment of iron-deficient patients. Some PECs offer intravenous iron onsite. Referrals to specialists for the treatment of other types of anemia may also be facilitated via the PEC. A comprehensive program should aim to minimize patient visits while maximizing the information obtained at each visit. This patient-centered diagnostic and treatment pathway can improve outcomes, which can be tracked by the hospital's quality assurance department. Transfusion rates and hospital length of stays are expected to decrease when this model is implemented.[29]

Obstructive sleep apnea is another common diagnosis that may be undiagnosed, yet associated with long-term health risks if left untreated. Screening the patient to determine their risk of obstructive sleep apnea, providing them with education about the long-term risks associated with the condition, and providing a referral for a sleep study are functions that a PEC may provide.

The pain catastrophizing scale is a validated tool used to identify patients who are at greatest risk of poor pain control in the acute postoperative period.[21] Patients who exhibit a higher level of catastrophization are at greater risk of poor pain control, and poor pain control leads to longer length of stay and higher levels of patient dissatisfaction. Furthermore, catastrophic thinking related to pain may increase the risk of chronicity.[21] Referrals to integrative health, pain management, and psychiatry are all useful components to optimizing the patient's postoperative course while potentially reducing the overall length of time that opioid pain medications are required.

POTENTIAL FOR REVENUE GENERATION IN PREOPERATIVE EVALUATION CLINIC

Some well-designed PECs are able to generate revenue for the institution by either providing preoperative optimization or prehabilitation services onsite, or through referrals to affiliated clinics. Examples include preoperative anemia screening and treatment, preoperative pain management assessment and counseling, referrals for physical therapy, nutritional counseling or integrative health services, smoking cessation counseling, osteoporosis screening and treatment, and counseling on shared decision-making. Fewer still are billing for the preoperative consultations provided in the PEC itself.

KNOW THE VALUE, SHOW THE VALUE: CREATING A VALUE PROPOSITION FOR THE PREOPERATIVE EVALUATION CLINIC

When designing a PEC, it is important to address the mission and scope of the PEC with all stakeholders early in the process. Ensure that all stakeholders agree on the role of the PEC within the perioperative process, as well as the metrics by which its success will be determined. The surgeons' view of what the PEC should accomplish may be very different than that of hospital administration, and those concepts may be different, or even contradict, the anesthesiologists' or patients' points of view.

Goals of the clinic must be delineated and the components of the preoperative process that PEC is not accountable for must also be established. This will likely be facilitated by the creation of a mission statement for the PEC that all stakeholders have a part in creating. Renaming of the PEC to reflect the current mission may be required. Creation of the mission statement is important because the role of the APPs who staff the PEC will be an extension of the anesthesiologist-director's role, and that will be defined by the PEC's mission. In turn, the mission statement should be driven by the value that the PEC is intended to add to the perioperative process. It may be useful to also create a vision statement. The mission statement will reflect the current state and the vision statement will represent future directions for the clinic.

To create a value proposition for the PEC, there are key questions to consider:
- Who are the decision-makers in this process? How does one demonstrate the PEC's value to them?
  - Consider emphasizing patient safety, improved patient outcomes, improved reimbursement through coding, and/or potential for revenue generation.
- Who are the end-users of this process? How does one improve the process for them and/or drive new value?
  - Consider emphasizing an improvement in efficiency, efficacy (initiation and adherence to enhanced recovery protocols), and the timeliness of care that is provided.

- What is the cost of switching to this solution? Why is it worthwhile?
  - Start with the changes that can be put into place with current staff and existing space. Can the workflow of existing staff be redesigned? Can the current space be used? When the current workflow is optimized for efficiency, one has to opportunity to best understand staffing needs and current space constraints.

The value proposition that is created for the PEC will determine which metrics the team decides to track. Certain measures may be more readily available and easier to follow through the generation of an automatic report, whereas others may require manual collection or require the distribution of patient and/or staff satisfaction surveys (**Box 2**).

TRAINING ADVANCED PRACTICE PROVIDERS TO PROVIDE HIGH QUALITY, COST-EFFECTIVE
Preoperative Care

Most of the efforts in a PEC that will improve the value of the care delivered will come from focusing on an improvement in the quality of the care.[1] APPs have the ability to positively affect all 6 dimensions through their defined roles in the PEC by applying evidence-based practice guidelines, health coaching,[2] improving care coordination, and participating in shared decision-making, as well as adhering to value-based protocols for reduction in preoperative testing.

A potential challenge may arise if the APPs who staff the PEC are under a different department and budget than its medical director. The medical director is still able to define the role of the APPs in the PEC; she or he should work collaboratively with the director of APPs or the advanced practice council to create the job descriptions and scope of practice for these clinicians (**Box 3**). Furthermore, the institution's advanced practice council likely has a position description for a nurse practitioner or physician assistant who works in an ambulatory clinic. This existing document may be able to be modified for APPs who practice in the ambulatory clinic

---

Box 2
Metrics to consider

- Clinical outcomes
  - Length of hospital stay
  - Readmission
  - Adverse events
  - Unanticipated intensive care unit admission, unexpected outpatients converted to inpatients
  - Incidence of postoperative delirium
  - Units of blood transfused

- Operational efficiency
  - Case cancellations: plan of care
  - Unindicated preoperative laboratory testing orders
  - Number of days before surgery chart is completed
  - Days between PEC visit and date of surgery
  - Patient wait times or length of appointment time

- Patient satisfaction
  - Survey results show satisfaction with pain management
  - Pediatric topical lidocaine cream (LMX 4%) orders

- Provider satisfaction
  - Avoidance of burnout, staff turnover

Box 3
Medical director of the preoperative evaluation clinic's responsibilities

- Define the role of the APP in the PEC: create a job description and a delineation of privileges document

- Establish preoperative evaluation protocols and pathways for use by APPs

- Mentor APPs to develop relevant quality and safety projects, as well as initiatives to improve the efficiency of the unit

- Coordinate the training of APPs responsible for the perioperative care of patients undergoing procedures outside the OR

---

environment to include language specific to the APP's role in the PEC, or to provide PEC-specific examples for the role expectations.[33,34]

Most APPs do not have direct personal experience in providing anesthesia. Therefore, the orientation for each APP will require a combination of didactic teaching covering major aspects of preoperative anesthesia assessments, shadowing an attending anesthesiologist (while conducting preoperative visits in PEC and providing anesthesia in the OR), and shadowing providers in the postanesthesia care unit (PACU). If possible, providing PACU cross-training is another valuable strategy to provide the APPs with ongoing, continued experience in the postoperative management of patients. Cross-rotating of APPs between the PEC and PACU also helps with communication by building relationships with team-members outside of the PEC. The presence of an onsite anesthesiologist-director in PEC whenever possible, or an anesthesiologist who is readily available to answer any questions that arise during the day, is also critical to the success of the PEC. Without continued feedback (positive and negative) to the APPs, growth and improvement will stall. Clearly establish a culture of safety when cultivating the relationship between the APP, PECs, and their collaborating physician.

Determining the correct staffing model requires a clear understanding of the role of the PEC, as well as the roles of the APPs who will staff the PEC. The medical director will need to consider whether the proposed roles and expectations of the APPs are realistic given the staff size and the number of patients seen each day. After roles are clearly established, it is important to measure the average length of appointment time, as well as times for the preanesthesia or APP consult itself. These data, along with the PEC's hours of operation, the number of examination rooms, and the expected patient volume are used to determine staffing needs. Takt time is a concept from Lean Management that describes the maximum amount of time that can be spent on a process yet still meet customer demand for the service.[35] In the context of the PEC, the Takt time is the maximum amount of time that can be allotted for each patient visit to be able to offer enough appointments to serve all patients who will require them. The cycle time is defined as the actual length of time required to complete all steps of a patient visit. An estimation of staff size can be assessed by comparing the Takt time to the cycle time, the number of available rooms, and the PEC's hours (**Box 4**).

Illustrative example

A PEC's hours are 8 AM to 6 PM. If there are no patient appointments scheduled at the 12 PM hour to accommodate staff lunch break, there are 9 hours per day available for patient appointments, or 540 minutes. This PEC has 7 examination rooms, so there are 3780 minutes per day available to provide patient care. This PEC sees an average of

> **Box 4**
> **Factors to measure when determining the correct staff model**
>
> - Average length of time patient spends in the PEC
> - Average time required to complete the preanesthesia or APP consult itself (APP cycle time)
> - Total amount of time to complete all components of the PEC visit (overall cycle time)
> - Number of hours that PEC is open per day
> - Number of patient examination rooms
> - Expected patient volume

45 patients per day. Therefore, the Takt time for this PEC is 84 minutes. Each patient visit will need to be completed within 84 minutes to remain on schedule and accommodate all patients. This hypothetical PEC currently measures its overall cycle time at 110 minutes with the components of each visit requiring the following times:

- Patient registration: 20 minutes
- Nursing assessment: 45 minutes
- APP assessment: 45 minutes.

In this scenario, the clinic could use this information in the following ways: the team may consider either shortening the length of time in 1 or more of the steps of the process, or use other areas to provide a portion of the assessment (eg, registration may need to take place virtually or in a reception area outside of the patient examination room).

To determine the number of APPs the clinic will need to staff the PEC on a daily basis, measure the cycle time for the APP assessment. The cycle time can help in assessing possible staffing options. Assuming each APP works a 10-hour shift, if the APPs are projected to see 45 patients per day for 45 minutes each, the PEC will need to plan to have approximately 4 APPs present in the PEC each day. Other options for this hypothetical PEC to consider (eg, seeing all PEC patients for a shorter length of time, as well as seeing fewer patients for a full-length assessment) are listed in **Table 1**.

After an orientation process and the scope-of-practice documents are established for APPs who work in the PEC, similar training and educational materials can be provided to APPs who work on services that care for patients who are anesthetized in locations outside the OR. The benefit of extending similar, if abbreviated, training in the preanesthesia evaluation to providers on these service lines lies in the ability to extend

Table 1
Measurement options to help determine the number of advanced practice providers needed on a daily basis

APP Cycle Time Options (Minutes per Cycle Time)	Number of Patients	Minutes with Patient	Total Minutes Needed per Day	Minutes Converted to Hours	Number of Providers per Day[a]
45	45	45	2025	33.75	3.75
30	45	30	1350	22.5	2.5
45	30	45	1350	22.5	2.5
30	30	30	900	15	1.66

[a] Crew size does not equal number of full-time equivalent staff needed.

the valuable patient care initiatives that PEC provides to patients who otherwise may not be seen in the PEC. Although their collaborating or supervising physician will most likely be a physician on their service line, the medical director of PEC should be readily available to consult on clinical issues and to answer questions.

Whenever possible, the APPs should have the opportunity to provide input in defining their goals for each calendar year, as well as the metrics that they will be measured by. A dry-erase board in a breakroom or other common area not used for patient care can be used to track the goals and metrics of the unit to improve team dynamics and commitment to the unit-based goals. Although most unit-specific goals should be quality initiatives created to improve the patient experience or efficiency on the unit, consideration should be given to reserving space for an initiative related to provider satisfaction and team-building.

TEACHING IN THE PREOPERATIVE EVALUATION CLINIC

The Accreditation Council for Graduate Medical Education (ACGME) requires a 2-week rotation in preoperative medicine, which may be best undertaken in a PEC. Although the components of the 2-week curriculum are not standardized, the ACGME emphasizes the importance of "the pre-operative preparation of the patient and their perioperative maintenance of normal physiology."[36,37] Residents are expected to incorporate a variety of skills from multiple specialties, including internal medicine, surgery, and obstetrics, that extend beyond the ability to perform a standard preoperative evaluation on the day of surgery.[37] Offering this rotation in a PEC provides a unique setting in which these specialties can be incorporated into anesthesia practice.

The ACGME identifies 6 core competencies that a resident is expected to master during their residency: medical knowledge, patient care, professionalism, interpersonal skills and communication, practice-based learning and improvement, and system-based practice.[38] Most of these competencies can be addressed during this 2-week rotation if a well-planned curriculum is established. During the preoperative evaluation rotation, residents not only have the opportunity to learn about evidence-based indications for appropriate preoperative testing and evaluation but also how to stratify risk and optimize the patient for the proposed anesthetic. They should participate in shared decision-making conversations with patients. The opportunity for teaching systems-based practice concepts presents itself when the anesthesiologist explains the importance of how the comorbidities of the patient will affect the anesthetic care, as well as appropriate assignment of surgical location (inpatient vs outpatient vs an off-site ambulatory surgery center). Their experience in the PEC should provide residents with an understanding of the most effective systems for patient assessment, staffing of a preoperative assessment program, and alternative methods for gathering and evaluating the preoperative data. Residents should also learn how to analyze preoperative data and make evidence-based decisions about anesthetic management.[39]

Each resident should have a sound base of medical knowledge before beginning this rotation. A rotation in preoperative assessment in the PEC will further expand this knowledge because the resident will be asked to apply this to patients in an anesthesia-specific manner. Central to this knowledge is a grasp of the cardiopulmonary changes that occur with anesthesia. Lectures on cardiac stent management, anticoagulation management, and airway anatomy and management should be part of any 2-week rotation. The ACGME stresses the importance of this clinical teaching by suggesting that faculty members with documented interest and expertise in these fields provide the lectures.[37] Management of antiplatelet and anticoagulation agents provides residents with the additional opportunity to improve their administrative and communication skills because coordination with multiple providers is needed. Clear communication with the patient about when to stop their anticoagulation is vital to their safety, and residents will gain confidence in patient-teaching techniques, such as the teach-back method.[40]

At times, senior anesthesiology residents may be participating in an advanced elective in preoperative medicine and/or surgical home topics. An individualized, self-directed learning approach that emphasizes the creation of defined objectives in advance of the rotation may be appropriate. All learners, especially those who are more advanced in their training, are likely to benefit from the exercise of following patients forward: consulting with the patient in the PEC, and then participating in their care throughout the entire perioperative journey. Advanced elective rotations may also concentrate on concepts of human systems engineering and business models such as Lean Management, as well as participation in PEC-related quality-improvement initiatives.

REFERENCES

1. Berwick DM, Nolan TW, Whittington J. The triple aim: care, health, and cost. Health Aff 2008;27(3):759–69.
2. Blitz JD, Kendale SM, Jain SK, et al. Preoperative evaluation clinic visit is associated with decreased risk of in-hospital postoperative mortality. Anesthesiology 2016;125:280–94.
3. Ferschl MB, Tung A, Sweitzer B, et al. Preoperative clinic visits reduce operating room cancellations and delays. Anesthesiology 2005;103:855–9.
4. Correll DJ, Bader AM, Hull MW, et al. Value of preoperative clinic visits in identifying issues with potential impact on operating room efficiency. Anesthesiology 2006;105:1254–9.
5. Kash BA, Zhang Y, Cline KM, et al. The perioperative surgical home (PSH): a comprehensive review of US and non-US studies shows predominantly positive quality and cost outcomes. Milbank Q 2014;92:796–821.
6. Grocott MP, Mythen MG. Perioperative medicine: the value proposition for anesthesia?: a UK perspective on delivering value from anesthesiology. Anesthesiol Clin 2015;33:617–28.
7. Grocott MPW, Plumb JOM, Edwards M, et al. Re-designing the pathway to surgery: better care and added value. Perioper Med (Lond) 2017;6:9.
8. Available at: https://www.cms.gov/ICD10Manual/version34-fullcode-cms/fullcode_cms/Defining_the_Medicare_Severity_Diagnosis_Related_Groups_(MS-DRGs)_PBL-038.pdf. Accessed March 10, 2018.
9. Matulis J, Liu S, Mecchella J, et al. Choosing Wisely: a quality improvement initiative to decrease unnecessary preoperative testing. BMJ Qual Improv Rep 2017;6:1–5.
10. Available at: http://www.choosingwisely.org/clinician-lists/#parentSociety=American_Society_of_Anesthesiologists. Accessed March 10, 2018.
11. Available at: https://www.cms.gov/Regulations-and-Guidance/Guidance/Transmittals/downloads/R1719B3.pdf. Accessed March 10, 2018.
12. Bader A, Sweitzer B, Kumar A. Nuts and Bolts of preoperative clinics: the view from three institutions. Cleve Clin J Med 2009;76(Suppl 4):S104–11.
13. Richardson WC. Improving the 21st-century health care system. Committee on the Quality ofHealth Care in America, Institute of Medicine, editor. Crossing the quality Chasm, a new health system for the 21st century, 4th printing. Washington, DC: National Academy Press; 2003. p. 39–60.

14. Wijeysundera DM, Austin PC, Beattie WS, et al. Outcomes and processes of care related to preoperative medical consultation. Arch Intern Med 2010;170:1365–74.
15. Vazirani S, Lankarani-Fard A, Liang LJ, et al. Perioperative processes and outcomes after implementation of a hospitalist-run preoperative clinic. J Hosp Med 2012;7:697–701.
16. Carlisle J, Swart M, Dawe EJ, et al. Factors associated with survival after resection of colorectal adenocarcinoma in 314 patients. Br J Anaesth 2012;108:430–5.
17. Kluger MT, Tham EJ, Coleman NA, et al. Inadequate preoperative evaluation and preparation: a review of 197 reports from the Australian incident monitoring study. Anaesthesia 2000;55:1173–8.
18. Vetter TR, Downing ME, Vanlandingham SC, et al. Predictors of patient medication compliance on the day of surgery and the effects of providing patients with standardized yet simplified medication instructions. Anesthesiology 2014; 121:29–35.
19. Auerbach AD, Rasic MA, Sehgal N, et al. Opportunity missed: medical consultation, resource use, and quality of care of patients undergoing major surgery. Arch Intern Med 2007;167:2338–44.
20. Katz RI, Cimino L, Vitkun SA. Preoperative medical consultations: impact on perioperative management and surgical outcome. Can J Anaesth 2005;52:697–702.
21. Sullivan MJL. The pain catastrophizing scale. User manual. Montreal (Canada): McGill University; 2009.
22. Porter M. What is value in healthcare? N Engl J Med 2010;363:2477–81.
23. Banugo P, Amoako D. Prehabilitation. BJA Educ 2017;17(12):401–5.
24. Wong J, Abrishami A, Riazi S, et al. A perioperative smoking cessation intervention with varenicline, counseling, and fax referral to a telephone quitline versus a brief intervention: a randomized controlled trial. Anesth Analg 2017;125:571–9.
25. Sprung J. Postoperative Delirium in elderly patients is associated with subsequent cognitive impairment. Br J Anaesth 2017;119(2):316–23.
26. Moskowitz EE. Postoperative delirium is associated with increased 5 -year mortality. Am J Surg 2017;214(6):1036–8.
27. Mantilla CB, Wass CT, Goodrich A, et al. Risk for perioperative myocardial infarction and mortality in patients undergoing hip or knee arthroplasty; the role of anemia. Transfusion 2011;51:82–91.
28. Wu WC, Schifftner TL, Henderson WG, et al. Preoperative hematocrit levels and postoperative outcomes in older patients undergoing noncardiac surgery. JAMA 2007;297:2481–8.
29. Guinn NR, Guercio JR, Hopkins TJ, et al. How do we develop and implement a preoperative anemia clinic designed to improve perioperative outcomes and reduce cost? Transfusion 2016;56:297–303.
30. Smilowitz NR, Oberweis BS, Nukala S, et al. Association between anemia, bleeding, and transfusion with long-term mortality following non-cardiac surgery. Am J Med 2016;129(3):315–23.e2.
31. Goodnough L, Maniatis A, Earnshaw P, et al. Detection, evaluation, and management of preoperative anaemia in the elective orthopaedic surgical patient: NATA guidelines. Br J Anaesth 2011;106:13–22.
32. Muñoz M, Acheson AG, Auerbach M, et al. International consensus statement on the peri-operative management of anaemia and iron deficiency. Anaesthesia 2017;72:233–47.
33. Lofgren MA, Berends SK, Reyes J, et al. Scope of practice barriers for advanced practice registered nurses: a state task force to minimize barriers. J Nurs Adm 2017;47:465–9.

34. Varughese AM, Byczowski TI, Wittkugel EP, et al. Impact of a nurse practitioner-assisted preoperative assessment program on quality. Paediatr Anaesth 2006;16: 723–33.

35. Abdelhadi A. Investigating emergency room service quality using lean manufacturing. Int J Health Care Qual Assur 2015;28(5):510–9.

36. Gerlach R, Blitz J, Sweitzer B. Teaching in the preanesthesia clinic. In: Bowe E, Schell R, DiLorenzo A, editors. Education in anesthesia: how to deliver the best learning experience. 1st edition. Cambridge (UK): Cambridge University Press; 2018. p. 41.

37. Accreditation Council for Graduate Medical Education and the American Board of Anesthesiology. ACGME anesthesia residency requirements. 2018. Available at: http://www.acgme.org/Specialities/Program-Requirements-and-FAQs-and-Applications/pfcatid/6/Anesthesiology. Accessed August 15, 2018.

38. Heard J, Allen R, Clardy J. Assessing the needs of residency program directors to meet the ACGME general competencies. Acad Med 2002;77(7):750.

39. Accreditation Council for Graduate Medical Education and the American Board of Anesthesiology. The Anesthesiology Milestone Project. 2015. Available at: www.acgme.org/Portals/0/PDFs/Milestones/AnesthesiologyMilestones.pdf. Accessed February 12, 2018.

40. Caplin M, Saunders T. Utilizing teach-back to reinforce patient education: a step-by-step approach. Orthop Nurs 2015;34:365–8 [quiz: 369–70].

Preoperative Laboratory Testing

Angela F. Edwards, MD[a],*, Daniel J. Forest, MD[b]

KEYWORDS

- Preoperative laboratory testing • Preprocedural laboratory testing • Preop testing
- Health care costs • Testing protocols

KEY POINTS

- Preoperative testing should occur following a targeted history and physical examination and review of medical record and relate to procedural risks. Evidence supports only that which is medically necessary to direct perioperative care.
- Avoid testing healthy ASA I or II type patients having low-risk, minimally invasive procedures. It is unnecessary to repeat recent testing without significant change in clinical condition.
- The more the tests ordered the higher the likelihood of an abnormal result. False-positive results increase with number of tests ordered with significant economic implications.
- Without specific testing guidelines, excessive ordering often results. Problems arise if tests are ordered based on protocol, not medical necessity.
- Available guidelines to support preoperative testing in specific populations are reviewed.
- Indications and limitations of preprocedural testing are described.

INTRODUCTION

In the United States, the number of patients seeking surgical intervention in the ambulatory setting continues to increase. As recently as 2012, elective surgery represented a major proportion of health care expenditures. With more than 36 million procedures performed annually, 22.5 million within the ambulatory surgery setting, health care costs across the country will continue to escalate as the population ages and requires surgical intervention. An opportunity for value enhancement may lie in more effectively managing preoperative testing decisions during the surgical phase of care. Early

Disclosures: Neither author has financial relations to disclose.
[a] Department of Anesthesiology, Wake Forest University School of Medicine, Medical Center Boulevard, 9 CSB Janeway Tower, Winston-Salem, NC 27157, USA; [b] Preoperative Assessment Clinic, Department of Anesthesiology, Wake Forest University School of Medicine, Medical Center Boulevard, 9 CSB Janeway Tower, Winston-Salem, NC 27157, USA
* Corresponding author.
E-mail address: afedward@wakehealth.edu

Anesthesiology Clin 36 (2018) 493–507
https://doi.org/10.1016/j.anclin.2018.07.002   **anesthesiology.theclinics.com**
1932-2275/18/© 2018 Elsevier Inc. All rights reserved.

adoption of best practice care designs using cost-effective testing may improve the management of complex patients and special populations.[1,2]

Obtaining routine or baseline preoperative laboratory tests increases health care costs and has been listed, by the Choosing Wisely Campaign, as one of the top 5 practices anesthesiologists should avoid.[3] At a time when age and medical complexity in those seeking surgical intervention continues to increase, the need for thorough preoperative evaluation is now more evident than ever. In many institutions, preoperative assessment clinics incorporate focused physical examinations, diagnostic and laboratory analysis, medical optimization, decision-making, patient education, and advanced care planning as a means of mitigating perioperative risk.[2] This comprehensive approach ensures preoperative testing is conducted in a manner that is both evidence based and targeted at identifying areas for medical optimization.

WHERE IS THE EVIDENCE?

Testing based on institutional protocols is unnecessary and could increase risk.[4] Performing any presurgical test should be directly related to comorbidities and risk of procedure, with the expectation that the results will alter management or improve outcomes.[5,6] Each preoperative test ordered needs to be carefully considered. Random testing, as with protocols, irrespective of medical evaluation, often results in abnormalities and subsequent investigations. The more the tests ordered, the greater the likelihood of obtaining false-positive results that could result in significant economic and emotional burden. False-positive results often lead to additional testing that may or may not affect surgical proceedings. Guidelines recommend, and evidence supports, selective testing based on recent history and physical examination and functional status.

Comorbidity-specific testing based on clinical findings during history and physical examination and following review of the medical record is most effective.[7–9] It has been estimated that 60% to 90% of presurgical patients have at least one unnecessary test ordered.[9] Recent evidence suggests almost all preoperative urine, liver function, or coagulation tests ordered lack support to justify the test.[6]

When adhering to evidence-based testing, diagnostic efficacy and effectiveness of the test must be considered. If the test correctly identifies abnormalities and changes the diagnosis to impact management, then the test is worth ordering. If the test has a high degree of therapeutic effectiveness and will change outcome, then the test is worth performing. Abnormal results and subsequent management must be weighed against the urgency for the surgery.[10,11]

General recommendations to consider before ordering preoperative tests include the following:

- Clinical findings from targeted history and physical examination should guide testing
- Consider ASA classification and risk of surgical procedure before testing
  - ASA I or II classification patients do not benefit; testing is not recommended[4,7]
  - ASA Class III or IV type patients may benefit depending on surgical comorbidities
- Relative risk of surgery must be considered (intermediate risk or high risk) before testing
  - Low-risk, ambulatory surgical procedures do not benefit (cataracts, inguinal hernia repair, etc.)
- Avoid if patient has results within 6 months to 1 year or if comorbidity management is stable

TESTING PROTOCOLS

Testing grids refer to a prescribed set of instructions for ordering specific tests based on age, anticipated procedure, or surgeon preference. Such protocols are adhered to irrespective of recent results or comorbidities. There is no value for ordering laboratory tests based solely on the anticipated surgical procedure. A large randomized controlled trial (RCT) and Cochrane meta-analysis demonstrated the lack of effectiveness of preoperative test grids for low-risk surgery.[4] Evidence exists to demonstrate routine preoperative testing will not affect outcomes in low-risk surgery and in fact may lead to significant harm and unnecessary costs.[12,13]

Reasons for automated testing protocols often include the following:

- Medical legal concerns
- Institutional rules
- Concern that another physician may find laboratory value necessary and delay or cancel case
- Patient satisfaction
- Lack of awareness of published guidelines

Concerns regarding automated testing include the following:

- Medicolegal implications of incidental findings
- Failure to review results
- Cost and inconvenience related to unnecessary delay to pursue abnormalities
- Patient anxiety regarding an abnormal result that may or may not affect future management

Preoperative testing should be based on the patient's history, review of medical records, physical examination, and type of procedure. Healthy, ASA I or II, patients undergoing minimally invasive procedures or those who have had recent laboratory evaluations do not need repeat testing. Preoperative testing in low-risk ambulatory surgery has not been demonstrated to affect perioperative care, decrease complications, cancellations, or delays.[9] It is unnecessary to repeat laboratory analysis if there has been no recent change in the patient's condition.

SPECIAL POPULATIONS
Advanced Age

Preoperative testing based on advanced age often occurs in patients older than 70 years and is associated with expected abnormalities.[14] It is anticipated that 7% to 12% of elderly patients will have an abnormal creatinine, hemoglobin (Hgb), and glucose.[14,15] Seventy-five percent of these patients will have abnormalities on their electrocardiogram (ECG). None of these findings predict adverse perioperative outcomes. To date, the predictors of adverse surgical outcomes predominately relate to ASA physical status, higher surgical risk, and heart failure.[16]

Obesity

Obesity, and its related comorbidities, has a significant impact on health care costs and outcomes. Obesity is associated with alterations in respiratory, cardiovascular, and endocrine physiology, which increase perioperative risk.[17,18] Restrictive lung disease is often present yet preoperative pulmonary function tests in asymptomatic patients have not been demonstrated to affect postoperative outcomes.[3,19] Screening tools to identify those at risk for obstructive sleep apnea or sleep disturbances prove beneficial.[20] Once identified, referral for further revaluation is reasonable but should not delay surgery. Screening tools seem beneficial in identifying at-risk patients in order to alter management using opioid sparing techniques, increased monitoring, and continuous positive airway pressure postoperatively.

Obese patients are at high risk for hypertension, hyperlipidemia, heart failure, and cardiomyopathy. Determination of functional status and cardiopulmonary signs could predict the need for additional cardiac testing. Obesity is not an absolute indication for echocardiography, stress testing, or ECG.[21]

Obesity can lead to increased insulin resistance, hyperglycemia, and diabetes mellitus. Poorly treated hyperglycemia can lead to impaired wound healing, osmotic diuresis, and dehydration postoperatively. In such patients, consideration should be given to obtaining fasting glucose, electrolytes, Hgb A1C, or fructosamine as a more immediate indicator of glycemic regulation.[22] These values will facilitate adjustments in perioperative management.

Pregnancy

In institutions where preoperative pregnancy testing is not required, obtaining an accurate menstrual history is essential. Testing should be offered, with risks and benefits discussed, and subsequently ordered if doubt remains.

It is appropriate to consider pregnancy testing in any woman of childbearing age because results will precipitate a change in decision-making and perioperative management.[23,24] In 2002, the Practice Advisory for Preanesthesia Testing acknowledged that a "standard history and physical examination may be inadequate to detect early pregnancy and pregnancy tests should be considered in women of childbearing age, especially if there is an uncertain pregnancy history." When updated, the investigators acknowledged the literature was inadequate to inform whether anesthesia causes harmful effects during early pregnancy. The recommendation was, again, to offer pregnancy testing to women of childbearing age in which case results would alter management.[11]

In many instances, serum human chorionic gonadotropin (beta-hCG [B-hCG]) performed within 7 to 10 days of procedure will reliably predict pregnancy.[25] Serum or urine tests may be repeated the day of surgery if there is significant concern regarding change since initial evaluation. Most urine tests detect B-hCG levels of 25 to 50 mIU/mL yet have a fairly high rate of false negatives at 6 to 7 days postconception. B-hCG levels are very low at that time (10 mIU/mL). Serum hCG levels double every 1.4 to 2 days during the early days of pregnancy.[26] So during the first trimester (especially <6 weeks postconceptual age), it is reasonable to obtain serum hCG level to detect occult pregnancy. Beyond 6 weeks after last menstrual period, a urine test is adequate to detect pregnancy.

Cardiovascular Testing in Noncardiac Surgery

Guidelines available for perioperative risk assessment include the 2017 Canadian Cardiovascular Society (CCS) guidelines for management of noncardiac surgery patients and the 2014 American College of Cardiology/American Heart Association (ACC/AHA) guidelines.[27–29] The CCS guidelines incorporate much evidence published since the ACC/AHA guidelines were released in 2014. Although some recommendations remain consistent between the 2, the CCS has significant differences regarding preoperative testing and risk stratification.

The 2014 ACC/AHA guidelines rely on functional capacity and recommended risk calculators to determine if a patient planning nonemergent surgery should have further testing. If a patient is considered high risk and has unknown functional capacity or poor exercise capacity (<4 metabolic equivalents [METS]), the patient may be referred for pharmacologic stress testing if results will change management. The CCS guidelines make no recommendation regarding the use of functional capacity, citing variability between studies in how data were collected, and in contrast to 2014 ACC/AHA guidelines, the CCS recommends against preoperative assessment of risk using echocardiography, exercise or pharmacologic stress testing, or coronary computed tomographic angiography. Instead, the CCS recommends the use of B-type natriuretic peptide (BNP) testing to assess cardiac risk in patients older than or equal to 65 years, having Revised Cardiac Risk Index score greater than or equal to 1, or aged 45 to 64 years with significant cardiovascular disease as defined earlier in their focus population. A comparison of these guidelines is outlined in **Table 1**.

The CCS guidelines recommend BNP and N-terminal fragment proBNP (NT-proBNP) testing for superior risk prediction compared with stress or echocardiographic testing.[27] Furthermore, they suggest patients older than or equal to 65 years or 45 to 64 years of age with cardiac risk factors planning elective surgery undergo BNP testing. Regardless of the result, the patient is recommended to proceed to surgery. However, postoperative daily troponin measurements and ECGs are recommended for patients with higher biomarker thresholds, NT-proBNP greater than or equal to 300 mg/L, or BNP greater than or equal to 92 mg/L.

Electrocardiograms

- Preoperative ECGs should not be ordered for asymptomatic patients undergoing low-risk surgical procedures regardless of age.
- Routine ECGs have low specificity with high prevalence of abnormalities and false positives. Testing does not add value beyond thorough history isolating risk factors and physical examination.[30]

Table 1
Comparison of 2017 Canadian Cardiovascular Society (CCS) and 2014 American College of Cardiology/American Heart Association (ACC/AHA) preoperative cardiac testing guidelines

Preoperative Test	CCS Guidelines (2017)	ACC/AHA Guidelines (2014)
Cardiac Risk Stratification		
Echocardiogram	Not recommended	Recommend if LV function or valves require evaluation
Exercise stress testing	Not recommended	Recommend when exercise tolerance is low or unknown
Pharmacologic stress testing	Not recommended	Recommend if high risk, <4 METS, changes management
CCTA	Not recommended	Not recommended
Postop Troponin	Recommended if any of the following: • Elevated preoperative BNP • RCRI $\geq$1 • Age $\geq$65 y • Significant cardiac risk	Not routinely recommended in any patient group (only when ischemia is suspected clinically)
BNP or NT-proBNP	Recommended if age $\geq$65 y, 45–65 y or older with significant cardiovascular disease, or RCRI score $\geq$1	Not recommended

Abbreviations: CCTA, coronary computed tomographic angiography; LV, left ventricular; NT-proBNP, N-terminal fragment of proBNP.
Data from Refs.[27–29]

- Preoperative ECGs can be considered in patients with coronary heart disease, significant arrhythmia, peripheral arterial disease, cerebrovascular disease, or other significant structural heart disease.[29,31]
- ST depression and baseline tachycardia are predictors of increased morbidity and mortality.[31]

Preoperative ECGs are often obtained in patients with a history of coronary artery disease, dysrhythmia, and cardiac risk factors scheduled for intermediate- to high-risk surgery. This practice has little impact on perioperative management or postoperative outcomes. Risk factors predictive of abnormal ECG findings include the following: age greater than 65 years, heart failure, high cholesterol, angina, myocardial infarction, and severe valvular disease.[30] Liu and colleagues[15] described the specificity of an ECG abnormality in predicting postoperative cardiac adverse events is only 26% and a normal ECG does negate the possibility of underlying cardiac disease. Advanced age has been suggested as a reason to obtain a preoperative ECG as rhythm abnormalities increase in older patients. Although ECG abnormalities are common in those older than 65 years, only functional capacity or symptomatic cardiac disease has effectively resulted in a change in preoperative medical management. In one prospective observational study, van Klei and colleagues[32] found that 45% of patients older than 50 years having noncardiac surgery had an abnormality on a preoperative ECG. Bundle branch blocks were associated with major adverse cardiac events and death, yet provided no additional predictive value beyond the revised cardiac risk index. Given the high likelihood that ECG abnormalities will be found in patients of advanced age and these are unlikely to affect management, using age-based criteria for ordering preoperative ECGs should not be performed. The 2014 ACC/AHA guidelines state that "preoperative ECG is reasonable for patients with known coronary heart disease, significant arrhythmia, peripheral arterial disease, CVA or other significant heart disease structural heart disease except for those undergoing low risk surgeries." The guidelines also state that "routine ECG is not useful for asymptomatic patients undergoing low risk surgery."[29] Although not specifically stated, it is reasonable to accept an ECG within 1 year if one available provided no changes in the patient's symptoms or if cardiac risk factors exist.

Echocardiogram

Echocardiograms identify valvular lesions, regional wall motion abnormalities, pulmonary hypertension, and ventricular function serving to guide perioperative management. A preoperative echocardiogram should be considered in patients who present with heart failure symptoms, dyspnea on exertion, orthopnea, or bilateral pedal edema. For patients with known heart failure, repeat echocardiogram is reasonable in those who have not had an evaluation for greater than 1 year scheduled for intermediate- or high-risk surgery. However, it has not been shown to reduce length of stay or improve survival.[33]

In patients with known valvular disease, it is recommended to obtain an echocardiogram if there is concern for worsening disease or in whom cardiology consultation may affect the perioperative anesthetic management.[28]

Cardiac Stress Test

Routine pharmacologic or exercise stress testing is not recommended preoperatively. When determining preoperative myocardial ischemic risk, consideration should be given to the patient's functional capacity, risk factors, and the complexity of the planned procedure. It is reasonable to proceed to surgery without further testing in patients who perform greater than or equal to 4 METS, seem medically optimized, and hemodynamically stable. In patients with increased cardiac risk and poor functional capacity (METS < 4), it is acceptable to perform cardiac stress testing before surgery if a positive test for inducible ischemia was likely to alter perioperative management.[29]

B-Type Natriuretic Peptide

BNP is synthesized in response to increased ventricular filling pressures and wall stress. BNP helps regulate blood pressure and fluid balance by effecting secretion of renin, aldosterone, and angiotensin. This biomarker has demonstrated utility diagnosing heart failure as elevations become evident in right heart failure, pulmonary hypertension, pulmonary embolism, as well as acute coronary syndromes.[34] Abnormalities are typically seen in volume-overloaded states and can be obtained in the preoperative period to help guide cardiac optimization before surgery.

BNP has shown prognostic value in both patients with heart failure and without heart failure predicting postoperative cardiac outcomes during noncardiac surgery.[35] There is good evidence to show that elevations may predict poor outcomes and mortality. Obtaining preoperative BNP in high-risk cardiac patients undergoing noncardiac surgery may demonstrate predictive utility.[36–38]

Troponins

During times of myocardial ischemia or decreased coronary perfusion, cardiac troponins released into circulation can be monitored for the presence of disease and also increased risk of short-term mortality.[37,39] Values are followed to determine peak concentrations because this relates to the extent of cellular damage. Historically, small elevations were evident with myocardial strain, but not direct injury. Strenuous exercise or proinflammatory states were described as subclinical leaks. Recent literature supports the fact that even small changes in troponin levels suggest adverse outcomes.[37,40]

In reviewing preoperative troponins in patients undergoing elective noncardiac surgery, Maile and colleagues[41] showed 30-day mortality was significantly increased in patients with elevated troponin levels preoperatively compared with those with normal levels.[40] Furthermore, they reported mortality was highest in those with the highest troponin level and shortest duration between the preoperative measurements and surgical encounter. Although consideration should be given to obtaining preoperative troponins in patients at high risk for cardiac morbidity, additional prospective studies are required before routine use can be recommended.

Chest Radiography

- Routine preoperative chest radiography is not indicated in asymptomatic patients.
- Chest radiography should be considered in patients with new or unstable cardiopulmonary signs or symptoms that would likely require additional medical management or delay of surgery.[42]

Once considered to be a part of every thorough preoperative evaluation, chest radiography in asymptomatic patients has demonstrated minimal effectiveness and very rarely leads to a change in perioperative management. One of the more expensive laboratory tests, preoperative chest radiography, has not demonstrated predictive value for postoperative pulmonary complications.[11] It is not uncommon to find unrelated abnormalities, and this increases with age. The findings are usually chronic in nature and often predicted by the information obtained from the history and physical examination.[43] Selective use of preoperative chest radiography may be reasonable in patients with signs or symptoms of acute or unstable cardiopulmonary disease.[44] However, the relationship between this test and patient outcomes, morbidity, and mortality is unknown.

Renal Function Testing

- ASA III or IV type patients should be considered for renal function testing, especially those with significant cardiovascular disease undergoing high-risk vascular surgery.
- Biomarkers for predicting acute kidney injury in order of appearance include neutrophil gelatinase-associated lipocalin (NGAL), Kim-1 (6–24 hours), cystatin C (22–48 hours), and creatinine (36 hours to weeks[45,46]).
- Baseline serum creatinine, blood urea nitrogen, and estimated glomerular filtration rate (eGFR) before contrast media administration and organ transplantation are appropriate.

Physiologic functions of the renal system include water balance, elimination of waste, erythropoiesis, hormonal regulations, acid-base system, and cardio circulatory functions. Many disease states disrupt the delicate homeostatic balance. Diabetes, arteriosclerosis, chronic heart failure, and coronary heart disease are some of the more prevalent disease states affecting surgical outcomes. Laboratory assessment of serum markers for preoperative renal function is in widespread use. The most common are serum creatinine, blood urea nitrogen, eGFR, and calculated creatinine clearance.[13,46,47] Serum creatinine is a waste product of metabolism, yet ineffective as a predictor of renal dysfunction because level directly depends on muscle mass, gender, and age. eGFR provides a better estimate because it calculates renal function by eliminating these variables.[48,49] A reduced eGFR (<60 mL/min/1.73 m^2) has been associated with a 3-fold increase in postoperative 30-day mortality after vascular and cardiac surgery and therefore represents a reasonable test for detecting subclinical renal failure.[50,51] Besides these well-known tests, new biomarkers, cystatin C and NGAL, are emerging in clinical utility.[45] Plasma cystatin C represents a functional damage biomarker and NGAL correlates with tubular damage. At present, the precise utility of these parameters remains unclear. However, that renal function tests are incorporated in various risk calculators and mentioned in numerous preoperative guidelines and practice advisories.[11,29,52–54] These parameters have been shown to predict adverse outcome in various surgical settings.

Preoperative Urinalysis

There is no evidence supporting routine urine analysis in asymptomatic patients without clinical suspicion. Common abnormalities found in urinalysis, including asymptomatic bacteriuria, do not seem to be associated with postoperative joint infections.[55] The ASA Task Force does not recommend routine preanesthesia urinalysis except for specific procedures including prosthesis implantation and urologic procedures or in the presence of urinary tract symptoms.[11] The decision to obtain should be made on an individual basis based on patient and procedure risk factor. There is no evidence supporting routine urinalysis in asymptomatic patients.

Diabetes

- Blood glucose testing should only be performed if there is a clinical suspicion of disturbance in glucose metabolism or diagnosis of diabetes mellitus.

- Preoperative hyperglycemia is a risk factor for increased 30-day mortality in patients undergoing noncardiac, nonvascular surgery and for increased long-term mortality in vascular surgery patients.[56–58]
- Glycosylated[59] Hgb A1C is a measure of long-term (3 months) glucose control. Elevated levels are associated with increased risk for cardiovascular events and postoperative infections.

Diabetes is included in several risk stratification measures as an indicator of poor surgical outcomes.[60] Because of the lack of RCTs, there is a little level of evidence to support routine preoperative screening in patients without a preexisting diagnosis or concern for dysregulated glucose metabolism. Two systematic reviews summarized the effects of preoperative testing in such patients. Both confirmed testing should only be performed only if clinical suspicion exists.[22,61] However, testing is reasonable in diabetics, obese patients, and those on long-term steroid therapy, because there is a correlation between elevated blood glucose, abnormal postoperative values, and poor outcomes.[62] In high-risk groups, those undergoing vascular, orthopedic, or spine surgery, preoperative testing for hyperglycemia may be justified.

In high-risk groups, elevated blood glucose concentrations have been associated with increased risk of infections among patients scheduled for spine surgery, knee or hip replacement, and orthopedic trauma surgery.[63–65] Vascular surgery patients with elevated blood glucose concentrations are at high risk for myocardial ischemia, infarction, release of markers for myocardial damage, and cerebrovascular ischemic events.[56,57] This population is also prone to undiagnosed diabetes mellitus,[66] so preoperative laboratory review is of critical importance.

Hgb A1C reflects intermediate-term glucose control and plays an important role. Preoperative values greater than 53 mmol/mol is a predictor of postoperative hyperglycemia in patients with diabetes undergoing elective noncardiac surgery.[67,68]

Even slightly elevated values have been associated with increased cardiac morbidity after elective and urgent vascular surgery.[69] Yet, elevated HbA1C did not predict increased postoperative 30-day mortality in patients scheduled for cardiac and major surgery.[70] Nonetheless, HbA1C is a risk factor for increased long-term mortality in vascular surgery patients.[70]

Liver Function Testing

Liver function testing is rarely indicated except in such instances as acute hepatitis, significant liver dysfunction, or cirrhosis. Testing is indicated if end-stage liver disease is suspected in order to calculate the Model for End-Stage Liver Disease score.

Patients with acute hepatitis, liver dysfunction, or cirrhosis are at increased risk of perioperative complications and death. In patients with visible ascites and associated infection-related comorbidities, liver function testing is reasonable. There are no data to suggest that patients with asymptomatic elevations in transaminases, bilirubin, or prothrombin time have adverse perioperative events. However, albumin level, an indicator of malnutrition or malabsorption, is incorporated in several risk calculators and as a predictor of poor outcomes.

Hemoglobin/Hematocrit

Preoperative Hgb should be obtained based on the likelihood of anemia, polycythemia, and increased blood loss with the surgical procedure. The Anesthesia Task Force recommends that type and invasiveness of procedure; extremes of age; and history of liver disease, anemia, bleeding, and other hematologic disorders be considered before determining the need for preprocedural hematocrit (HCT).[11] With preprocedural Hgb and HCT levels, only about one-third of the tests ordered turn out to be necessary. Occasionally an abnormality results that affects medical management if the planned procedure has a high anticipated blood loss. Preoperative HCT, surgical procedure, and surgeon can predict the risk for perioperative transfusion and guide need for Type and Screen or crossmatch. It is reasonable to order in patients with liver disease, extremes of age, history of anemia, or other hematologic disorders and occasionally helpful in patients who seem elderly, frail, or have higher risk surgery planned. However, routine preoperative Hgb or HCT testing is not supported by the literature.

Coagulation Studies (Prothrombin Time/Partial Thromboplastin Time)

Coagulation studies may be beneficial if patient currently taking anticoagulants (warfarin) has a history of coagulopathy or chronic liver disease. A systematic review of the literature suggests routine coagulation screening is unlikely to predict bleeding risk. A thorough patient history has a higher sensitivity for the detection of bleeding.[71–74] Reviewing patient history looking for bleeding abnormalities is more effective if it includes a family history of coagulation issues, history of excess bleeding with prior surgical procedures, and use of anticoagulants. Clinical conditions that predispose patients to bleeding, such as liver and renal dysfunction, should also be noted. Results of partial thromboplastin time (PTT) and prothrombin time should be put into the context of the patient's clinical status, prior bleeding challenges, and family history. The presence of lupus anticoagulant will prolong the PTT results and is not predictive of increased bleeding. In general, preoperative coagulation studies are costly and should be reserved for patients on anticoagulants, history of bleeding abnormality, or medical condition that predisposes to coagulopathy (liver disease, malnutrition). Testing is also reasonable in patients with suspected bleeding disorders or undergoing craniotomy where bleeding would be devastating.

Genetic Testing

Pharmacogenetic testing is available to tailor treatment based on a patient's genetic composition. This information can guide therapy for postoperative pain, postoperative nausea and vomiting, and thrombosis prevention. With patients demonstrating a high variability in their response to various pharmacologic agents, there is increasing evidence to suggest that genetic variations have a major impact on the pharmacokinetics and the pharmacodynamics of some commonly used medications, including warfarin, nonsteroidal antiinflammatory drugs, benzodiazepines, opioids, antiemetics, and proton pump inhibitors.[75] Genetic variations of the cytochrome (CYP) 450 enzyme system, a microsomal drug metabolism supergroup involved in the biotransformation of most analgesics, antibiotics, antiarrhythmic agents, antiplatelet drugs, and psychiatric agents is often implicated. More specifically, the CYP enzymes CYP3A4 and CYP2D6 are highly prone to genetic variability, resulting in either hypermetabolism of prodrugs inducing toxic levels of analgesics or reduced metabolism of already biologically effective drugs.[75]

In 2006, the US Food and Drug Administration approved genetic testing for CYP2D6[76] for families with a suspicious history for genetic variability of the CYP system.[76] The test, which takes 7 days to perform, may be reasonable in patients undergoing elective major surgery.[77]

SUMMARY

1. Evidence does not support routine preoperative testing even for high-risk surgical procedures. Decisions should be based on comorbidities after a targeted history and physical examination.
2. Preoperative laboratory testing based on protocols, not medical necessity, is expensive and results in false positives that potentiate harm and increase medical costs. Testing protocols, as with age-based criteria, are unnecessary, expensive, and have higher likelihood of abnormal results.
3. Preoperative guidelines should be the same for all perioperative physicians: anesthesiologists, surgeons, hospitalists, and primary care providers. Valid justification for preoperative testing occurs if the benefit of the test outweighs the potential health risks, surgical delays and cost and will result in a change in management.

REFERENCES

1. Porter ME. What is value in health care? N Engl J Med 2010;363(26):2477–81.
2. Correll DJ, Bader AM, Hull MW, et al. Value of preoperative clinic visits in identifying issues with potential impact on operating room efficiency. Anesthesiology 2006;105(6):1254–9 [discussion: 1256A].
3. Cassel CK, Guest JA. Choosing wisely: helping physicians and patients make smart decisions about their care. JAMA 2012;307(17):1801–2.
4. Schein OD, Katz J, Bass EB, et al. The value of routine preoperative medical testing before cataract surgery. Study of Medical Testing for Cataract Surgery. N Engl J Med 2000;342(3):168–75.
5. Hepner DL. The role of testing in the preoperative evaluation. Cleve Clin J Med 2009;76(Suppl 4):S22–7.
6. Bock M, Fritsch G, Hepner DL. Preoperative laboratory testing. Anesthesiol Clin 2016;34(1):43–58.
7. Kirkham KR, Wijeysundera DN, Pendrith C, et al. Preoperative testing before low-risk surgical procedures. CMAJ 2015;187(11):E349–58.
8. Kirkham KR, Wijeysundera DN, Pendrith C, et al. Preoperative laboratory investigations: rates and variability prior to low-risk surgical procedures. Anesthesiology 2016;124(4):804–14.
9. Chung F, Yuan H, Yin L, et al. Elimination of preoperative testing in ambulatory surgery. Anesth Analg 2009;108(2):467–75.
10. Fritsch G, Flamm M, Hepner DL, et al. Abnormal pre-operative tests, pathologic findings of medical history, and their predictive value for perioperative complications. Acta Anaesthesiol Scand 2012;56(3):339–50.
11. Committee on Standards and Practice Parameters, Apfelbaum JL, Connis RT, Nickinovich DG, et al. Practice advisory for preanesthesia evaluation: an updated report by the American Society of Anesthesiologists task force on preanesthesia evaluation. Anesthesiology 2012;116(3):522–38.
12. Martin SK, Cifu AS. Routine preoperative laboratory tests for elective surgery. JAMA 2017;318(6):567–8.
13. Johansson T, Fritsch G, Flamm M, et al. Effectiveness of non-cardiac preoperative testing in non-cardiac elective surgery: a systematic review. Br J Anaesth 2013;110(6):926–39.
14. Dzankic S, Pastor D, Gonzalez C, et al. The prevalence and predictive value of abnormal preoperative laboratory tests in elderly surgical patients. Anesth Analg 2001;93(2):301–8, 2nd contents page.

15. Liu LL, Dzankic S, Leung JM. Preoperative electrocardiogram abnormalities do not predict postoperative cardiac complications in geriatric surgical patients. J Am Geriatr Soc 2002;50(7):1186–91.
16. Benarroch-Gampel J, Sheffield KM, Duncan CB, et al. Preoperative laboratory testing in patients undergoing elective, low-risk ambulatory surgery. Ann Surg 2012;256(3):518–28.
17. Smetana GW, Lawrence VA, Cornell JE. Preoperative pulmonary risk stratification for noncardiothoracic surgery: systematic review for the American College of Physicians. Ann Intern Med 2006;144(8):581–95.
18. Nelson JA, Fischer JP, Chung CU, et al. Obesity and early complications following reduction mammaplasty: an analysis of 4545 patients from the 2005-2011 NSQIP datasets. J Plast Surg Hand Surg 2014;48(5):334–9.
19. Sun LY, Gershon AS, Ko DT, et al. Trends in pulmonary function testing before noncardiothoracic surgery. JAMA Intern Med 2015;175(8):1410–2.
20. Nagappa M, Patra J, Wong J, et al. Association of STOP-bang questionnaire as a screening tool for sleep apnea and postoperative complications: a systematic review and bayesian meta-analysis of prospective and retrospective cohort studies. Anesth Analg 2017;125(4):1301–8.
21. Ramaswamy A, Gonzalez R, Smith CD. Extensive preoperative testing is not necessary in morbidly obese patients undergoing gastric bypass. J Gastrointest Surg 2004;8(2):159–64 [discussion: 164–5].
22. Bock M, Johansson T, Fritsch G, et al. The impact of preoperative testing for blood glucose concentration and haemoglobin A1c on mortality, changes in management and complications in noncardiac elective surgery: a systematic review. Eur J Anaesthesiol 2015;32(3):152–9.
23. Kahn RL, Stanton MA, Tong-Ngork S, et al. One-year experience with day-of-surgery pregnancy testing before elective orthopedic procedures. Anesth Analg 2008;106(4):1127–31. Table of contents.
24. Hennrikus WL, Shaw BA, Gerardi JA. Prevalence of positive preoperative pregnancy testing in teenagers scheduled for orthopedic surgery. J Pediatr Orthop 2001;21(5):677–9.
25. Maher JL, Mahabir RC. Preoperative pregnancy testing. Can J Plast Surg 2012; 20(3):e32–4.
26. Wingfield M, McMenamin M. Preoperative pregnancy testing. Br J Surg 2014; 101(12):1488–90.
27. Duceppe E, Parlow J, MacDonald P, et al. Canadian cardiovascular society guidelines on perioperative cardiac risk assessment and management for patients who undergo noncardiac surgery. Can J Cardiol 2017;33(1):17–32.
28. Fleisher LA, Fleischmann KE, Auerbach AD, et al. 2014 ACC/AHA guideline on perioperative cardiovascular evaluation and management of patients undergoing noncardiac surgery: executive summary: a report of the American College of Cardiology/American Heart Association Task Force on practice guidelines. Developed in collaboration with the American College of Surgeons, American Society of Anesthesiologists, American Society of Echocardiography, American Society of Nuclear Cardiology, Heart Rhythm Society, Society for Cardiovascular Angiography and Interventions, Society of Cardiovascular Anesthesiologists, and Society of Vascular Medicine Endorsed by the Society of Hospital Medicine. J Nucl Cardiol 2015;22(1):162–215.
29. Fleisher LA, Fleischmann KE, Auerbach AD, et al. 2014 ACC/AHA guideline on perioperative cardiovascular evaluation and management of patients undergoing noncardiac surgery: a report of the American College of Cardiology/American

Heart Association Task Force on practice guidelines. J Am Coll Cardiol 2014; 64(22):e77–137.

30. Correll DJ, Hepner DL, Chang C, et al. Preoperative electrocardiograms: patient factors predictive of abnormalities. Anesthesiology 2009;110(6):1217–22.

31. Jeger RV, Probst C, Arsenic R, et al. Long-term prognostic value of the preoperative 12-lead electrocardiogram before major noncardiac surgery in coronary artery disease. Am Heart J 2006;151(2):508–13.

32. van Klei WA, Bryson GL, Yang H, et al. The value of routine preoperative electrocardiography in predicting myocardial infarction after noncardiac surgery. Ann Surg 2007;246(2):165–70.

33. Wijeysundera DN, Beattie WS, Karkouti K, et al. Association of echocardiography before major elective non-cardiac surgery with postoperative survival and length of hospital stay: population based cohort study. BMJ 2011;342:d3695.

34. Troughton R, Michael Felker G, Januzzi JL Jr. Natriuretic peptide-guided heart failure management. Eur Heart J 2014;35(1):16–24.

35. Simmers D, Potgieter D, Ryan L, et al. The use of preoperative B-type natriuretic peptide as a predictor of atrial fibrillation after thoracic surgery: systematic review and meta-analysis. J Cardiothorac Vasc Anesth 2015;29(2):389–95.

36. Bayes-Genis A, Barallat J, Galan A, et al. Multimarker strategy for heart failure prognostication. value of neurohormonal biomarkers: neprilysin vs NT-proBNP. Rev Esp Cardiol (Engl Ed) 2015;68(12):1075–84.

37. Bayes-Genis A, Lupon J, Jaffe AS. Can natriuretic peptides be used to guide therapy? EJIFCC 2016;27(3):208–16.

38. Rodseth RN, Biccard BM, Le Manach Y, et al. The prognostic value of preoperative and post-operative B-type natriuretic peptides in patients undergoing noncardiac surgery: B-type natriuretic peptide and N-terminal fragment of pro-B-type natriuretic peptide: a systematic review and individual patient data meta-analysis. J Am Coll Cardiol 2014;63(2):170–80.

39. Aimo A, Januzzi JL Jr, Vergaro G, et al. Prognostic value of high-sensitivity troponin T in chronic heart failure: an individual patient data meta-analysis. Circulation 2018;137(3):286–97.

40. Eggers KM, Venge P, Lindahl B, et al. Cardiac troponin I levels measured with a high-sensitive assay increase over time and are strong predictors of mortality in an elderly population. J Am Coll Cardiol 2013;61(18):1906–13.

41. Maile MD, Jewell ES, Engoren MC. Timing of preoperative troponin elevations and postoperative mortality after noncardiac surgery. Anesth Analg 2016; 123(1):135–40.

42. Loggers SAI, Giannakopoulos GF, Vandewalle E, et al. Preoperative chest radiographs in hip fracture patients: is there any additional value? Eur J Orthop Surg Traumatol 2017;27(7):953–9.

43. Joo HS, Wong J, Naik VN, et al. The value of screening preoperative chest x-rays: a systematic review. Can J Anaesth 2005;52(6):568–74.

44. Young EM, Farmer JD. Preoperative chest radiography in elective surgery: review and update. S D Med 2017;70(2):81–7.

45. Martensson J, Martling CR, Bell M. Novel biomarkers of acute kidney injury and failure: clinical applicability. Br J Anaesth 2012;109(6):843–50.

46. Shavit L, Dolgoker I, Ivgi H, et al. Neutrophil gelatinase-associated lipocalin as a predictor of complications and mortality in patients undergoing non-cardiac major surgery. Kidney Blood Press Res 2011;34(2):116–24.

47. Cho E, Kim SC, Kim MG, et al. The incidence and risk factors of acute kidney injury after hepatobiliary surgery: a prospective observational study. BMC Nephrol 2014;15:169.
48. Cockcroft DW, Gault MH. Prediction of creatinine clearance from serum creatinine. Nephron 1976;16(1):31–41.
49. Levey AS, Bosch JP, Lewis JB, et al. A more accurate method to estimate glomerular filtration rate from serum creatinine: a new prediction equation. Modification of diet in renal disease study group. Ann Intern Med 1999;130(6):461–70.
50. Mooney JF, Ranasinghe I, Chow CK, et al. Preoperative estimates of glomerular filtration rate as predictors of outcome after surgery: a systematic review and meta-analysis. Anesthesiology 2013;118(4):809–24.
51. Huynh TT, van Eps RG, Miller CC 3rd, et al. Glomerular filtration rate is superior to serum creatinine for prediction of mortality after thoracoabdominal aortic surgery. J Vasc Surg 2005;42(2):206–12.
52. Lee TH, Marcantonio ER, Mangione CM, et al. Derivation and prospective validation of a simple index for prediction of cardiac risk of major noncardiac surgery. Circulation 1999;100(10):1043–9.
53. Hoste EA, Clermont G, Kersten A, et al. RIFLE criteria for acute kidney injury are associated with hospital mortality in critically ill patients: a cohort analysis. Crit Care 2006;10(3):R73.
54. Bishop MJ, Souders JE, Peterson CM, et al. Factors associated with unanticipated day of surgery deaths in Department of Veterans Affairs hospitals. Anesth Analg 2008;107(6):1924–35.
55. Drekonja DM, Zarminski B, Johnson JR. Preoperative urine cultures at a veterans affairs medical center. JAMA Intern Med 2013;173(1):71–2.
56. Feringa HH, Vidakovic R, Karagiannis SE, et al. Impaired glucose regulation, elevated glycated haemoglobin and cardiac ischaemic events in vascular surgery patients. Diabet Med 2008;25(3):314–9.
57. McGirt MJ, Woodworth GF, Brooke BS, et al. Hyperglycemia independently increases the risk of perioperative stroke, myocardial infarction, and death after carotid endarterectomy. Neurosurgery 2006;58(6):1066–73 [discussion: 1066–73].
58. Noordzij PG, Boersma E, Schreiner F, et al. Increased preoperative glucose levels are associated with perioperative mortality in patients undergoing noncardiac, nonvascular surgery. Eur J Endocrinol 2007;156(1):137–42.
59. Mutter TC, Bryson GL. Choosing wisely and preoperative hemoglobin A1c testing: what should it mean? Can J Anaesth 2016;63(12):1307–13.
60. Krolikowska M, Kataja M, Poyhia R, et al. Mortality in diabetic patients undergoing non-cardiac surgery: a 7-year follow-up study. Acta Anaesthesiol Scand 2009; 53(6):749–58.
61. Routine preoperative tests for elective surgery. 2016. Available at: https://www.nice.org.uk/guidance/ng45. Accessed May 7, 2018.
62. Akhtar S, Barash PG, Inzucchi SE. Scientific principles and clinical implications of perioperative glucose regulation and control. Anesth Analg 2010;110(2):478–97.
63. Jamsen E, Nevalainen P, Kalliovalkama J, et al. Preoperative hyperglycemia predicts infected total knee replacement. Eur J Intern Med 2010;21(3):196–201.
64. Olsen MA, Nepple JJ, Riew KD, et al. Risk factors for surgical site infection following orthopaedic spinal operations. J Bone Joint Surg Am 2008;90(1):62–9.
65. Richards JE, Kauffmann RM, Zuckerman SL, et al. Relationship of hyperglycemia and surgical-site infection in orthopaedic surgery. J Bone Joint Surg Am 2012; 94(13):1181–6.

66. van Kuijk JP, Dunkelgrun M, Schreiner F, et al. Preoperative oral glucose tolerance testing in vascular surgery patients: long-term cardiovascular outcome. Am Heart J 2009;157(5):919–25.

67. Moitra VK, Greenberg J, Arunajadai S, et al. The relationship between glycosylated hemoglobin and perioperative glucose control in patients with diabetes. Can J Anaesth 2010;57(4):322–9.

68. Gustafsson UO, Thorell A, Soop M, et al. Haemoglobin A1c as a predictor of postoperative hyperglycaemia and complications after major colorectal surgery. Br J Surg 2009;96(11):1358–64.

69. O'Sullivan CJ, Hynes N, Mahendran B, et al. Haemoglobin A1c (HbA1C) in non-diabetic and diabetic vascular patients. Is HbA1C an independent risk factor and predictor of adverse outcome? Eur J Vasc Endovasc Surg 2006;32(2):188–97.

70. Acott AA, Theus SA, Kim LT. Long-term glucose control and risk of perioperative complications. Am J Surg 2009;198(5):596–9.

71. Harris NS, Bazydlo LAL, Winter WE. Coagulation tests: a primer on hemostasis for clinical chemists. 2012. Available at: https://www.aacc.org/publications/cln/articles/2012/january/coagulation-tests. Accessed May 8, 2018.

72. Chee YL, Crawford JC, Watson HG, et al. Guidelines on the assessment of bleeding risk prior to surgery or invasive procedures. British Committee for Standards in Haematology. Br J Haematol 2008;140(5):496–504.

73. Seicean A, Schiltz NK, Seicean S, et al. Use and utility of preoperative hemostatic screening and patient history in adult neurosurgical patients. J Neurosurg 2012; 116(5):1097–105.

74. Burk CD, Miller L, Handler SD, et al. Preoperative history and coagulation screening in children undergoing tonsillectomy. Pediatrics 1992;89(4 Pt 2):691–5.

75. Trescot AM. Genetics and implications in perioperative analgesia. Best Pract Res Clin Anaesthesiol 2014;28(2):153–66.

76. Kitzmiller JP, Groen DK, Phelps MA, et al. Pharmacogenomic testing: relevance in medical practice: why drugs work in some patients but not in others. Cleve Clin J Med 2011;78(4):243–57.

77. Meyer UA. Pharmacogenetics and adverse drug reactions. Lancet 2000; 356(9242):1667–71.

Preoperative Cardiac Evaluation for Noncardiac Surgery

Vahé S. Tateosian, MD*, Deborah C. Richman, MBChB, FFA (SA)

KEYWORDS

- Cardiac risk assessment • RCRI (revised cardiac risk index)
- CAD (coronary artery disease) • PCI (percutaneous coronary interventions)
- Congestive heart failure • Congenital heart disease • Valvular heart disease
- Surgical risk

KEY POINTS

- Risk stratification provides patients and health care providers with information for shared decision-making.
- The foundation of a preoperative cardiovascular evaluation is the history and physical examination, including accurate assessment of exercise tolerance.
- Published guidelines serve as a major outline for preoperative cardiac risk assessment as well as perioperative management in noncardiac surgery.
- Risk/benefit of bleeding/thrombosis prevention is key in deciding on cardiac intervention and timing of surgery.
- Expert cardiology input can be very informative, especially regarding specific details of patients' status (eg, stent type, position, and deployment) as well as recently published cardiology management updates.

INTRODUCTION

Perioperative cardiac complications are a significant concern for nearly 230 million individuals undergoing surgery worldwide.[1] Surgical safety is a substantial global health concern. The risks are based on both patient- and procedure-related factors. Stratification of risk presents the patients and health care providers with information for shared decision-making that tailors perioperative care and helps understand the risk-to-benefit ratio of a procedure as well as potential preoperative interventions. Efforts in surveillance and assessment of patients are the cornerstone to establishing

Disclosure Statement: Neither author has any financial conflicts of interest.
Department of Anesthesiology, Stony Brook Medicine, 101 Nicolls Road, Stony Brook, NY 11794-8480, USA
* Corresponding author.
E-mail address: Vahe.Tateosian@stonybrookmedicine.edu

Anesthesiology Clin 36 (2018) 509–521
https://doi.org/10.1016/j.anclin.2018.07.003
1932-2275/18/© 2018 Elsevier Inc. All rights reserved.
anesthesiology.theclinics.com

preoperative optimization of individuals undergoing surgery. Anesthesiologists are increasingly being called on to serve as consultants in the preoperative care of individuals, particularly those with multiple comorbidities. Dogan and colleagues[2] found that preoperative cardiology consultations for individuals undergoing intermediate-risk, noncardiac, nonvascular surgery offered no change in perioperative management or improved outcome of surgery. Nevertheless, primary care physicians, internists, cardiologists, and anesthesiologists collectively play an integral role in preoperative cardiac risk assessment.[3] One of the most crucial objectives of preoperative patients' experience is to outline the optimal and most cost-effective method for a cardiovascular evaluation that strives to improve outcomes in patient care. The perioperative cardiovascular care for noncardiac surgery is continually evolving; assessments and strategies to improve clinical outcomes are increasingly sought.[4] The focus is on overall value of the care provided, as defined by quality/cost. The preoperative evaluation of high-risk patients may also serve to reduce unnecessary testing, case cancellations, delays on the day of surgery, and mortality.[5,6] Ultimately, it allows patients the opportunity to make a truly informed decision regarding treatment.

GENERAL CONSIDERATIONS

All patients scheduled for noncardiac surgery should have a cardiovascular risk assessment performed preoperatively. The foundation of a preoperative cardiovascular evaluation is the history and physical examination. An anesthesiologist must inquire about symptoms, such as dyspnea, angina, anginal equivalents, palpitations, as well as comorbidities, such as a history of heart disease, including ischemic, valvular, or cardiomyopathy; hypertension; diabetes; chronic kidney disease; and cerebrovascular or peripheral artery disease. Cardiac functional status should also be assessed and is most commonly expressed in metabolic equivalents (METs), whereby 1 MET is defined as 3.5 mL O_2 uptake per kilogram per minute, which is the resting oxygen uptake in a sitting position.[7] An independent risk factor and a sign of poor functional status has been described as the inability to climb 2 flights of stairs or walk 4 blocks.[8,9] However, accurately assessing function may prove difficult, particularly in patients with orthopedic conditions or those with the inability to exert themselves physically. Practically, it may be difficult at times to assess and differentiate between benign deconditioning and an actual decline in functional status. The physical examination should focus on the cardiovascular system and include blood pressure measurements, auscultation of the heart and lungs, abdominal palpation, and examination of the extremities for edema and vascular integrity. Important findings include evidence of heart failure or a murmur suspicious for hemodynamically significant valvular heart disease. All of the aforementioned symptoms and signs allow the anesthesiologist to gain insight into possible unstable cardiac disease, such as myocardial ischemia, active congestive heart failure, valvular disease, or significant cardiac arrhythmias.

The American College of Cardiology/American Heart Association's (AHA/ACC) 2014 guidelines continue to serve as a major outline for preoperative cardiac risk assessment as well as perioperative management in noncardiac surgery.[10] These guidelines, along with several other reviews, have sought to address preoperative optimization of patients with coronary artery disease (CAD), active heart failure, perioperative use of beta-blockers, angiotensin-converting enzyme inhibitors, and the use of antiplatelet therapy for post–percutaneous coronary intervention (PCI) patients undergoing noncardiac surgery.[11–13] The preoperative evaluation is set to perform several functions, including (1) assessment of risk, (2) determining the changes in management, and (3) identification of cardiovascular conditions or risk factors that necessitate longer-term management. Changes in management may lead to decisions regarding changes in medical therapies, further preoperative cardiovascular interventions, or recommendations about intraoperative and postoperative monitoring. They may also lead to recommendations and discussions regarding the optimal timing of surgery or use of alternate procedural or nonsurgical strategies.

Occasionally, this assessment uncovers previously undiagnosed conditions that place patients at untoward risk for the proposed procedure and may necessitate further management or intervention. The clinician should use information elicited from the history, physical examination, and type of surgery to estimate the overall perioperative risk associated with the intended procedure. Risk models estimate the risk based on information obtained from the history, physical examination, electrocardiogram, and type of surgery. When assessing preoperative cardiac risk, one can use either the revised cardiac risk index (RCRI) or the American College of Surgeons National Surgical Quality Improvement Program (NSQIP) risk model.[14,15] Both models provide the clinician with an overall percentage of risk of cardiac complications. Higher-risk patients should weigh the risk-to-benefit ratio of preoperative interventions and focus on improved long-term outcomes rather than simply perioperative outcomes. High-risk individuals include those with recent (<60 days) myocardial infarction (MI), unstable angina, decompensated heart failure, high-grade arrhythmias, or hemodynamically important valvular heart disease (aortic stenosis in particular). Insulin-dependent diabetes mellitus, advanced age, American Society of Anesthesia class III and greater, and poor preoperative functional status have also been linked to high-risk perioperative outcomes.[16] Although not included in the risk factors discussed earlier, obesity and atrial fibrillation have also been associated with greater perioperative risks.[17,18] Patients with all of these risk factors are at increased risk for perioperative MI, heart failure, ventricular fibrillation, complete heart block, cardiac arrest, and cardiac death. When undergoing nonemergent procedures, these patients should be medically optimized before the induction of anesthesia. Patients who require emergency surgery are at increased risk of perioperative cardiovascular events at even lower levels of baseline risk; however, comprehensive cardiac assessment may still have value as a risk assessment tool. In those situations, the clinician must evaluate the risks and benefits of the procedure and may attempt to optimize the status of patients after the procedure.

CORONARY ARTERY DISEASE AND PERCUTANEOUS CORONARY INTERVENTION

The ACC/AHA's 2014 guidelines state that it is reasonable to obtain a preoperative electrocardiogram (ECG) in many patients with known cardiovascular disease, significant arrhythmia, or significant structural heart disease unless the patients are undergoing low-risk surgery, that is, surgery associated with less than 1% morbidity/ mortality, such as surgery that has been traditionally considered ambulatory. This guideline may not apply to known intermediate-risk surgeries like total knee arthroplasty, which are now being performed on an ambulatory basis. An ECG obtained in asymptomatic patients without cardiac disease is rarely helpful. In higher-risk patients, a rationale for obtaining a preoperative ECG is to allow the clinician to have a baseline ECG should a postoperative ECG be abnormal. A preoperative ECG should be evaluated for the presence of Q waves or significant ST-segment elevation or depression, which increases the possibility of myocardial ischemia, left ventricular (LV) hypertrophy, QTc prolongation, bundle-branch block, or clinically significant arrhythmias.[19] Patients who present with signs of ischemia or significant coronary artery disease should follow the guidelines on perioperative management of those with known or significant disease (**Fig. 1**). Increased coronary risk associated with noncardiac surgery in patients with previous MI has previously been shown to have an increased incidence of reinfarction, if the previous MI was less than 6 months preoperatively. Improvements in the management of patients who have had an MI, as well as in perioperative care, have shortened this time interval. The AHA/ACC Task Force on Perioperative Evaluation of the Cardiac Patient Undergoing Noncardiac Surgery has suggested the highest-risk patients are those within 30 days of the most recent MI, during which time plaque and myocardial healing and remodeling occur. Risk continues to decrease over time, and 60 days is the preferred waiting period after an MI for elective surgery. Coronary revascularization in stable patients has been shown to have limited value in affecting patient outcomes beyond optimal medical therapy.[20] Several studies have assessed the benefit of PCI before noncardiac surgery. The "2014 [European Society of Cardiology/ European Society of Anaesthesiology] ESC/ ESA Guidelines on Noncardiac Surgery: Cardiovascular Assessment and Management," noted a significantly lower rate of 30 day cardiac complications in patients who underwent PCI at least 90 days before the noncardiac surgery. However, PCI within 90 days of the procedure did not improve the outcome.[21] The advent of drug-eluting stents (DES), requiring prolonged antiplatelet therapy, may promote operative bleeding complications or increase the incidence of in-stent thrombosis if antiplatelet therapy is stopped perioperatively, especially prematurely.

PCI with stent implants, bare-metal stents (BMS), and especially DES is the most common form of coronary revascularization procedure performed in patients with both stable ischemic heart disease and acute coronary syndrome (ACS).[22] Of the nearly 3 million individuals who undergo PCI worldwide each year, approximately 7% to 17% require noncardiac surgery within a year of stent insertion.[23,24] Antiplatelet agents are prescribed following PCI to lower the risk of future ischemic and thrombotic events; however, their use also poses potential risks during the perioperative period. Antiplatelet therapy interruption exposes patients to the potential risk of in-stent thrombosis and perioperative MI, whereas continuation of these agents often leads to increased bleeding perioperatively. Thrombotic risk may be defined by (1) type of implanted stent (BMS vs DES), (2) timing of noncardiac surgery after PCI, (3) angiographic features of the coronary lesions and complexity of PCI, and (4) clinical presentation and characteristics. Determination of hemorrhagic risk focuses mainly on perioperative bleeding related to the noncardiac surgery. Surgical interventions may be classified as either high, medium, or low risk for bleeding complications. Thus, what is the best revascularization strategy for symptomatic patients or someone with unstable angina with a high-grade lesion that needs urgent noncardiac surgery? Early invasive intervention with the intent to revascularize severe proximal stenosis in the setting of unstable angina, new ST-segment depression, and elevated biomarker evidence of myonecrosis has been shown to be a reasonable approach.[25]

Discontinuation of dual-antiplatelet therapy (DAPT) after stent implantation is one of the strongest predictors of stent thrombosis, and the magnitude of risk is inversely proportional to the timing of noncardiac surgery after PCI.[26] PCI for ACS was an independent predictor of perioperative ischemic complications. Furthermore, data from previous observational studies suggest that the timeframe for stent-related thrombotic complications in the perioperative period is approximately 6 months, irrespective of stent type, DES or BMS.[27] However, a meta-

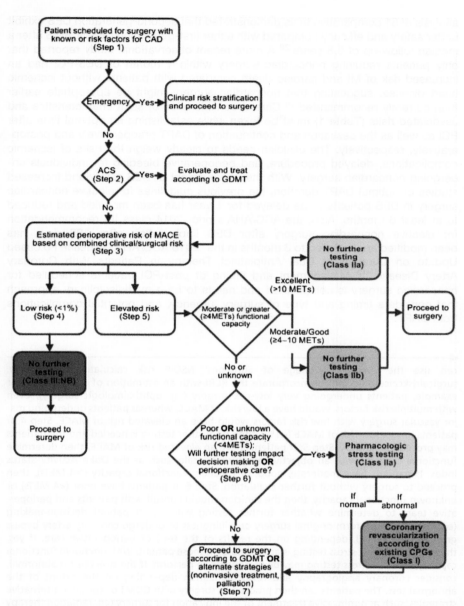

Fig. 1. Stepwise approach to perioperative cardiac assessment for CAD. Step 1: In patients scheduled for surgery with risk factors for or known CAD, determine the urgency of surgery. If an emergency, then determine the clinical risk factors that may influence perioperative management and proceed to surgery with appropriate monitoring and management strategies based on the clinical assessment. Step 2: If the surgery is urgent or elective, determine if patients have an acute coronary syndrome. If yes, then refer patients for cardiology evaluation and management according to guideline-directed therapy (GDMT) according to the unstable angina/non-ST elevation MI and ST elevation MI clinical practice guidelines. Step 3: If patients have risk factors for stable CAD, then estimate the perioperative risk of a major adverse cardiac event (MACE) from the combined clinical/surgical risk. This estimate

analysis of 51 comparative trials demonstrated that second-generation DES exhibit better safety and efficacy compared with either first-generation DES or BMS after a median follow-up of 3.8 years.[28] A more recent observational study reported that only patients requiring noncardiac surgery within 1 month of DES-PCI had an increased risk of MI and cardiac death compared with patients without ischemic heart disease, suggesting that noncardiac surgery might be appropriate earlier than currently recommended.[29] Careful consideration of stent characteristics and associated risks (**Table 1**) must be taken while establishing an optimal time after PCI as well as the cessation and continuation of DAPT preoperatively and postoperatively, respectively. The clinician needs to clearly weigh the risks of ischemic complications, delayed procedure, and perioperative bleeding for individuals undergoing noncardiac surgery. With the improvement of DES safety and increased studies of optimal DAPT duration, the previous guidelines for elective noncardiac surgery in DES patients to be delayed for 1 year has been modified and reduced to at least 6 months. Also, the ACC/AHA's prior 2014 class IIb recommendation for elective noncardiac surgery after DES implantation after 180 days has been modified and reduced to 3 months in the "2016 ACC/AHA Guideline Fo'cused Update on Duration of Dual Antiplatelet Therapy in Patients With Coronary Artery Disease."[13] Management and timing of post-PCI patients scheduled for noncardiac surgery is complicated and needs to be a multidisciplinary approach that considers timing and type of surgery, urgency, and potential complications from DAPT.

---

can use the American College of Surgeons' NSQIP risk calculator (http://www.surgicalriskcalculator.com) or incorporate the RCRI with an estimation of surgical risk. For example, patients undergoing very low-risk surgery (eg, ophthalmologic surgery), even with multiple risk factors, would have a low risk of MACE, whereas patients undergoing major vascular surgery with few risk factors would have an elevated risk of MACE. Step 4: If patients have a low risk of MACE (<1%), then no further testing is needed and the patients may proceed to surgery. Step 5: If patients have an elevated risk of MACE, then determine functional capacity with an objective measure or scale, such as the Duke Activity Status Index. If patients have moderate, good, or excellent functional capacity ($\geq$4 METs), then proceed to surgery without further evaluation. Step 6: If patients have poor (<4 METs) or unknown functional capacity, then the clinician should consult with patients and perioperative team to determine whether further testing will impact patient decision-making (eg, decision to perform original surgery or willingness to undergo coronary artery bypass graft surgery or PCI, depending on the results of the test) or perioperative care. If yes, then pharmacologic stress testing is appropriate. In those patients with unknown functional capacity, exercise stress testing may be reasonable to perform. If the stress test is abnormal, consider coronary angiography and revascularization depending on the extent of the abnormal test. The patients can then proceed to surgery with GDMT or consider alternative strategies, such as noninvasive treatment of the indication for surgery (eg, radiation therapy for cancer) or palliation. If the test is normal, proceed to surgery according to GDMT. Step 7: If testing will not impact decision-making or care, then proceed to surgery according to GDMT or consider alternative strategies, such as noninvasive treatment of the indication for surgery (eg, radiation therapy for cancer) or palliation. ACS, acute coronary syndrome; CABG, coronary artery bypass graft surgery; CPG, clinical practice guideline; DASI, Duke Activity Status Index; GDMT, guideline-directed therapy; HF, heart failure; MACE, major adverse cardiac event; MET, metabolic equivalent; NB, no benefit; STEMI, ST elevation myocardial infarction; UA/NSTEMI, unstable angina/non-ST elevation MI; VHD, valvular heart disease. (*Reprinted with permission* Circulation 2014;130e278–e333© 2014 American Heart Association, Inc.)

Table 1
Development of percutaneous coronary intervention and associated risk/solutions

PCI	Decade	Early Risk	Solution	Late Risk	Solution	Comments
Balloon angioplasty	1980s	3% Artery collapse/rupture	Stent	25% Restenosis	—	—
BMS	1990s	Minimal	—	25% Restenosis	Antineoplastic drug (DES)	—
DES	2002/2003 in United States	Minimal	—	Minimal restenosis + thrombosis	DAPT	70% Off-label use • Affect flow characteristics • Delayed washout of drug
DES	Second/third generation 2007 onwards	Minimal	—	Less thrombosis	Shorter DAPT duration	Strut polymer less irritating to coronary artery

VALVULAR DISEASES

According to the ACC/AHA's 2014 guidelines, patients with suspected moderate or greater degree of valvular stenosis or regurgitation should undergo preoperative echocardiography, unless there was echocardiography within 1 year and no clinically significant change in health status or physical examination since that last assessment. For patients who met the criteria for a valve intervention, either replacement or repair, before elective noncardiac surgery, a clinically significant perioperative risk reduction was seen.[30] The guidelines also suggest that in patients with severe asymptomatic valvular disease (severe aortic stenosis, severe mitral regurgitation, and severe aortic regurgitation with normal LV ejection fraction) it is appropriate to proceed with elevated-risk, elective noncardiac surgery. They caution about appropriate careful intraoperative and postoperative hemodynamic monitoring in these patients. More recently, the "2017 AHA/ACC Focused Update of the 2014 AHA/ACC Guideline for the Management of Patients with Valvular Heart Disease" addressed the current principles of endocarditis prophylaxis.[30] Universal agreement regarding prophylaxis against infective endocarditis (IE) is yet to be achieved, and protection from endocarditis for those undergoing high-risk procedures is not guaranteed. Mougeot and colleagues[31] demonstrated that prophylaxis given to patients for what are typically considered high-risk dental procedures reduced but did not eliminate the incidence of bacteremia. Epidemiologic data are conflicting with regard to the incidence of IE after the adoption of more limited prophylaxis by the AHA. There is currently no evidence for the use of prophylaxis in gastrointestinal procedures or genitourinary procedures, in the absence of known infection. The risk of developing IE is higher in individuals with preexisting valvular heart disease; however, even in patients with high risk, the evidence for the efficacy of prophylaxis for complete elimination of IE is lacking. The 2017 consensus is that antibiotic prophylaxis is reasonable for the subset of individuals at increased risk of developing IE and at high risk for developing complications from IE. These individuals include patients with a history of prosthetic heart valve, prior IE, cardiac transplant recipients, and patients with congenital heart disease (CHD) peri-repair (see section on CHD later.) IE has also been reported to occur with patients after transcatheter aortic valve replacement at rates equal to or exceeding those associated with surgical aortic valve replacement and is associated with a 1-year mortality of approximately 75%.[32,33] Persons at risk of developing IE should also attempt to practice the best oral health to reduce the potential sources of bacterial seeding.

CONGESTIVE HEART FAILURE

Active heart failure is an independent risk for perioperative morbidity.[34] There was a substantial risk as well as increased 30-day all-cause readmission rate associated with patients with heart failure undergoing major noncardiac surgery in the United States. The outcomes analysis from surgical procedures of varying risk showed evidence that elderly patients with heart failure remained a significantly higher risk of morbidity and mortality, even after adjusting for all other risk factors. To put heart failure–associated risk in context, only nonelective admission status as well as renal disease conferred a higher risk for mortality and no other factors, including surgical urgency, were as correlated with readmission as was heart failure. Interestingly, there was no increased risk of readmission for heart failure and CAD, suggesting that the increased risk was related to the diagnosis of heart failure. Patients with CAD were at higher risk for perioperative mortality as compared with those without CAD; however, the risk conferred was much smaller to that compared with patients with heart failure. The impact of comorbidities in patients with heart failure also needs to be considered; however, even after the adjustment for and in the absence of important comorbid conditions, heart failure remained a significant predictor of adverse cardiovascular events. According to the ACC/AHA's 2014 guidelines, it is reasonable for patients with dyspnea of unknown origin as well as those with a history of heart failure with worsening dyspnea or other change in clinical status to undergo preoperative evaluation of LV function. Reassessment of LV function in clinically stable patients with previously documented LV dysfunction may be considered if there has been no assessment within the past year. Routine evaluation of LV function is not recommended and has shown no outcome benefit. The type and degree of heart failure are important factors and may necessitate preoperative optimization and individualized monitoring within the perioperative timeframe. Heart failure is not only a low ejection fraction. Current evidence acknowledges this and heart failure with preserved ejection fraction recognizes the importance of diastolic heart failure in causing symptoms and increasing the risk of morbidity.

CONGENITAL HEART DISEASE

Our understanding of CHD has improved significantly over the past few decades. Major advances have been made in surgical techniques and skill, long-term medical treatments, percutaneous interventions, intraoperative and perioperative care, as well as critical care management. An increasing number of patients with CHD are surviving to adulthood. Given the modern surgical mortality rates and perioperative management, by 2020, according to the "ACC/AHA 2008 Guidelines for the Management of Adults with Congenital Heart Disease," it is expected that 1 in 150 young adults will have some form of CHD.[35] These adults and children will present to operating rooms for surgical procedures involving noncardiac systems as well as various other settings, such as pregnancy and labor; anesthesiologists are expected to provide them with appropriate care.

Although many consider the patients who survive to adulthood as palliated or cured, they experience an exceedingly disproportionate morbidity burden.[35] A list of cardiovascular complications they are afflicted with include pulmonary hypertension, left and right heart failure, systemic heart failure, cyanosis, residual shunts, dysrhythmias, and valvular lesions. The probability of developing heart failure increases with age in all patients with congenital cardiac disease, with the probabilities increasing based on the degree of severity of the lesion. The evaluation of an adult with CHD can be extremely complex. They represent a wide variety of lesions at different stages of repair that present different comorbidities. They may present with an uncorrected lesion, partially corrected, in between repair stages, or a failed repair. No single best risk index assessment exists to stratify perioperative risk in these patients presenting for noncardiac surgery. The ACC/AHA categorized the severity of lesion to the risk status of patients and considered low-risk lesions to include a small atrial septal defect (ASD), patent ductus arteriosus (PDA), a small ventricular septal defect (VSD), or those after complete repair of ASD, PDA, or VSD.[35] Moderate risk included aortic coarctation, Ebstein anomaly, and tetralogy of Fallot, whereas high-risk lesions included any of the cyanotic heart lesions, Eisenmenger syndrome, single ventricular physiology, and transposition of the great arteries, among others. Preoperative evaluation and preparation should include a thorough history and detailed knowledge of current anatomy and physiology at rest as well as changes in pulmonary and peripheral vascular resistances. Preoperative exercise tolerance and conditional status is an extremely important indicator of cardiovascular reserve. IE prophylaxis is restricted only to patients at highest risk undergoing highest-risk procedures. Aside from the previously mentioned criteria, within patients with CHD those include heart transplant patients, patients within the first 6 months after complete repair of their cardiac lesion, and those with unrepaired cyanotic heart disease. Also included are patients who have a repaired lesion but exhibit a residual defect at or near the prosthetic valve or patch that may inhibit proper endothelialization. IE prophylaxis has also been deemed appropriate for all of these patients undergoing invasive dental procedures to minimize the incidence of bacteremia.

THE IMPORTANCE OF THE SURGICAL PROCEDURE

Surgical procedures themselves carry inherent risks beyond patient comorbidities for a multitude of reasons, including blood loss, fluid dynamics, inflammation, patient positioning, mismatches of ventilation/perfusion, and other such acute physiologic changes. Anesthesiologists recognize that different procedures carry different inherent risks of perioperative mortality. Traditionally, ambulatory procedures are seen as relatively low risk, whereas vascular surgery has been denoted as high risk. The RCRI labels intraperitoneal, intrathoracic, and suprainguinal vascular operations as high risk; however, a laparoscopic cholecystectomy may have a different intrinsic risk associated than a pancreaticoduodenectomy. Recently, Liu and colleagues[36] sought to improve preoperative risk assessments by recognizing the intrinsic cardiac risk of each procedure when performing preoperative cardiac risk assessments. Accurate estimation of risk allows for patients to make informed decisions and clinicians to formulate intraoperative and postoperative plans individualized for patients. Instead of grouping operations into anatomic or physiologic categories, their approach derived the intrinsic cardiac risk of each individual surgery. They cited an example from the AHA/ACC's 2014 guidelines that labels plastic surgery as low risk; however, the authors understand that a 12-hour free flap with microvascular anastomosis carries a different cardiac risk when compared with a mastectomy with tissue expanders. A few examples of their cited low-intrinsic-cardiac-risk surgeries were simple mastectomy, laparoscopic appendectomy, and laparoscopic cholecystectomy. Intermediate risk included total hip arthroplasty, transurethral resection of bladder tumor, and open appendectomy, whereas high-risk surgeries included breast reconstruction with free flap, open cholecystectomies, and pylorus-sparing Whipple procedures. One must recognize that there exist varied perioperative cardiac risks associated with specific surgical procedures. Sophisticated risk calculators seek to stratify preoperative cardiac risks for noncardiac surgery; however, anesthesiologists must be equipped with more specific data, understand the differences in risks associated with various surgeries, and be prepared to inform their patients as well as collaborate with surgeons as perioperative consultants with respect to surgery-specific risks.

SUMMARY

Preexisting cardiac disease carries significant perioperative risk for cardiovascular complications and death. Careful assessment starting with an excellent history and physical examination is essential to risk stratification. Exercise tolerance is a very important component of the history to accurately elicit. Further testing may be justified if it will change management and/or outcomes. Available guidelines from various societies can guide us on when to ask for further testing or management advice; however, those guidelines are published only every 5 to 8 years and new literature may change practice in the interim. Therefore, in certain situations, it may also be valuable to appreciate cardiology recommendations for perioperative medication management and optimization are part of the multidisciplinary approach to the perioperative patient.

REFERENCES

1. Weiser TG, Regenbogen SE, Thompson KD, et al. An estimation of the global volume of surgery: a modelling strategy based on available data. Lancet 2008; 372(9633):139–44.
2. Dogan V, Biteker M, Ozlek E, et al. Impact of pre-operative cardiology consultation prior to intermediate-risk surgical procedures. Eur J Clin Invest 2017. https://doi.org/10.1111/eci.12794.
3. Thilen SR, Wijeysundera DN, Treggiari MM. Preoperative consultations. Anesthesiol Clin 2016;34(1):17–33.
4. Fleisher LA. The value of preoperative assessment before noncardiac surgery in the era of value-based care. Circulation 2017;136(19):1769–71.
5. Partridge JS, Harari D, Martin FC, et al. Randomized clinical trial of comprehensive geriatric assessment and optimization in vascular surgery. Br J Surg 2017; 104(6):679–87.
6. van Klei WA, Moons KG, Rutten CL, et al. The effect of outpatient preoperative evaluation of hospital inpatients on cancellation of surgery and length of hospital stay. Anesth Analg 2002;94(3):644–9. Table of contents.
7. Eagle KA, Berger PB, Calkins H, et al. ACC/AHA guideline update for perioperative cardiovascular evaluation for noncardiac surgery–executive summary: a report of the American College of Cardiology/American Heart Association Task Force on practice guidelines (committee to update the 1996 guidelines on perioperative cardiovascular evaluation for noncardiac surgery). J Am Coll Cardiol 2002;39(3):542–53.
8. Girish M, Trayner E Jr, Dammann O, et al. Symptom-limited stair climbing as a predictor of postoperative cardiopulmonary complications after high-risk surgery. Chest 2001;120(4):1147–51.
9. Reilly DF, McNeely MJ, Doerner D, et al. Self-reported exercise tolerance and the risk of serious perioperative complications. Arch Intern Med 1999;159(18): 2185–92.
10. Fleisher LA, Fleischmann KE, Auerbach AD, et al. 2014 ACC/AHA guideline on perioperative cardiovascular evaluation and management of patients undergoing noncardiac surgery: a report of the American College of Cardiology/American Heart Association Task Force on practice guidelines. J Am Coll Cardiol 2014; 64(22):e77–137.
11. Wijeysundera DN, Duncan D, Nkonde-Price C, et al. Perioperative beta blockade in noncardiac surgery: a systematic review for the 2014 ACC/AHA guideline on perioperative cardiovascular evaluation and management of patients undergoing noncardiac surgery: a report of the American College of Cardiology/American Heart Association Task Force on practice guidelines. Circulation 2014;130(24): 2246–64.
12. Roshanov PS, Rochwerg B, Patel A, et al. Withholding versus continuing angiotensin-converting enzyme inhibitors or angiotensin II receptor blockers before noncardiac surgery: an analysis of the vascular events in noncardiac surgery patients cohort evaluation prospective cohort. Anesthesiology 2017;126(1): 16–27.
13. Levine GN, Bates ER, Bittl JA, et al. 2016 ACC/AHA guideline focused update on duration of dual antiplatelet therapy in patients with coronary artery disease: a report of the American College of Cardiology/American Heart Association Task Force on clinical practice guidelines: an update of the 2011 ACCF/AHA/SCAI guideline for percutaneous coronary intervention, 2011 ACCF/AHA guideline for

coronary artery bypass graft surgery, 2012 ACC/AHA/ACP/AATS/PCNA/SCAI/ STS guideline for the diagnosis and management of patients with stable ischemic heart disease, 2013 ACCF/AHA guideline for the management of st-elevation myocardial infarction, 2014 AHA/ACC guideline for the management of patients with non-ST-Elevation acute coronary syndromes, and 2014 ACC/AHA guideline on perioperative cardiovascular evaluation and management of patients undergoing noncardiac surgery. Circulation 2016;134(10):e123–55.

14. Lee TH, Marcantonio ER, Mangione CM, et al. Derivation and prospective validation of a simple index for prediction of cardiac risk of major noncardiac surgery. Circulation 1999;100(10):1043–9.

15. Bilimoria KY, Liu Y, Paruch JL, et al. Development and evaluation of the universal ACS NSQIP surgical risk calculator: a decision aid and informed consent tool for patients and surgeons. J Am Coll Surg 2013;217(5):833–42.e1-3.

16. Tashiro T, Pislaru SV, Blustin JM, et al. Perioperative risk of major non-cardiac surgery in patients with severe aortic stenosis: a reappraisal in contemporary practice. Eur Heart J 2014;35(35):2372–81.

17. van Diepen S, Bakal JA, McAlister FA, et al. Mortality and readmission of patients with heart failure, atrial fibrillation, or coronary artery disease undergoing noncardiac surgery: an analysis of 38 047 patients. Circulation 2011;124(3):289–96.

18. Poirier P, Alpert MA, Fleisher LA, et al. Cardiovascular evaluation and management of severely obese patients undergoing surgery: a science advisory from the American Heart Association. Circulation 2009;120(1):86–95.

19. van Klei WA, Bryson GL, Yang H, et al. The value of routine preoperative electrocardiography in predicting myocardial infarction after noncardiac surgery. Ann Surg 2007;246(2):165–70.

20. Bangalore S, Pursnani S, Kumar S, et al. Percutaneous coronary intervention versus optimal medical therapy for prevention of spontaneous myocardial infarction in subjects with stable ischemic heart disease. Circulation 2013;127(7): 769–81.

21. Kristensen SD, Knuuti J, Saraste A, et al. 2014 ESC/ESA guidelines on non-cardiac surgery: cardiovascular assessment and management: the joint task force on non-cardiac surgery: cardiovascular assessment and management of the European Society of Cardiology (ESC) and the European Society of Anaesthesiology (ESA). Eur J Anaesthesiol 2014;31(10):517–73.

22. Mozaffarian D, Benjamin EJ, Go AS, et al. Heart disease and stroke statistics–2015 update: a report from the American Heart Association. Circulation 2015; 131(4):e29–322.

23. Alshawabkeh LI, Prasad A, Lenkovsky F, et al. Outcomes of a preoperative "bridging" strategy with glycoprotein IIb/IIIa inhibitors to prevent perioperative stent thrombosis in patients with drug-eluting stents who undergo surgery necessitating interruption of thienopyridine administration. EuroIntervention 2013;9(2): 204–11.

24. van Diepen S, Tricoci P, Podder M, et al. Efficacy and safety of vorapaxar in non-ST-segment elevation acute coronary syndrome patients undergoing noncardiac surgery. J Am Heart Assoc 2015;4(12) [pii:e002546].

25. Amsterdam EA, Wenger NK, Brindis RG, et al. 2014 AHA/ACC guideline for the management of patients with non-ST-Elevation acute coronary syndromes: a report of the American College of Cardiology/American Heart Association Task Force on practice guidelines. J Am Coll Cardiol 2014;64(24):e139–228.

26. Spertus JA, Kettelkamp R, Vance C, et al. Prevalence, predictors, and outcomes of premature discontinuation of thienopyridine therapy after drug-eluting stent placement: results from the PREMIER registry. Circulation 2006;113(24):2803–9.
27. Hawn MT, Graham LA, Richman JS, et al. Risk of major adverse cardiac events following noncardiac surgery in patients with coronary stents. JAMA 2013; 310(14):1462–72.
28. Palmerini T, Sangiorgi D, Valgimigli M, et al. Short- versus long-term dual anti-platelet therapy after drug-eluting stent implantation: an individual patient data pairwise and network meta-analysis. J Am Coll Cardiol 2015;65(11):1092–102.
29. Egholm G, Kristensen SD, Thim T, et al. Risk associated with surgery within 12 months after coronary drug-eluting stent implantation. J Am Coll Cardiol 2016;68(24):2622–32.
30. Nishimura RA, Otto CM, Bonow RO, et al. 2017 AHA/ACC focused update of the 2014 AHA/ACC guideline for the management of patients with valvular heart disease: a report of the American College of Cardiology/American Heart Association Task Force on clinical practice guidelines. J Am Coll Cardiol 2017;70(2):252–89.
31. Mougeot FK, Saunders SE, Brennan MT, et al. Associations between bacteremia from oral sources and distant-site infections: tooth brushing versus single tooth extraction. Oral Surg Oral Med Oral Pathol Oral Radiol 2015;119(4):430–5.
32. Amat-Santos IJ, Messika-Zeitoun D, Eltchaninoff H, et al. Infective endocarditis after transcatheter aortic valve implantation: results from a large multicenter registry. Circulation 2015;131(18):1566–74.
33. Mangner N, Woitek F, Haussig S, et al. Incidence, predictors, and outcome of patients developing infective endocarditis following transfemoral transcatheter aortic valve replacement. J Am Coll Cardiol 2016;67(24):2907–8.
34. Hammill BG, Curtis LH, Bennett-Guerrero E, et al. Impact of heart failure on patients undergoing major noncardiac surgery. Anesthesiology 2008;108(4): 559–67.
35. Warnes CA, Williams RG, Bashore TM, et al. ACC/AHA 2008 guidelines for the management of adults with congenital heart disease: a report of the American College of Cardiology/American Heart Association Task Force on practice guidelines (writing committee to develop guidelines on the management of adults with congenital heart disease). developed in collaboration with the American Society of Echocardiography, Heart Rhythm Society, International Society for Adult Congenital Heart Disease, Society for Cardiovascular Angiography and Interventions, and Society of Thoracic Surgeons. J Am Coll Cardiol 2008;52(23): e143–263.
36. Liu JB, Liu Y, Cohen ME, et al. Defining the intrinsic cardiac risks of operations to improve preoperative cardiac risk assessments. Anesthesiology 2018;128(2): 283–92.

Preoperative Evaluation
Estimation of Pulmonary Risk Including Obstructive Sleep Apnea Impact

Yamini Subramani, MD[a], Mahesh Nagappa, MD[b],
Jean Wong, MD, FRCPC[c], Talha Mubashir, MD[c],
Frances Chung, MBBS, FRCPC[c],*

KEYWORDS

- Preoperative evaluation • Pulmonary risk • Risk factors • Obstructive sleep apnea
- Pulmonary complications • Surgery • Anesthesia

KEY POINTS

- Postoperative pulmonary complications are common and are associated with significant morbidity and increased cost of care.
- Increased risk may be recognized by preoperative evaluation and may be mitigated by preventive measures.
- The clinical and laboratory predictors of perioperative pulmonary risk are reviewed in this article, with special emphasis on obstructive sleep apnea.

INTRODUCTION

Postoperative pulmonary complications (PPCs) after major surgery are common and are associated with significant morbidity and high cost of care. In a recent analysis of the National Surgical Quality Improvement Program (NSQIP) of the 165,196 patients

Disclosure: F. Chung has received research grants from Ontario Ministry of Health and Long-Term Care Innovation Fund, University Health Network Foundation, Acacia, Medtronic; STOP-Bang tool, proprietary to University Health Network; royalties from Up-To-Date. J. Wong has received research grants from the Ontario Ministry of Health and Long-Term Care, Anesthesia Patient Safety Foundation, and Acacia Pharma outside of the submitted work.
[a] Department of Anesthesia and Perioperative Medicine, London Health Science Centre, St. Joseph Health Care, Western University, Centre, Victoria Hospital, 800 Commissioners Road East, London, Ontario N6A 5W9, Canada; [b] Department of Anesthesia and Perioperative Medicine, London Health Science Centre, St. Joseph Health Care, Western University, University Hospital, 339 Windermere Road, London, Ontario N6A 5A5, Canada; [c] Department of Anesthesiology, Toronto Western Hospital, University Health Network, University of Toronto, 399 Bathurst street, Toronto, Ontario M5T2S8, Canada
* Corresponding author. Department of Anesthesiology, Room 405, 2McL, 399 Bathurst Street, Toronto, Ontario M5T2S8, Canada.
E-mail address: frances.chung@uhn.ca

Anesthesiology Clin 36 (2018) 523–538
https://doi.org/10.1016/j.anclin.2018.07.004
1932-2275/18/© 2018 Elsevier Inc. All rights reserved.

undergoing major abdominal surgery, the incidence of PPCs was 5.8%.[1] PPCs have been shown to be one of the most significant factors associated with poor patient outcomes, leading to longer duration of hospital stay, increased likelihood of rehospitalization, and increased mortality.[2] PPCs can predict long-term mortality more accurately than cardiac complications.[3]

Clinical PPCs include respiratory failure, reintubation within 48 hours, weaning failure, pneumonia, atelectasis, bronchospasm, exacerbation of chronic obstructive pulmonary disease (COPD), pneumothorax, pleural effusion, and various forms of upper airway obstruction.[2] Predictions of PPCs are based on patient characteristics, risks linked to comorbidities, as well as to the type of surgical procedure. Increased risk may be recognized with preoperative evaluation and may be mitigated by preventive measures.

This article reviews the clinical and laboratory predictors of perioperative pulmonary risk before noncardiothoracic surgery, with special emphasis on obstructive sleep apnea (OSA). The commonly used pulmonary risk indices to predict PPCs are also described.

The risk factors for predicting PPC can be divided into 3 aspects: patient-related, procedure-related, and laboratory testing–related risk factors.

Patient-Related Risk Factors for Postoperative Pulmonary Complications

The patient-related risk factors can be classified as modifiable and non-modifiable. The non-modifiable risk factors include age, COPD, congestive heart failure (CHF), functional dependence, American Society of Anesthesiologists (ASA) classification, low preoperative blood hemoglobin oxygen saturation (Spo_2), impaired sensorium, and OSA.[2] The modifiable patient-related risk factors include smoking, obesity, respiratory infection in the last month, alcohol use, and weight loss.[2] These risk factors are further elaborated here.

Age

Advanced age is an important predictor of PPCs, even after adjustment for comorbid conditions. A population-based cohort study identified that age more than 80 years was associated with a 5.6 times higher risk of developing PPCs.[4] Another multivariable analysis indicated that age 80 years or older was one of the most important predictors of PPC rates.[1] Older patients carry a substantial risk of pulmonary complications after surgery, even if healthy. In contrast, reports have indicated that young, healthy, athletic, adult male patients may be at increased risk of postoperative pulmonary edema secondary to postextubation laryngospasm. These events were likely caused by excessive negative intrathoracic pressure generated by forced inspiration against a closed glottis.[5]

Chronic lung disease

Patients with COPD have an increased risk for PPCs, although there seems to be no prohibitive level of the pulmonary function below which surgery is absolutely contraindicated. A recent study showed that COPD was one of the independent predictors for postoperative respiratory failure and reintubation (odds ratio [OR], 1.74; 95% confidence interval [CI], 1.01–3.00; $P = .04$).[6] The onset of an acute pulmonary disorder or a recent exacerbation of a preexisting lung condition are considered important risk factors for developing PPCs and are valid reasons to postpone elective surgery.[7] Patients with COPD who are particularly high risk based on effort tolerance or spirometric values warrant aggressive preoperative treatment to reduce risk. A low body mass index (BMI) is associated with a poor prognosis in patients with COPD independent of the degree of ventilatory impairment.[8] Lower BMI is often associated with protein depletion, which in turn can lead to impairment of respiratory muscle strength, reduction in diaphragmatic muscular mass, and maximum voluntary ventilation, predisposing the patient to pulmonary complications.[9]

Congestive heart failure
CHF is an important predictor of PPCs. A recent study showed that CHF is a significant risk factor for postoperative respiratory failure and reintubation (OR, 2.36 [1.58–5.92]; $P = .005$).[6]

Functional dependence
In a recent National Surgical Quality Improvement data analysis, dependent functional status was one of the highest nonmodifiable predictors for PPCs, with a risk ratio of more than 2 times.[1] A multicenter prospective data analysis also identified dependent functional status as an important preoperative predictor of PPCs.[10]

American Society of Anesthesiologists classification
A recent study showed that an ASA score of greater than or equal to 3 is a significant risk factor for postoperative respiratory failure and reintubation (OR, 5.32 [2.85–9.95]; $P<.0001$).[6] A 7-year database analysis showed that ASA score of greater than or equal to 3 was associated with 2 to 4 times higher risk of PPCs.[1]

Low preoperative blood oxygen saturation
A population-based cohort study showed that a low preoperative Spo_2 in patients breathing room air was the strongest patient-related PPC risk factor.[4] This finding may be highly useful because Spo_2 can be easily obtained preoperatively and can predict unforeseen hypoxic events.[4]

Altered sensorium
Impaired sensorium has been associated with an increased risk of PPCs.[11] This increased risk may be secondary to an increased risk of occurrence of aspiration of gastric or pharyngeal secretions.[2,12,13]

Obstructive sleep apnea
Obstructive sleep apnea and postoperative respiratory complications Postoperative respiratory complications, including hypoventilation with hypercapnic respiratory arrest, are well documented in patients with OSA.[14] In patients with OSA, operative risks depend on the severity of the underlying OSA and the invasiveness of the surgical procedure.[15,16] Risk factors that predispose individuals with OSA to critical postoperative complications include morbid obesity, male sex, undiagnosed/untreated OSA, suboptimal use of postoperative continuous positive airway pressure (CPAP), need for opioid analgesia, and lack of appropriate postoperative monitoring.[17] Preoperative recognition of diagnosed or undiagnosed OSA allows the tailoring of perioperative management to minimize its impact on the postoperative course.[18,19]

Sedation and anesthesia have been shown to increase the upper airway collapsibility, increasing the risk of postoperative complications in these patients. Surgical patients with OSA are at increased risk of having perioperative respiratory complications, including hypoxemia, pneumonia, difficult intubation, pulmonary embolism, atelectasis, and unanticipated admission to the ICU.[14] Moreover, an increased incidence of postoperative pulmonary edema has been noted in patients who are at high risk for OSA.[20] Memtsoudis and colleagues[21] reported that patients with OSA had a 5-fold increase in intubation and mechanical ventilation after orthopedic surgery (OR, 5.2; 95% CI, 5.05–5.37) and a 2-fold increase after general surgery (OR, 1.95; 95% CI, 1.91–1.98) compared with controls without OSA. Similarly, a large database study of 1 million patients using the national inpatient sample showed a strong association between postoperative respiratory failure and OSA in patients undergoing orthopedic or urologic surgery.[22] In a recent meta-analysis of 3942 patients with polysomnography (PSG)-diagnosed OSA, Kaw and colleagues[23] found an increased incidence of respiratory failure compared with patients without OSA (OR, 2.43; 95% CI, 1.34–4.39; P = .003). Moreover, an analysis of the Canadian health administrative database in Manitoba confirmed the increased postoperative respiratory complications in patients with OSA, regardless of early diagnosis and prescription of CPAP. Patients with OSA are also considered to be at a higher risk for opioid-induced ventilatory impairment (OIVI), which is a potentially catastrophic complication of opioid therapy that can be fatal.[24] Two recent studies highlight the association between OIVI and OSA, reporting that 30% of patients with postoperative opioid-related life-threatening respiratory events had OSA[25] and that 40% of postoperative opioid-related deaths in an ASA closed claims registry analysis had known or suspected OSA.[26] A recent systematic review identified that OSA, elderly, female sex, COPD, cardiac disease, diabetes mellitus, hypertension, neurologic disease, renal disease, obesity, 2 or more comorbidities, opioid dependence, use of patient-controlled analgesia, and concomitant administration of sedatives are significant risk factors for postoperative opioid-induced respiratory depression.[27]

A subset of patients with OSA can have obesity hypoventilation syndrome (OHS). OHS is defined as a combination of:

1. Obesity with BMI greater than 30 kg/m^2
2. Daytime hypercapnia with $Paco_2$ more than 45 mm Hg during wakefulness
3. Sleep disordered breathing[28]

Note that 90% of patients with OHS have concomitant OSA.[29] The prevalence of OHS is approximately 0.15% to 0.6% in the general population[30] and has been shown to increase more than 50% with an increase in BMI of greater than 50 kg/m^2.[31] Patients with hypercapnia from OHS and overlap syndrome are more likely to experience postoperative respiratory failure (OR, 10.9; 95% CI, 3.7–32.3; $P<.0001$)[32] and therefore may not be suited for ambulatory surgery.

Preoperative evaluation of obstructive sleep apnea A preoperative evaluation of suspected OSA should include a comprehensive review of the patient's medical records for a history of difficulty in airway management, a physical examination, and a focused interview with the patient and/or a family member asking questions related to snoring, apneic episodes, frequent arousals from sleep, nocturia, gastroesophageal reflux disease, daytime headache, somnolence, and impaired memory.[33]

Laboratory PSG is currently considered the gold standard for diagnosing patients with OSA. A recent study on patients with OSA undergoing upper airway surgery identified 2 polysomnographic variables that were significantly associated with short-term operative complications: lowest oxygen desaturation (OR, 1.03; 95% CI, 0.96–1.45; P = .04) and longest apnea duration (OR, 1.03; 95% CI, 0.99–1.08; P = .02).[31] Forty-three percent of the surgical patients had serious pulmonary complications, such as aspiration, atelectasis, pulmonary edema, postoperative tracheal reintubation or tracheostomy, oxygen desaturation of 85% or less in the postoperative period, bronchospasm, and respiratory arrest.[34] Oxygen desaturation index (ODI) from high-resolution nocturnal oximetry is a sensitive and specific tool to detect undiagnosed sleep disordered breathing in surgical patients.[35] Patients with preoperative mean overnight Spo_2 less than 93%, or ODI greater than 29 events per hour, or cumulated overnight oxygen desaturation less than 7% were shown to be at higher risk for postoperative adverse events.[36] Hwang and colleagues[37] showed that the rate of postoperative complications was increased in proportion to episodes of overnight desaturation during home nocturnal oximetry.

Although PSG can delineate and predict patients with OSA at high risk of operative complications, it may be difficult to implement PSG in the perioperative setting because of the short duration between preoperative evaluation at a clinic and date of surgery. Moreover, some patients may be being evaluated on the same day, especially in ambulatory surgery. Screening questionnaires, nocturnal pulse oximetry, and home sleep testing are more commonly used to evaluate for OSA perioperatively.

The STOP-Bang (snoring, tiredness, observed apnea, high blood pressure, BMI, age, neck circumference, and male gender) questionnaire (**Box 1**) is widely used as

---

Box 1
STOP-Bang questionnaire

STOP-Bang scoring model:

1. Snoring?
   Do you snore loudly (loud enough to be heard through closed doors or your bed-partner elbows you for snoring at night)?
   Yes/no

2. Tired?
   Do you often feel tired, fatigued, or sleepy during the daytime (such as falling asleep during driving or talking to someone)?
   Yes/no

3. Observed?
   Has anyone observed you stop breathing or choking/gasping during your sleep?
   Yes/no

4. Pressure?
   Do you have, or are you being treated for, high blood pressure?
   Yes/no

5. BMI more than 35 kg/m²?
   Yes/no

6. Age older than 50 years?
   Yes/no

7. Neck size large? (Measured around Adam's apple.)
   For men, is your shirt collar 43 cm (17 inches) or larger?
   For women, is your shirt collar 41 cm (16 inches) or larger?
   Yes/no

8. Gender: male?
   Yes/no

Scoring criteria for general population:

Low risk of OSA: yes to 0 to 2 questions

Intermediate risk of OSA: yes to 3 to 4 questions

High risk of OSA: yes to 5 to 8 questions
Or yes to 2 or more of 4 STOP questions + male gender
Or yes to 2 or more of 4 STOP questions + BMI greater than 35 kg/m²
Or yes to 2 or more of 4 STOP questions + neck circumference (43 cm/17 inches in men, 41 cm/16 inches in women).

Adapted from Nagappa M, Wong J, Singh M, et al. An update on the various practical applications of the STOP-Bang questionnaire in anesthesia, surgery, and perioperative medicine. Curr Opin Anaesthesiol 2017;30(1):120; with permission.

a screening tool for OSA.[38,39] It has the highest methodological validity and reasonable accuracy in predicting a diagnosis of OSA[18] and a STOP-Bang score of 5 to 8 identifies patients with moderate to severe OSA with a fairly high probability.[40] The addition of serum HCO_3^- levels of 28 mmol/L or greater to a STOP-Bang score of 3 or more improves the specificity for preoperative recognition of severe OSA.[41] For obese or morbidly obese patients, a STOP-Bang score of 4 or greater can be used as a cutoff.[42] A modified STOP-Bang score with additional points for BMI (1 point for BMI 35–40 kg/m[2], 2 points for BMI 40–45 kg/m[2], 3 points for BMI 45 kg/m[2]) and HCO_3^- (1 point for HCO_3^- 26–28 mmol/L, 2 points for HCO_3^- 28 mmol/L) was compared with the original STOP-Bang score for predicting OHS. A modified score of at least 6 showed an increase in sensitivity and a decrease in specificity (89.2% and 47.6%) compared with the original STOP-Bang score of 6 or greater (71.6% and 59.1%).[43]

The STOP-Bang questionnaire can be used as a preoperative risk stratification tool to predict the risk of intraoperative and early postoperative adverse events.[15,44] A recent systematic review and meta-analysis of 10 cohort studies noted that postoperative complications were almost 4-fold higher and the duration of the hospital stay was 2 days longer in high-risk patients with OSA (with STOP-Bang score 3 or greater) versus low-risk patients with OSA.[15] Similarly, another prospective study of 3452 patients showed that patients identified as high risk for OSA by the STOP-Bang questionnaire had a higher rate of postoperative complications (9% vs 2%), difficult intubation (20% vs 9%), and difficult mask ventilation (23% vs 7%).[45] STOP-Bang scores of 3, 4, and 5 were associated with 2-fold, 3-fold, and 5-fold risk of critical care admission, respectively.[46] Perioperative respiratory events were more frequent in patients with risk of OSA (STOP-Bang score $\geq$3).[47,48]

The Society of Anesthesia and Sleep Medicine guidelines suggests that additional evaluation for preoperative cardiopulmonary optimization should be considered in patients who have a high probability of OSA and in whom there is an indication of uncontrolled systemic conditions or additional problems with ventilation or gas exchange, such as (1) hypoventilation syndromes, (2) severe pulmonary hypertension, and (3) resting hypoxemia not attributable to other cardiopulmonary disease.[49] Hillman and colleagues[50] proposed a pathway for the perioperative assessment and management of patients with OSA (**Fig. 1**).

Cigarette use

Smoking has been identified as one of the few modifiable risk factors for PPCs in several studies.[4,13] A study found that 30-day postoperative respiratory events were more frequent in current smokers versus former smokers/nonsmokers (OR, 1.45 vs 1.13).[51] PPC rates are higher for patients with at least a 20-pack-year smoking history than for those with a lesser pack-year smoking history.[7] It is important to assess current smoking status and encourage smoking cessation early in the preparation for elective surgery. Smoking cessation for at least 4 weeks before surgery reduces the risk of PPCs, and longer periods of smoking cessation may be even more effective.[52] A lesser duration of preoperative cessation confers less protection against PPCs, although it does not increase PPC risk, in contrast with an earlier report.[7,53] A recent prospective multicenter study of a brief, multifaceted intervention featuring a patient e-learning program for smoking cessation reported that 22% of the patients quit smoking on the day of surgery and remained abstinent 6 months after surgery.[51] This study supports the evidence that preoperative smoking cessation interventions are valuable to help patients quit smoking.[54]

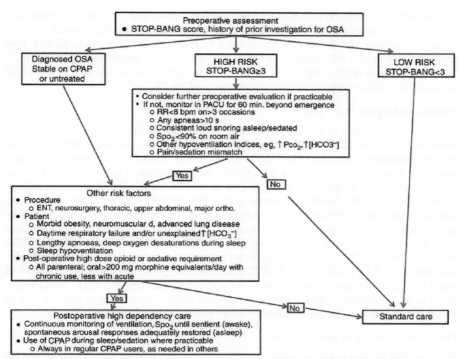

Fig. 1. Principles for perioperative management of adult patients with sleep-disordered breathing. bpm, breaths per minute; CPAP, continuous positive airway pressure; d, disease; ENT, ear, nose, and throat; HCO_3^-, serum bicarbonate; ortho, orthopedic surgery; PACU, postanesthesia care unit; RR, respiration rate. (*From* Hillman DR, Chung F. Anaesthetic management of sleep-disordered breathing in adults. Respirology 2017;22:236; with permission.)

Obesity
Studies evaluating PPCs have generally found no increased risk attributable to obesity or morbid obesity.[55,56] A recent review of the National Surgical Quality Improvement database showed that obesity (BMI>35 kg/m²) was not associated with an increase in PPCs.[1] BMI greater than or equal to 60 kg/m² and truncal obesity in combination with OHS and/or OSA were identified as risk factors for postoperative pulmonary embolism.[57] Obesity has long been associated with possible difficult airway management. A thorough upper airway examination of obese patients should include a measurement of the neck circumference, mouth opening, and neck range of motion. A neck circumference of approximately 44 cm of an obese patient increases the difficulty in intubation compared with the general population. Moreover, this risk increases to 35% at a neck circumference of 60 cm.[58] Interesting, a study found that excessive abdominal fat measured by computed tomography conferred a risk of PPCs, which was independent of the patient's BMI.[59] Hence, some obese patients may be at risk of PPCs.

Respiratory infection in the last month
A history of upper/lower respiratory infection in the month before surgery is another avoidable risk factor for PPCs. Delaying elective surgery in some cases may be a reasonable choice.[4] Recent respiratory infection increases bronchial reactivity and the risk of laryngospasm, bronchospasm, and/or transient perioperative hypoxemia.[60]

In summary, it is recommended that all patients undergoing noncardiothoracic surgery should be evaluated for the following 5 significant risk factors that predict PPCs in order to institute perioperative interventions to reduce pulmonary risk: COPD, age older than 60 years, ASA class of II or greater, functionally dependency, and CHF.[61] In addition, there is also significant evidence in a systematic review of more than 60 studies that OSA is associated with increased risk for PPCs.[14]

Procedure-Related Risk Factors

Surgical site, duration of surgery, anesthetic technique, and emergency surgery have been shown to predict PPCs. Major upper abdominal surgeries play a significant role in diaphragmatic dysfunction and can predispose to PPCs.[62] Yang and colleagues[1] identified that 25.6% of patients undergoing esophagectomy had PPCs and it was associated with more than 5-fold risk of combined PPCs on their multivariate analysis. There is fair amount of evidence showing that the following surgeries are associated with a higher rate of PPCs: aortic aneurysm repair, thoracic surgery, abdominal surgery, upper abdominal surgery, neurosurgery, prolonged surgery, head and neck surgery, emergency surgery, and vascular surgery.[61] A recent study showed that an ASA score of 3 or 4 is a significant risk factor for postoperative respiratory failure and reintubation (OR, 4.21 [2.29–7.73]; $P<.0001$).[6] Moreover, prolonged surgery duration of more than 2 hours was shown to be an independent predictor of PPCs.[4] In addition, there is some evidence that general anesthesia is associated with a greater risk of PPCs,[61] but this has not been confirmed by recent studies.[4]

Laboratory Testing to Estimate Risk

Preoperative testing could provide valuable information that would otherwise not be easily extracted from a patient's history and physical examination. Moreover, these tests can help identify patients who are more prone to developing PPCs. The most commonly available preoperative tests for pulmonary risk assessment include spirometry, chest radiograph, arterial blood gas (ABG), and serum albumin measurement.

Spirometry
Studies that have compared spirometric data with clinical data have not consistently shown spirometry to be superior to history and physical examination in predicting PPCs.[61,63] Spirometry should be reserved for patients who are thought to have undiagnosed COPD for diagnostic purposes.[61] The current evidence suggests that the results of pulmonary function test should not be used as a primary factor to deny surgery.

Chest radiograph
In a recent literature review, 23.1% of preoperative chest radiographs were abnormal but only 3% had findings clinically important enough to influence management.[64] The existing evidence suggests that radiographs only rarely provide unexpected information that influences preoperative management and are not recommended for clinical evaluation in identifying healthy patients at risk for PPCs.[7] There is reasonable evidence to obtain a chest radiograph in patients with known cardiopulmonary disease and those older than 50 years of age who are undergoing a high-risk surgical procedure like upper abdominal, esophageal, thoracic, or aortic surgery.[61]

Arterial blood gas
ABG has been used to identify hypoxemia and hypercapnia preoperatively, but neither hypoxemia or hypercapnia has been identified as significant independent predictors of the risk for PPCs.[7] ABG may be useful to diagnose patients with OHS. The definitive test to identify daytime hypercapnia with OHS is blood gas analysis. Because ABG is

invasive, a higher serum HCO_3^- level caused by metabolic compensation with chronic respiratory acidosis can be used as a surrogate marker of hypercapnia, and a serum HCO_3- threshold of 27 mEq/L showed a 92% sensitivity in predicting hypercapnia on ABG.[65]

Serum albumin measurement

Serum albumin concentration is considered a measure of nutritional status. A serum albumin level of 3.5 g/dL or less was associated with a higher rate of respiratory failure (OR, 1.485; 95% CI, 1.34–1.64).[7,66]

PULMONARY RISK INDICES

Numerous pulmonary risk indices have been developed to predict the risk of respiratory failure or developing pneumonia for patients undergoing surgery. Risk scores can be useful if they can provide an estimate of the probability of a perioperative complication. This information can be used to advise patients regarding perioperative risks and expectations and to optimize patients at high risk.

Risk indices that provide a numerical estimate of the risk, such as that presented by Arozullah and colleagues[13,67] and the assess respiratory risk in surgical patients in catalonia (ARISCAT) risk indices,[4] rather than a qualitative category, are more useful at predicting PPCs. Furthermore, in contrast with many pulmonary risk indices that were based on small numbers of patients, these risk indices developed risk factors based on the analysis from thousands of patients from the Veterans' Affairs patient database[13,67] or from a large surgical cohort.[4] The commonly used risk indices are described here.

RISK INDICES FOR POSTOPERATIVE RESPIRATORY FAILURE

In a large multicenter observational cohort study of subjects undergoing major noncardiac surgery, Arozullah and colleagues[67] developed and validated a respiratory failure risk index to identify patients at risk for developing PPCs (**Table 1**). The index included abdominal aortic aneurysm repair, thoracic surgery, neurosurgery, upper abdominal surgery, peripheral vascular surgery, neck surgery, emergency surgery, albumin level less than 30 g/L, blood urea nitrogen level more than 30 mg/dL, dependent functional status, COPD, and age. The type of surgery performed had the highest associated risk for developing postoperative respiratory failure and the major patient-specific risk factors were related to general health, respiratory, renal, and fluid status.[67] Point scores are assigned based on the strength of association in the multivariate analysis, and patients are stratified into 5 classes with respiratory failure ranging from 0.5% to 26.6% (**Table 2**).[67]

The ARISCAT risk index (**Table 3**) includes 7 independent risk factors: advanced age, preoperative oxygen saturation, respiratory infection in the last month, preoperative anemia, type of surgical incision, duration of surgery, and emergent surgery. Each factor is assigned a weighted score and patients are stratified as low, intermediate, and high risk for developing pulmonary complications.[4]

RISK INDICES FOR POSTOPERATIVE PNEUMONIA

Arozullah and colleagues[13] also developed a postoperative pneumonia risk index to identify patients at risk for postoperative pneumonia. It includes the type of surgery performed and several patient-specific risk factors related to general health and immune status, respiratory status, neurologic status, and fluid status. These risk factors were used to develop a preoperative risk assessment model for predicting postoperative pneumonia, called the postoperative pneumonia risk index.[13]

Table 1
Arozullah respiratory failure index

Preoperative Predictor	Point Value
Type of surgery	
Abdominal aortic aneurysm	27
Thoracic	21
Neurosurgery, upper abdominal, or peripheral vascular	14
Neck	11
Emergency surgery	11
Albumin (<30 g/L)	9
Blood urea nitrogen (>30 mg/dL)	8
Partially or fully dependent functional status	7
History of chronic obstructive pulmonary disease	6
Age (y)	
≥70	6
60–69	4

From Arozullah AM, Daley J, Henderson WG, et al. Multifactorial risk index for predicting postoperative respiratory failure in men after major noncardiac surgery. Ann Surg 2000;232(2):250; with permission.

Gupta and colleagues[68] developed a validated risk calculator to provide a risk estimate for postoperative pneumonia to aid in surgical decision making. Preoperative variables associated with an increased risk of postoperative pneumonia include age, the ASA classification, COPD, dependent functional status, preoperative sepsis, smoking before operation, and type of operation.[68]

PREOPERATIVE STRATEGIES TO DECREASE POSTOPERATIVE PULMONARY COMPLICATIONS

After identifying patients at high risk for PPC, there is a scope for preoperative strategies to minimize risks and prevent complications. Preoperative interventions that have proved to reduce PPC rates in high-risk patients include the following:

1. Smoking cessation
   Smoking cessation for at least 4 weeks before surgery reduces the risk of PPCs,[52] although stopping for 8 weeks is optimal.[7]

Table 2
Performance of the Arozullah respiratory failure index

Class	Point Total	Incidence of Respiratory Failure (%)
1	≤10	0.5
2	11–19	1.8
3	20–27	4.2
4	28–40	10.1
5	>40	26.6

Adapted from Arozullah AM, Daley J, Henderson WG, et al. Multifactorial risk index for predicting postoperative respiratory failure in men after major noncardiac surgery. Ann Surg 2000;232(2):250; with permission.

Table 3
ARISCAT risk index

Factor	Adjusted Odds Ratio (95% CI)	Risk Score
Age (y)		
≤50	1	—
51–80	1.4 (0.6–3.3)	3
>80	5.1 (1.9–13.3)	16
Preoperative Oxygen Saturation (%)		
≥96	1	—
91–95	2.2 (1.2–4.2)	8
≤90	10.7 (4.1–28.1)	24
Respiratory infection in the last month	5.5 (2.6–11.5)	17
Preoperative anemia (hemoglobin ≤10 g/dL)	3.0 (1.4–6.5)	11
Surgical Incision		
Upper abdominal	4.4 (2.3–8.5)	15
Intrathoracic	11.4 (1.9–26.0)	24
Duration of Surgery (h)		
≤2	1	—
2–3	4.9 (2.4–10.1)	16
>3	9.7 (2.4–19.9)	23
Emergency surgery	2.2 (1.0–4.5)	8

Risk Class	Number of Points in Risk Score	PPC Incidence (Validation Sample) (%)
Low	<26	1.6
Intermediate	26–44	13.3
High	≥45	42.1

Adapted from Canet J, Gallart L, Gomar C, et al. Prediction of postoperative pulmonary complications in a population-based surgical cohort. Anesthesiology 2010;113(6):1346; with permission.

2. Decreasing bronchial hyper-reactivity in patients with COPD and asthma

Inhaled β2-adrenergic agonists may protect against reflex bronchoconstriction during intubation and general anesthesia.[69] Preoperative administration of corticosteroids, alone or in combination with β2 agonists, may be beneficial, although it is unclear whether it is necessary for all patients with asthma or COPD.[69] Patients already receiving steroid therapy should continue therapy perioperatively.[70]

3. Treat any existing lower respiratory tract infections

4. High-flow nasal cannula (HFNC) oxygen therapy

HFNC reduces arousals and apnea hypopnea index in adult patients with OSA.[71] There is evidence that HFNCs reduced breathing frequency and carbon dioxide levels and increased the tidal volume in patients with COPD.[72,73] HFNC also increases exercise capacity for stable patients with COPD, providing better oxygenation than spontaneous breathing.[74]

5. Lung expansion techniques

Lung expansion techniques include incentive spirometry; chest physical therapy, including deep breathing exercises; cough; postural drainage; percussion and vibration; suctioning and ambulation; intermittent positive-pressure breathing; and CPAP. The literature suggests that, for patients undergoing abdominal surgery, any type of lung expansion intervention is better than no prophylaxis at all.[61,75]

SUMMARY

As many as 1 in 4 deaths occurring within a week of surgery are related to PPCs, making it the second most common serious morbidity after cardiovascular event. The most significant predictors of the PPCs are ASA physical status, advanced age, dependent functional status, surgical site, and duration of surgery. Once risk is estimated, there is scope to prevent PPCs by targeting the modifiable risk factors. There is no evidence to routinely perform pulmonary function tests and ABGs before elective noncardiac surgery. The overall risk of PPCs can be predicted using scores that incorporate readily available clinical data.

REFERENCES

1. Yang CK, Teng A, Lee DY, et al. Pulmonary complications after major abdominal surgery: National Surgical Quality Improvement Program analysis. J Surg Res 2015;198:441–9.
2. Sabaté S, Mazo V, Canet J. Predicting postoperative pulmonary complications: implications for outcomes and costs. Curr Opin Anaesthesiol 2014;27:201–9.
3. Ferguson MK. Preoperative assessment of pulmonary risk. Chest 1999;115:58S–63S.
4. Canet J, Gallart L, Gomar C, et al. Prediction of postoperative pulmonary complications in a population-based surgical cohort. Anesthesiology 2010;113:1338–50.
5. Holmes JR, Hensinger RN, Wojtys EW. Postoperative pulmonary edema in young, athletic adults. Am J Sports Med 1991;19:365–71.
6. Brueckmann B, Villa-Uribe JL, Bateman BT, et al. Development and validation of a score for prediction of postoperative respiratory complications. Anesthesiology 2013;118:1276–85.
7. Lakshminarasimhachar A. Preoperative evaluation: estimation of pulmonary risk. Anesthesiol Clin 2016;34:71–88.
8. Landbo C, Prescott E, Lange P, et al. Prognostic value of nutritional status in chronic obstructive pulmonary disease. Am J Respir Crit Care Med 1999;160:1856–61.
9. Windsor JA, Hill GL. Risk factors for postoperative pneumonia. The importance of protein depletion. Ann Surg 1988;208:209–14.
10. Gupta H, Gupta PK, Fang X, et al. Development and validation of a risk calculator predicting postoperative respiratory failure. Chest 2011;140:1207–15.
11. Arozullah AM, Conde MV, Lawrence VA. Preoperative evaluation for postoperative pulmonary complications. Med Clin North Am 2003;87:153–73.
12. Smetana GW, Lawrence VA, Cornell JE. Annals of internal medicine clinical guidelines preoperative pulmonary risk stratification for noncardiothoracic surgery: systematic review for the American College of Physicians. Ann Intern Med 2006;144:581–95.

13. Arozullah AM, Khuri SF, Henderson WG, et al. Development and validation of a multifactorial risk index for predicting postoperative pneumonia after major noncardiac surgery. Ann Intern Med 2001;135:847–57.

14. Opperer M, Cozowicz C, Bugada D, et al. Does obstructive sleep apnea influence perioperative outcome? A qualitative systematic review for the Society of Anesthesia and Sleep Medicine Task Force on preoperative preparation of patients with sleep-disordered breathing. Anesth Analg 2016;122:1321–34.

15. Nagappa M, Patra J, Wong J, et al. Association of STOP-Bang questionnaire as a screening tool for sleep apnea and postoperative complications: a systematic review and bayesian meta-analysis of prospective and retrospective cohort studies. Anesth Analg 2017;125:1301–8.

16. Nagappa M, Ho G, Patra J, et al. Postoperative outcomes in obstructive sleep apnea patients undergoing cardiac surgery. Anesth Analg 2017;125:2030–7.

17. Subramani Y, Nagappa M, Wong J, et al. Death or near-death in patients with obstructive sleep apnoea: a compendium of case reports of critical complications. Br J Anaesth 2017;119:885–99.

18. Nagappa M, Liao P, Wong J, et al. Validation of the STOP-Bang questionnaire as a screening tool for obstructive sleep apnea among different populations: a systematic review and meta-analysis. PLoS One 2015;10(12):e0143697.

19. Subramani Y, Wong J, Nagappa M, et al. The benefits of perioperative screening for sleep apnea in surgical patients. Sleep Med Clin 2017;12:123–35.

20. Shin CH, Grabitz SD, Timm FP, et al. Development and validation of a score for preoperative prediction of obstructive sleep apnea (SPOSA) and its perioperative outcomes. BMC Anesthesiol 2017;17:1–12.

21. Memtsoudis S, Liu SS, Ma Y, et al. Perioperative pulmonary outcomes in patients with sleep apnea after noncardiac surgery. Anesth Analg 2011;112:113–21.

22. Mokhlesi B, Hovda MD, Vekhter B, et al. Sleep-disordered breathing and postoperative outcomes after elective surgery: analysis of the nationwide inpatient sample. Chest 2013;144:903–14.

23. Kaw R, Chung F, Pasupuleti V, et al. Meta-analysis of the association between obstructive sleep apnoea and postoperative outcome. Br J Anaesth 2012;109:897–906.

24. Lam KK, Kunder S, Wong J, et al. Obstructive sleep apnea, pain, and opioids: is the riddle solved? Curr Opin Anaesthesiol 2016;29:134–40.

25. Ramachandran SK, Haider N, Saran KA, et al. Life-threatening critical respiratory events: a retrospective study of postoperative patients found unresponsive during analgesic therapy. J Clin Anesth 2011;23:207–13.

26. Lee LA, Caplan RA, Stephens LS, et al. Postoperative opioid-induced respiratory depression: a closed claims analysis. Anesthesiology 2015;122:659–65.

27. Gupta K, Prasad A, Nagappa M, et al. Risk factors for opioid-induced respiratory depression and failure to rescue. Curr Opin Anaesthesiol 2018;31(1):110–9.

28. Chau EHL, Mokhlesi B, Chung F. Obesity hypoventilation syndrome and anesthesia. Sleep Med Clin 2013;8:135–47.

29. Chau EHL, Lam D, Wong J, et al. Obesity hypoventilation syndrome: a review of epidemiology, pathophysiology, and perioperative considerations. Anesthesiology 2012;117:188–205.

30. Balachandran JS, Masa JF, Mokhlesi B. Obesity hypoventilation syndrome epidemiology and diagnosis. Sleep Med Clin 2014;9:341–7.

31. Banerjee D, Yee BJ, Piper AJ, et al. Obesity hypoventilation syndrome. Chest 2007;131:1678–84.

32. Kaw R, Bhateja P, Paz Y Mar H, et al. Postoperative complications in patients with unrecognized obesity hypoventilation syndrome undergoing elective non-cardiac surgery. Chest 2016;149:84–91.

33. Gross JB, Apfelbaum JL, Caplan RA, et al. Practice guidelines for the perioperative management of patients with obstructive sleep apnea an updated report by the American Society of Anesthesiologists Task Force on Perioperative Management of Patients with Obstructive Sleep Apnea. Anesthesiology 2014;120: 268–86.

34. Asha'ari ZA, Rahman J, Mohamed AH, et al. Association between severity of obstructive sleep apnea and number and sites of upper airway operations with surgery complications. JAMA Otolaryngol Head Neck Surg 2017;143:239–46.

35. Chung F, Liao P, Elsaid H, et al. Oxygen desaturation index from nocturnal oximetry: a sensitive and specific tool to detect sleep-disordered breathing in surgical patients. Anesth Analg 2012;114:993–1000.

36. Chung F, Zhou L, Liao P. Parameters from preoperative overnight oximetry predict postoperative adverse events. Minerva Anestesiol 2014;80:1084–95.

37. Hwang D, Shakir N, Limann B, et al. Association of sleep-disordered breathing with postoperative complications. Chest 2008;133:1128–34.

38. Chung F, Yegneswaran B, Liao P, et al. STOP questionnaire: a tool to screen patients for obstructive sleep apnea. Anesthesiology 2008;108:812–21.

39. Nagappa M, Wong J, Singh M, et al. An update on the various practical applications of the STOP-Bang questionnaire in anesthesia, surgery, and perioperative medicine. Curr Opin Anaesthesiol 2017;30:118–25.

40. Chung F, Subramanyam R, Liao P, et al. High STOP-Bang score indicates a high probability of obstructive sleep apnoea. Br J Anaesth 2012;108:768–75.

41. Chung F, Chau E, Yang Y, et al. Serum bicarbonate level improves specificity of STOP-Bang screening for obstructive sleep apnea. Chest 2013;143:1284–93.

42. Chung F, Yang Y, Liao P. Predictive performance of the STOP-Bang score for identifying obstructive sleep apnea in obese patients. Obes Surg 2013;23: 2050–7.

43. Bingol Z, Pıhtılı A, Kıyan E. Modified STOP-BANG questionnaire to predict obesity hypoventilation syndrome in obese subjects with obstructive sleep apnea. Sleep Breath 2016;20:495–500. Available at: http://www.ncbi.nlm.nih.gov/pubmed/26047651. Accessed February 16, 2018.

44. Seet E, Chua M, Liaw CM. High STOP-BANG questionnaire scores predict intraoperative and early postoperative adverse events. Singapore Med J 2015;56: 212–6.

45. Corso RM, Petrini F, Buccioli M, et al. Clinical utility of preoperative screening with STOP-Bang questionnaire in elective surgery. Minerva Anestesiol 2014;80: 877–84.

46. Chia P, Seet E, Macachor JD, et al. The association of pre-operative STOP-BANG scores with postoperative critical care admission. Anaesthesia 2013;68:950–2.

47. Pereira H, Xará D, Mendonça J, et al. Patients with a high risk for obstructive sleep apnea syndrome: postoperative respiratory complications. Rev Port Pneumol 2013;19:144–51.

48. Gali B, Whalen FX, Schroeder DR, et al. Identification of patients at risk for postoperative respiratory complications using a preoperative obstructive sleep apnea screening tool and postanesthesia care assessment. Anesthesiology 2009;110: 869–77.

49. Chung F, Memtsoudis S, Ramachandran SK, et al. Society of Anesthesia and Sleep Medicine guidelines on preoperative screening and assessment of adult patients with obstructive sleep apnea. Anesth Analg 2016;123(2):452–73.
50. Hillman DR, Chung F. Anaesthetic management of sleep-disordered breathing in adults. Respirology 2017;22:230–9.
51. Musallam KM, Rosendaal FR, Zaatari G, et al. Smoking and the risk of mortality and vascular and respiratory events in patients undergoing major surgery. JAMA Surg 2013;148:755.
52. Grønkjær M, Eliasen M, Skov-Ettrup LS, et al. Preoperative smoking status and postoperative complications. Ann Surg 2014;259:52–71.
53. Wong J, Lam DP, Abrishami A, et al. Short-term preoperative smoking cessation and postoperative complications: a systematic review and meta-analysis. Can J Anesth 2012;59:268–79.
54. Wong J, Raveendran R, Chuang J, et al. Utilizing patient e-learning in an intervention study on preoperative smoking cessation. Anesth Analg 2018;126(5): 1646–53, e-publishe:1.
55. Smetana GW. Preoperative pulmonary evaluation. N Engl J Med 1999;340: 937–44.
56. Sterling RK. Management of gastrointestinal disease in liver transplant recipients. Gastrointest Endosc Clin North Am 2001;11:185–97.
57. Sapala JA, Wood MH, Schuhknecht MP, et al. Fatal pulmonary embolism after bariatric operations for morbid obesity: a 24-year retrospective analysis. Obes Surg 2003;13:819–25.
58. Cartagena R. Preoperative evaluation of patients with obesity and obstructive sleep apnea. Anesthesiol Clin North America 2005;23:463–78.
59. Shimizu A, Tani M, Kawai M, et al. Influence of visceral obesity for postoperative pulmonary complications after pancreaticoduodenectomy. J Gastrointest Surg 2011;15:1401–10.
60. Nandwani N, Raphael JH, Langton JA. Effect of an upper respiratory tract infection on upper airway reactivity. Br J Anaesth 1997;78:352–5.
61. Qaseem A, Snow V, Fitterman N, et al. Annals of Internal Medicine clinical guidelines risk assessment for and strategies to reduce perioperative pulmonary complications for patients undergoing noncardiothoracic surgery: a guideline from the American College of Physicians. Ann Intern Med 2006;144:575–80.
62. Ferreyra G, Long Y, Ranieri VM. Respiratory complications after major surgery. Curr Opin Crit Care 2009;15:342–8.
63. Kundra P, Vitheeswaran M, Nagappa M, et al. Effect of preoperative and postoperative incentive spirometry on lung functions after laparoscopic cholecystectomy. Surg Laparosc Endosc Percutan Tech 2010;20:170–2.
64. Hamoui N, Kim K, Anthone G, et al. The significance of elevated levels of parathyroid hormone in patients with morbid obesity before and after bariatric surgery. Arch Surg 2003;138:891. Available at: http://www.ncbi.nlm.nih.gov/pubmed/12912749. Accessed January 25, 2018.
65. Mokhlesi B, Tulaimat A, Faibussowitsch I, et al. Obesity hypoventilation syndrome: prevalence and predictors in patients with obstructive sleep apnea. Sleep Breath 2007;11:117–24.
66. Gupta H, Ramanan B, Gupta PK, et al. Impact of COPD on postoperative outcomes: results from a national database. Chest 2013;143:1599–606.
67. Arozullah AM, Daley J, Henderson WG, et al. Multifactorial risk index for predicting postoperative respiratory failure in men after major noncardiac surgery. Ann Surg 2000;232:242–53.

68. Gupta H, Gupta PK, Schuller D, et al. Development and validation of a risk calculator for predicting postoperative pneumonia. Mayo Clin Proc 2013;88:1241–9.
69. Silvanus M-T, Groeben H, Peters J. Corticosteroids and inhaled salbutamol in patients with reversible airway obstruction markedly decrease the incidence of bronchospasm after tracheal intubation. Anesthesiology 2004;100:1052–7.
70. Haeck PC, Swanson JA, Iverson RE, et al. Evidence-based patient safety advisory: patient assessment and prevention of pulmonary side effects in surgery. Part 1—obstructive sleep apnea and obstructive lung disease. Plast Reconstr Surg 2009;124:45S–56S.
71. McGinley BM, Patil SP, Kirkness JP, et al. A nasal cannula can be used to treat obstructive sleep apnea. Am J Respir Crit Care Med 2007;176:194–200.
72. Nilius G, Franke K-J, Domanski U, et al. Effects of nasal insufflation on arterial gas exchange and breathing pattern in patients with chronic obstructive pulmonary disease and hypercapnic respiratory failure. Adv Exp Med Biol 2013;755:27–34.
73. Bräunlich J, Beyer D, Mai D, et al. Effects of nasal high flow on ventilation in volunteers, COPD and idiopathic pulmonary fibrosis patients. Respiration 2013;85: 319–25.
74. Chatila W, Nugent T, Vance G, et al. The effects of high-flow vs low-flow oxygen on exercise in advanced obstructive airways disease. Chest 2004;126:1108–15.
75. Kundra P, Subramani Y, Ravishankar M, et al. Cardiorespiratory effects of balancing PEEP with intra-abdominal pressures during laparoscopic cholecystectomy. Surg Laparosc Endosc Percutan Tech 2014;24:232–9.

Stratification and Risk Reduction of Perioperative Acute Kidney Injury: An Update

Sheela Pai Cole, MD*

KEYWORDS

- Kidney injury • Renal dysfunction • Perioperative period • Dialysis
- Perioperative hypotension • Nephrotoxins • Cardiac surgery
- Urgent or emergent surgery

KEY POINTS

- Perioperative kidney injury is associated with significant morbidity and mortality.
- Patients with perioperative acute kidney injury are at increased risk of developing chronic kidney disease.
- Many sets of criteria are available to predict perioperative kidney injury after cardiac surgery.
- Modifiable risk factors such hemodynamic management and anemia treatment may mitigate the course of acute renal injury.

BACKGROUND

Perioperative renal injury is associated with significant morbidity and mortality. Increased duration of hospital stay, ventilator dependence, and cardiovascular events are commonly seen in patients who have renal injury in the perioperative period. Furthermore, even with resolution of acute kidney injury (AKI), the patient may have increased risk of development acute and chronic kidney disease (CKD) in the future.

DEFINITIONS

Until recently, a lack of standardized criteria for classification of renal injury has been a challenge to defining the incidence and prevalence of perioperative kidney injury. However, in the past 20 years, the Kidney Disease: Improving Global Outcomes (KDIGO) organization has unified definitions and developed consensus guidelines for AKI and CKD. These new guidelines are now being used in research and clinical

Conflicts: Medscape Editor, not relevant to this article.
Anesthesiology, Perioperative and Pain Medicine, Stanford University, 300 Pasteur Dr, H3580, Stanford, CA 94305, USA
* 300 Pasteur Dr, H3580, Stanford, CA 94305.
E-mail address: spaicole@stanford.edu

Anesthesiology Clin 36 (2018) 539–551
https://doi.org/10.1016/j.anclin.2018.07.005
1932-2275/18/© 2018 Elsevier Inc. All rights reserved.

anesthesiology.theclinics.com

practice, allowing for the accurate assessment of the problem. AKI is defined as an abrupt decline in kidney function that occurs over a period of 7 days or less. In contrast, CKD is defined by abnormalities in kidney structure or function that persist beyond 90 days. Since the consensus definitions, it has become evident that AKI and CKD are not discrete entities, but most likely represent a continuum whereby patients with AKI have an increased risk of development of CKD or worsening preexisting CKD. Furthermore, it seems that risk factors for AKI and CKD such as advanced age, hypertension, and diabetes overlap. A related term that needs to be defined is acute kidney disease, which is characterized by the course of pathophysiologic processes in the kidney that follows AKI before the 90-day time course of CKD.[1,2]

Clarifying Concepts

Health care providers commonly use the terms prerenal azotemia and acute tubular necrosis (ATN) interchangeably with AKI. Bellomo and colleagues suggest this practice is inaccurate. ATN is a histologic diagnosis based on renal tissue biopsy, which is rarely performed nowadays and, thus, scientifically difficult to prove, whereas prerenal azotemia refers to kidney disease as a function of persistent hypoperfusion. We know now that AKI is a continuum of disease and it seems that the recognition of terms such as ATN and prerenal azotemia obviates that conclusion. As awareness of AKI grows, it is likely that the terms ATN and prerenal azotemia will become obsolete.[1]

INCIDENCE AND PREVALENCE

The incidence of AKI is a diagnostic challenge owing to the use of varying definitions until the recent KDIGO consensus guidelines. Furthermore, the prevalence of AKI differs when factoring in the need for dialysis. Among hospitalized patients, the incidence of AKI is 8% to 16% and carries a high financial cost as well as personal burden for these patients. Moreover, among hospitalized patients, admission to the intensive care unit is associated with an increased risk of development of AKI.[1] In 2014, a cross-sectional global study by the International Society of Nephrology demonstrated an incidence of 10% to 12% worldwide across a spectrum of incomes with a slightly increased 7-day mortality among lower income communities (12%) versus higher income communities (10%).[3] Additionally, older individuals are disproportionately affected by AKI; among US Medicare patients aged 66 to 69 years, mortality was 14.9 per 1000 persons, increasing with age to 18.8 per 1000 individuals aged 70 to 74, 26.4 per 1000 persons aged 75 to 79, 35.9 per 1000 persons aged 80 to 84, and 49.6 per 1000 persons aged 85 years of age or older. Although the mortality risk across age groups remains similar, it seems that older patients who develop AKI have a lower overall survival and are less likely to have renal recovery.[4]

DIAGNOSIS

The 3 recent sets of criteria to describe renal dysfunction include the Renal Injury, Failure, Loss and End Organ (RIFLE) consensus guidelines, the Acute Kidney Injury Network (AKIN) criteria, and the KDIGO AKI guidelines (**Fig. 1**). Although the KDIGO AKI guidelines are the widely accepted guidelines currently, all 3 sets of criteria play a role in describing the concept of AKI. Furthermore, recent research has used all 3 sets of criteria in their findings.

The RIFLE criteria set forth by the Acute Dialysis Quality Initiative Group identify 3 grades of severity (risk, injury, and failure) as well as 2 outcome classifications (loss and end-stage failure) on the basis of change in glomerular filtration rate estimated by the Modification of Diet in Renal Disease formula and serum creatinine.[5] Similarly,

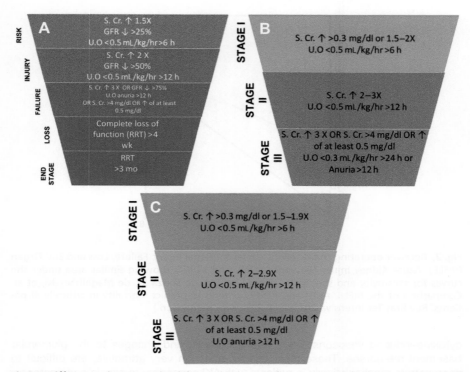

Fig. 1. Differences between the (*A*) Renal Injury, Failure, Loss and End Organ (RIFLE), (*B*) Acute Kidney Injury Network (AKIN), and (*C*) KDIGO criteria for AKI. GFR, glomerular filtration rate; RRT, renal replacement therapy; S. Cr., serum creatinine; U. O, urinary output. (*Courtesy of* S. Pai Cole, MD, FASE, Stanford, CA.)

AKIN criteria are also based on changes in the glomerular filtration rate, but serve to describe severity of AKI. AKIN describes worsening Stages I, II and III based on the increases in serum creatinine or decreases in the glomerular filtration rate.[6,7]

The KDIGO in 2012 simplified the process whereby AKI was diagnosed by either an increase in serum creatinine by 0.3 mg/dL over a 48-hour period, an increase in serum creatinine by more than 1.5 times the baseline over a 7-day period, or a decrease in urine output to less than 0.5 mL/kg/h over a 6-hour period.[8]

It is important to state that all 3 criteria use the same laboratory values to determine preestablished severity scores of renal injury (**Fig. 2**). As a result, all 3 criteria are subject to the same biases and are equivalent in predicting morbidity and mortality in critically ill patients.[9]

OVERALL PATHOPHYSIOLOGY OF ACUTE KIDNEY INJURY

Mechanisms of renal parenchymal diseases such as glomerulonephritis and vasculitis are beyond the purview of this review. Perioperative and intensive care–related AKI are most often secondary to prerenal factors. However, much of the data demonstrating prerenal AKI is from animal models using acute renal artery occlusion, which is often not the mechanism of hospital-acquired AKI.[10] Other animal models have implicated activation of the coagulation cascade and leukocytic injury to vascular endothelium,[11]

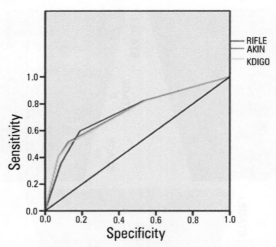

Fig. 2. Receiver operating characteristic curves for Renal Injury, Failure, Loss and End Organ (RIFLE), Acute Kidney Injury Network (AKIN), and KDIGO showing similar area under the curves for sensitivity and specificity. (*From* Levi TM, de Souza SP, de Magalhães JG, et al. Comparison of the RIFLE, AKIN and KDIGO criteria to predict mortality in critically ill patients. Rev Bras Ter Intensiva 2013;25(4):293; with permission.)

cytokine-induced vasoconstriction and apoptosis, and changes to the glomerular basement membrane. These mechanisms, although very attractive, are difficult to demonstrate mechanistically in patients with AKI secondary to sepsis and postoperative and acute decompensated heart failure, the 3 most common causes of hospital acquired AKI. Furthermore, although acute complete renal artery occlusion might be implicated experimentally in AKI, hypoperfusion owing to an 80% occlusion of the renal artery for up to 2 hours (as might happen in the perioperative period) is unlikely to be the cause of renal dysfunction.[12]

PERIOPERATIVE ACUTE KIDNEY INJURY AND RISK FACTORS

Depending on the type of surgery, the incidence of AKI and the modifiable factors may vary. It is worthwhile to examine the major types of surgery and factors contributing to postoperative renal dysfunction. Various predictive models stratifying risk associated with the different surgical specialties are also ascribed in this section.

Cardiac Surgery

Patients presenting for cardiac surgery have one of the greatest risks of development of AKI in the perioperative period. The risk of perioperative AKI varies between 1% and 3% for patients undergoing coronary artery bypass grafting (CABG)[13] and 27% and 29% among patients undergoing aortic valve replacement.[14] With recent successes of transcatheter aortic valve replacement, it seems that the risk of AKI remains similar despite certain advantages seen with transcatheter aortic valve replacement.[14] Although no large, randomized, controlled studies have been performed in patients undergoing combined cardiac surgical procedures, it seems that the risk of AKI remains between 1% and 29%. Preexisting risk factors for AKI after cardiac surgery include advanced age, female gender, anemia, preoperative renal dysfunction, left ventricular systolic dysfunction, peripheral arterial disease, race, type of surgery, diabetes mellitus requiring insulin, emergency surgery, preoperative intraaortic balloon pump support, and congestive heart or shock.

Prediction models for perioperative risk of acute kidney injury after cardiac surgery
Various indices have been proposed for predicting postoperative AKI, especially in patients undergoing cardiac surgery. The Berg index, from a single-center observational study, is one such model that factors in 11 preoperative variables including body mass index, age, hyperlipidemia, hypertension, peripheral vascular disease, chronic obstructive pulmonary disease, hemoglobin concentration, serum creatinine concentration, previous cardiac surgery, emergency operation, and operation type. It is suggested that this index would have improved accuracy if serum creatinine was used instead of glomerular filtration rate at diagnosing AKI.[15]

Thakar and colleagues[16] have proposed a risk assessment model to predict acute renal failure needing dialysis after cardiac surgery: the Cleveland Clinic risk score. The Cleveland Clinic risk score is a point-based score that is frequently used to assess the risk of renal dysfunction after cardiac surgery. Furthermore, this score has been validated in several studies and remains the most widely quoted risk assessment tool to date. The Cleveland Clinic risk score values similar preoperative characteristics as discussed, giving 1 point each for female gender, congestive heart failure, left ventricular ejection fraction of less than 35%, chronic obstructive pulmonary disease, diabetes needing insulin, previous cardiac surgery, and valve surgery; 2 points each for preoperative use of intraaortic balloon pump, combined CABG and valve surgery, emergency surgery, non-CABG or valve cardiac surgery (ie, aortic root or ascending aortic procedures), and a preoperative creatinine of 1.2 to 2.1 mg/dL. A creatinine of greater than 2.1 mg/dL receives 5 points. The acute renal failure/Cleveland Score allows a maximum score of 17, deeming maximal risk of developing acute renal failure. Interestingly, the use of deep hypothermic circulatory arrest, as is required for complex aortic procedures, is not an independent risk factor for AKI.[17]

A recent predictive model by Demirjian and colleagues[18] examined the role of preoperative as well as intraoperative factors in predicting postoperative AKI. This model used preoperative variables such as age, body mass index, gender, prior cardiac surgery, emergent surgery, and so on, as described in other models and for the first time included intraoperative variables such as cardiopulmonary bypass (CPB) time, aortic cross-clamp time, use of transfusions, and urine output, as well as use of diuretics. The type of surgery such as CABG alone versus CABG/valve was also included. Furthermore, the authors compared their model with the Cleveland clinic risk score described elsewhere in this article and proved equivalence. As expected, this model is focused more on AKI than prior models. It also highlights that patients with low intraoperative urine output and needing diuretics as more likely to have renal injury.

Pathogenesis of acute kidney injury after cardiac surgery
Cardiac surgical procedures, especially those requiring CPB, are unique. CPB has been implicated in a multitude of processes in renal dysfunction, including the release of proinflammatory cytokines, mounting a sympathomimetic response, and the release of vasoconstrictor hormones such as vasopressin. Additionally, a few modifiable factors on CPB have been associated with AKI, including hyperthermic perfusion during rewarming on CPB, hemodilution on CPB, mean arterial pressure (MAP) limits during nonpulsatile flow on CPB, and the influence of surgical technique.

Temperature and cardiopulmonary bypass
A multicenter study by Newland and colleagues[19] found an association between hyperthermic perfusion (temperature >37°C) during rewarming and AKI. Just before

the publication of this 2015 study, the Society of Thoracic Surgeons, the Society of Cardiovascular Anesthesiologists, and the American Society of Extracorporeal Technology temperature guidelines recommend limiting CPB arterial outlet blood temperature to less than 37°C to avoid cerebral hyperthermia and decrease stroke risk.[20]

Anemia and cardiopulmonary bypass

During CPB, moderate hemodilution decreases blood viscosity and plasma oncotic pressure, which can improve regional blood flow in the setting of hypothermia and hypoperfusion. However, this benefit is offset by an increased risk of adverse events and in-hospital deaths at extremely low hematocrits. In an observational study by DeFoe and colleagues[21] of patients undergoing isolated CABG, the mortality rate of patients with a single hematocrit value of 19% was twice that of those with a hematocrit of 25%, especially in small sized patients. Swaminathan and colleagues[22] examined the role of intraoperative anemia (hematocrit of <22%) and discovered a higher risk of AKI in patients with extremely low hematocrits. On the basis of these findings, the American College of Cardiology/American Heart Association guidelines recommend that a hematocrit of greater than 19% should be maintained on CPB.[23]

Mean arterial pressure and cardiopulmonary bypass

With nonpulsatile flow on CPB and widely varying temperature management on CPB, MAP targets remain very variable among perioperative personnel. Most centers manage MAP based on patient's age, presence of prior cerebrovascular events, and presence of carotid disease. Furthermore, there are few large, multicenter, randomized studies recommending goal MAPs while on CPB. One single-center, randomized, controlled trial studied high MAP (75–85 mm Hg) versus a low MAP (50–60 mm Hg) and found no difference in postoperative AKI.[24]

Surgical technique

The use of CPB has been primarily been implicated in morbidity after cardiac surgery. Some types of cardiac surgical procedure such as certain CABG cases can be performed without CPB, or off-pump CABG (OPCAB). Although there is no CPB use in OPCAB, the heart is often placed in nonanatomic positions to allow surgical access, resulting in hemodynamic instability. The ROOBY trial, a large multicenter trial examining OPCAB versus the use of CPB in patients presenting for CABG, demonstrated that in patients with normal kidney function preoperatively there was no protective benefit with OPCAB on postoperative kidney function.[25] However, in a recent 5-year follow-up study, OPCAB patients had a shorter survival than those undergoing CABG with CPB.[26] Furthermore, Chawla and colleagues[27] demonstrated that in patients with preexisting CKD use of OPCAB techniques is renoprotective.

Vascular Surgery

Although discussing the risk of AKI with every vascular surgical procedure is beyond the scope of this review, it is worth discussing the risk of AKI with descending aortic aneurysm repairs specifically Endovascular aortic aneurysm repair (EVAR), thoracic EVAR and open descending aortic repair (**Box 1**).

As with cardiac surgery, renal injury after vascular surgery remains a serious complication and carries a higher morbidity and mortality. Endovascular repair of the aortic and associated branch pathology has increasingly replaced open surgical repair. This minimally invasive repair is now used routinely for the treatment of abdominal aortic aneurysms, both in elective and emergency repair situations. Furthermore, randomized, controlled trials have shown superior results with endovascular surgery than with open surgery both in the short- and medium-term periods.[28–30] As with estimation

---

Box 1
Recommendations from the American College of Cardiology/American Heart Association to decrease the risk of acute kidney injury after cardiac surgery include (all Class IIb)

1. In patients with preoperative renal dysfunction (creatinine clearance <60 mL/min), off-pump coronary artery bypass grafting may be reasonable to reduce the risk of acute kidney injury (Level of Evidence: B).

2. In patients with preexisting renal dysfunction undergoing on-pump coronary artery bypass grafting, maintenance of a perioperative hematocrit of greater than 19% and mean arterial pressure of greater than 60 mm Hg may be reasonable (Level of Evidence: C).

3. In patients with preexisting renal dysfunction, a delay of surgery after coronary angiography may be reasonable until the effect of radiographic contrast material on renal function is assessed. (Level of Evidence: B).

4. The effectiveness of pharmacologic agents to provide renal protection during cardiac surgery is uncertain (Level of Evidence: B).

From Hillis LD, Smith PK, Anderson JL, et al. 2011 ACCF/AHA guideline for coronary artery bypass graft surgery. A report of the American College of Cardiology Foundation/American Heart Association Task Force on Practice Guidelines. Developed in collaboration with the American Association for Thoracic Surgery, Society of Cardiovascular Anesthesiologists, and Society of Thoracic Surgeons. J Am Coll Cardiol 2011;58(24):e123–210; with permission.

---

of AKI in cardiac surgery, until the new KDIGO guidelines were established, there was a wide discrepancy of reporting in this subset of patients.

Open Vascular Repair

It seems that the incidence of AKI in nonruptured aneurysm patients presenting for open repair is 5.4%[31]; dialysis need in patients undergoing open suprarenal aortic repair is significantly higher than those undergoing infrarenal aortic aneurysm repair at 5.4% versus 0.6%.[32] Mechanistically, AKI after open vascular surgery is secondary to renal ischemia, which definitely occurs in suprarenal abdominal aortic aneurysm repair; however, even in infrarenal abdominal aortic aneurysm repair, it seems that the process of aortic clamping does decrease the renal blood flow by 38% accompanied by a concomitant 75% increase in renovascular resistance.[32,33] Furthermore, limb ischemia from aortic clamping and unclamping causes the release of cytokines and inflammatory mediators and subsequent nephrotoxicity, resulting in renal injury or failure.[32,34]

Endovascular abdominal aneurysm repair

In comparison with open repair, endovascular techniques have a much lower incidence of AKI. However, EVAR requires a greater amount of contrast exposure periprocedurally. Furthermore, endovascular procedures have embolic potential during stent and wire placement. Both of these processes have been implicated in the occurrence of AKI after EVAR.[29,30,35,36]

Thoracic endovascular aneurysm repair

The ability to repair descending thoracic aortic aneurysms via an endovascular approach has markedly decreased morbidity and mortality in this patient population. Drews and colleagues[37] published a single-center study depicting saccular aneurysms, the use of red blood cell transfusion, nontraumatic rupture at presentation, and aortic arch involvement as independent risk factors for AKI after thoracic EVAR. This study demonstrated a 17% risk of AKI after thoracic EVAR; of note, the RIFLE criteria were used to describe kidney dysfunction.

Prediction Models for Perioperative Risk of Acute Kidney Injury After Vascular Surgery

In contrast with cardiac surgery, there are fewer predictive models for AKI after vascular surgery. The Berg index described elsewhere in this article has been explored by Fogagnolo and colleagues[38] in patients undergoing major vascular surgery and has not been found as accurate in predicting AKI. Perhaps an index that takes into consideration intraoperative details would help in this matter.

Other Types of Surgery

Grams and colleagues[39] studied the Veterans Administration database for postoperative AKI (by AKIN criteria) and were able to identify some key markers of AKI. Among the 161,185 patients found in the database, it seems that after cardiac surgical procedures (18.2%), general and thoracic surgeries had the highest incidence of AKI at 13.2% and 12.0%, respectively. Additional significant findings included a protective benefit for laparoscopic procedures and a higher incidence of AKI if the patient had been hospitalized for more than 5 days before the surgery. Although it houses a large cohort of patients, the limitations of this study remain a predominantly male cohort, which comprises the Veterans Administration database for now. Furthermore, although the surgeries included were cardiac, thoracic, general, ENT, urologic, and orthopedic procedures, the complexity of the cases remains unknown. Risk factors for development of AKI among the veterans included older age, African American race, and higher body mass index; the use of angiotensin-converting enzyme inhibitors, angiotensin receptor blockers, and diuretics were independently associated with a higher risk of AKI. Another study of abdominal surgical procedures demonstrated that patients undergoing exploratory laparotomy, hepatic and biliary tract procedures (not including cholecystectomy), and major esophageal procedures were more likely to be complicated by postoperative AKI.[40] Another study of colorectal surgery identified preexisting congestive heart failure, ischemic cardiac disease, and anemia, along with longer anesthetic exposure and intraoperative hypotension as risk factors for postoperative AKI.[41]

Prediction Models for Perioperative Risk of Acute Kidney Injury After Surgery

No specific risk predictive models have been identified to predict the risk of AKI after noncardiac, nonvascular surgery.

HEMODYNAMIC FACTORS IMPLICATED IN ACUTE KIDNEY INJURY

Renal perfusion depends on an adequate mean perfusion pressure, which is the difference between the MAP and venous back pressure, most often measured by the central venous pressure (CVP). The 2 main modifiable factors in the perioperative period are MAP and CVP.

Hypotension

Decreased blood pressure, specifically MAP, has been implicated in renal ischemia and AKI. Walsh and colleagues[42,43] describe a strong correlation between a MAP of less than 55 mm Hg for even a short duration and perioperative AKI after noncardiac surgery. The intraoperative concept of triple low(low MAP, low bispectral index, and low anesthetic gas requirement) was originally described as a marker of generalized illness. Specifically, perioperative myocardial events and AKI were ascribed to the phenomenon of triple low.[44,45] Although the concept of triple low maybe a symptom of generalized critical illness, Kertai and colleagues[46] found no association between triple low and AKI. Hypotension, especially in the elderly, is deleterious because aging is associated with renal senescence, and exposure to nephrotoxic drugs such as nonsteroidal antiinflammatory drugs.[47]

Elevated Central Venous Pressure

Data from patients with decompensated heart failure suggest that an elevated CVP signals end-organ congestion, including renal congestion, increasing the risk of renal ischemia and dysfunction. This situation is especially compounded by antecedent hypotension.[48] Furthermore, low mean perfusion pressure (the difference between the MAP and the CVP) is likely to increase the severity of kidney injury in the critically ill.[49] Randomized studies in the perioperative setting are lacking.

BIOMARKER RESEARCH IN ACUTE KIDNEY INJURY

Serum creatinine is a poor marker of AKI and a delay in instituting treatment may propel AKI into CKD. Over the past decade, research into renal biomarkers has yielded some options that need to be discussed. The ideal biomarker would be one that is easy to quantify rapidly and both sensitive and specific to AKI, much like troponin is to myocardial injury. However, unlike myocardial injury, which is secondary to ischemia, AKI remains multifactorial; hence, the challenge in biomarker research for AKI.[50] A variety of biomarkers have been linked to AKI with varying degrees of success. Most of these biomarkers may be found in plasma or excreted in the urine. It is important to discern whether plasma or urinary biomarkers are being discussed. A brief discussion on key biomarkers follows.

Neutrophil Gelatinase–Associated Lipocalin

Neutrophil gelatinase–associated lipocalin (NGAL) is expressed after ischemic or nephrotoxic kidney injury within 3 hours of injury, peaks at 6 hours, and is found in the circulation until 5 days after injury. Both plasma and urinary NGAL have been found in kidney dysfunction. Originally, NGAL showed promising results in pediatric cardiac surgery patients in a landmark publication[51]; however, in a large study of adult patients undergoing cardiac surgery using both urinary and plasma NGAL, the results were underwhelming.[52] In adults, NGAL has been studied extensively in patients presenting for cardiac surgery with limited results. Efficacy in other perioperative cases remains unknown. Finally, because plasma NGAL is a byproduct of neutrophils, it serves as an inflammatory biomarker, with limited use as a biomarker for AKI in patients with a proinflammatory state or sepsis.[53]

Kidney Injury Molecule 1

Urinary kidney injury molecule-1 is released from the proximal tubules during renal ischemia–reperfusion. It plays a role in renal recovery as well as it has phagocytic properties.[54] In the clinical setting, kidney injury molecule-1 has had modest success in early detection of AKI in the perioperative period.[50]

Tissue Inhibitor of Metalloproteinase-2 and Insulin-Like Growth Factor Binding Factor 7

Tissue inhibitor of metalloproteinase-2 and insulin-like growth factor binding factor-7 were among the first few biomarkers approved by the US Food and Drug Administration for the study of AKI. Both of these markers are generated during cell cycle arrest in the renal tubules. It seems that, when the product of multiplying urinary concentrations of the 2 biomarkers was greater than a predetermined cutoff value of 0.3 $(ng/mL)^2/1000$, there was a 7-fold increase in risk of AKI. Furthermore, this product was shown to be associated with a moderate to severe AKI.[55] Tissue inhibitor of metalloproteinase-2 alone was identified in a promising 2-part study by Kashani and colleagues.[56] Tissue inhibitor of metalloproteinase-2 was able to predict AKI and severity within 12 hours of occurrence in all patients, including those presenting for cardiac surgery. Perioperative use of these molecules remains under investigation.

Angiotensinogen

Angiotensinogen is a biomarker that has prognostic significance in severity of AKI. Especially in cardiac surgery patients, elevated levels of angiotensinogen have been associated with worse outcomes, an increased hospital duration of stay, and an increased need for renal replacement therapy.[57] Interestingly, it is one of the few current biomarkers that may be able to predict the onset of CKD after an AKI incident.[50] Furthermore, urinary angiotensinogen may be reflective of intrarenal renin angiotensin activity, offering novel interventional opportunities in the future as intrarenal renin angiotensin activation contributes to CKD.[58]

Although research on biomarkers is encouraging, it seems that a "renal troponin" is yet to be discovered; the presence of some of these molecules may imply transition to CKD, but there is a long way to go before incorporating them into routine perioperative practice.

SUMMARY

Perioperative AKI is a devastating injury and increases morbidity and mortality. Even with resolution of the injury, the occurrence of AKI may portend future CKD. Patients undergoing cardiac surgery have the highest incidence of AKI, followed by patients undergoing vascular surgery. Steps to mitigate AKI may include the management of intraoperative hypotension and anemia while minimizing vascular congestion secondary to an elevated CVP. Biomarker research into early identification of AKI is ongoing, but it seems that the presence of certain biomarkers in AKI signals the development of CKD.

REFERENCES

1. Bellomo R, Kellum JA, Ronco C. Acute kidney injury. Lancet 2012;380(9843): 756–66.
2. Chawla LS, Eggers PW, Star RA, et al. Acute kidney injury and chronic kidney disease as interconnected syndromes. N Engl J Med 2014;371(1):58–66.
3. Mehta RL, Burdmann EA, Cerdá J, et al. Recognition and management of acute kidney injury in the International Society of Nephrology 0by25 Global Snapshot: a multinational cross-sectional study. Lancet 2016;387(10032):2017–25.
4. Kane-Gill SL, Sileanu FE, Murugan R, et al. Risk factors for acute kidney injury in older adults with critical illness: a retrospective cohort study. Am J Kidney Dis 2015;65(6):860–9.
5. Bellomo R, Ronco C, Kellum JA, et al, Acute Dialysis Quality Initiative Workgroup. Acute renal failure - definition, outcome measures, animal models, fluid therapy and information technology needs: the Second International Consensus Conference of the Acute Dialysis Quality Initiative (ADQI) Group. Crit Care 2004;8: R204–12.
6. Uchino S, Bellomo R, Goldsmith D, et al. An assessment of the RIFLE criteria for acute renal failure in hospitalized patients. Crit Care Med 2006;34(7):1913–7.

7. Kellum JA, Bellomo R, Ronco C, et al. The 3rd international consensus conference of the Acute Dialysis Quality Initiative (ADQI). Int J Artif Organs 2005; 28(5):441–4.
8. Khwaja A. KDIGO clinical practice guidelines for acute kidney injury. Nephron Clin Pract 2012;120(4):c179–84.
9. Levi TM, de Souza SP, de Magalhães JG, et al. Comparison of the RIFLE, AKIN and KDIGO criteria to predict mortality in critically ill patients. Rev Bras Ter Intensiva 2013;25(4):290–6.
10. Lameire N, Van Biesen W, Vanholder R. Acute kidney injury. Lancet 2008; 372(9653):1863–5.
11. Thuillier R, Favreau F, Celhay O, et al. Thrombin inhibition during kidney ischemia-reperfusion reduces chronic graft inflammation and tubular atrophy. Transplantation 2010;90(6):612–21.
12. Saotome T, Ishikawa K, May CN, et al. The impact of experimental hypoperfusion on subsequent kidney function. Intensive Care Med 2010;36(3):533–40.
13. Hillis LD, Smith PK, Anderson JL, et al. 2011 ACCF/AHA guideline for coronary artery bypass graft surgery: a report of the American College of Cardiology Foundation/American Heart Association Task Force on Practice Guidelines. Circulation 2011;124:e652–735.
14. Thongprayoon C, Cheungpasitporn W, Srivali N, et al. AKI after transcatheter or surgical aortic valve replacement. J Am Soc Nephrol 2016;27(6):1854–60.
15. Berg KS, Stenseth R, Wahba A, et al. How can we best predict acute kidney injury following cardiac surgery? A prospective observational study. Eur J Anaesthesiol 2013;30(11):704–12.
16. Thakar CV, Arrigain S, Worley S, et al. A clinical score to predict acute renal failure after cardiac surgery. J Am Soc Nephrol 2005;16(1):162–8.
17. Englberger L, Suri RM, Greason KL, et al. Deep hypothermic circulatory arrest is not a risk factor for acute kidney injury in thoracic aortic surgery. J Thorac Cardiovasc Surg 2011;141(2):552–8.
18. Demirjian S, Schold JD, Navia J, et al. Predictive models for acute kidney injury following cardiac surgery. Am J Kidney Dis 2012;59(3):382–9.
19. Newland RF, Baker RA, Mazzone AL, et al, Perfusion Downunder Collaboration. Rewarming temperature during cardiopulmonary bypass and acute kidney injury: a multicenter analysis. Ann Thorac Surg 2016;101(5):1655–62.
20. Engelman R, Baker RA, Likosky DS, et al. The Society of Thoracic Surgeons, The Society of Cardiovascular Anesthesiologists, and The American Society of Extra-Corporeal Technology: clinical practice guidelines for cardiopulmonary bypass-temperature management during cardiopulmonary bypass. J Extra Corpor Technol 2015;47(3):145–54.
21. DeFoe GR, Ross CS, Olmstead EM, et al. Lowest hematocrit on bypass and adverse outcomes associated with coronary artery bypass grafting. Northern New England Cardiovascular Disease Study Group. Ann Thorac Surg 2001; 71(3):769–76.
22. Swaminathan M, Phillips-Bute BG, Conlon PJ, et al. The association of lowest hematocrit during cardiopulmonary bypass with acute renal injury after coronary artery bypass surgery. ATS 2003;76(3):784–91 [discussion: 792].
23. Hillis LD, Smith PK, Anderson JL, et al. 2011 ACCF/AHA guideline for coronary artery bypass graft surgery. J Am Coll Cardiol 2011;58(24):e123–210.
24. Azau A, Markowicz P, Corbeau JJ, et al. Increasing mean arterial pressure during cardiac surgery does not reduce the rate of postoperative acute kidney injury. Perfusion 2014;29(6):496–504.

25. Shroyer AL, Grover FL, Hattler B, et al. On pump versus off-pump coronary artery bypass grafting. N Engl J Med 2009;361:1827–37.
26. Shroyer AL, Hattler B, Grover FL. Five-year outcomes after on-pump and off-pump coronary-artery bypass. N Engl J Med 2017;377(19):1898–9.
27. Chawla LS, Zhao Y, Lough FC, et al. Off-pump versus on-pump coronary artery bypass grafting outcomes stratified by preoperative renal function. J Am Soc Nephrol 2012;23(8):1389–97.
28. Greenhalgh RM. Comparison of endovascular aneurysm repair with open repair in patients with abdominal aortic aneurysm (EVAR trial 1), 30-day operative mortality results: randomised controlled trial. Lancet 2004;364(9437):843–8.
29. Stather PW, Sidloff D, Dattani N, et al. Systematic review and meta-analysis of the early and late outcomes of open and endovascular repair of abdominal aortic aneurysm. Br J Surg 2013;100(7):863–72.
30. Jhaveri KD, Saratzis AN, Wanchoo R, et al. Endovascular aneurysm repair (EVAR)- and transcatheter aortic valve replacement (TAVR)-associated acute kidney injury. Kidney Int 2017;91(6):1312–23.
31. Johnston KW. Multicenter prospective study of nonruptured abdominal aortic aneurysm. Part II. Variables predicting morbidity and mortality. J Vasc Surg 1989;9(3):437–47.
32. Yang B, Fung A, Pac-Soo C, et al. Vascular surgery-related organ injury and protective strategies: update and future prospects. Br J Anaesth 2016;117:ii32–43.
33. Gamulin Z, Forster A, Morel D, et al. Effects of infrarenal aortic cross-clamping on renal hemodynamics in humans. Anesthesiology 1984;61(4):394–9.
34. Holt S, Moore K. Pathogenesis and treatment of renal dysfunction in rhabdomyolysis. Intensive Care Med 2001;27(5):803–11.
35. de Bruin JL, Vervloet MG, Buimer MG, et al. Renal function 5 years after open and endovascular aortic aneurysm repair from a randomized trial. Br J Surg 2013;100(11):1465–70.
36. Gray DE, Eisenack M, Gawenda M, et al. Repeated contrast medium application after endovascular aneurysm repair and not the type of endograft fixation seems to have deleterious effect on the renal function. J Vasc Surg 2017;65(1):46–51.
37. Drews JD, Patel HJ, Williams DM, et al. The impact of acute renal failure on early and late outcomes after thoracic aortic endovascular repair. Ann Thorac Surg 2014;97(6):2027–33 [discussion: 2033].
38. Fogagnolo A, Tartaglione M, Verri M, et al. Predictors of acute kidney injury in patients undergoing vascular surgery: a retrospective analysis. Eur J Anaesthesiol 2014;31:7–8.
39. Grams ME, Sang Y, Coresh J, et al. Acute kidney injury after major surgery: a retrospective analysis of veterans health administration data. Am J Kidney Dis 2016;67(6):872–80.
40. Long TE, Helgason D, Helgadottir S, et al. Acute kidney injury after abdominal surgery: incidence, risk factors, and outcome. Anesth Analg 2016;122(6):1912–20.
41. Teixeira C, Rosa R, Rodrigues N, et al. Acute kidney injury after major abdominal surgery: a retrospective cohort analysis. Crit Care Res Pract 2014;2014(1):132175–8.
42. Walsh M, Devereaux PJ, Garg AX, et al. Relationship between intraoperative mean arterial pressure and clinical outcomes after noncardiac surgery: toward an empirical definition of hypotension. Anesthesiology 2013;119(3):507–15.

43. Walsh M, Devereaux PJ, Garg AX, et al. Relationship between intraoperative mean arterial pressure and clinical outcomes after noncardiac surgery. Anesthesiology 2014;58(4):184–5.
44. Sessler DI, Sigl JC, Kelley SD, et al. Hospital stay and mortality are increased in patients having a "Triple Low" of low blood pressure, low bispectral index, and low minimum alveolar concentration of volatile anesthesia. Anesthesiology 2013;57(2):71–2.
45. Sessler DI, Sigl JC, Kelley SD, et al. Hospital stay and mortality are increased in patients having a "triple low" of low blood pressure, low bispectral index, and low minimum alveolar concentration of volatile anesthesia. Anesthesiology 2012; 116(6):1195–203.
46. Kertai MD, White WD, Gan TJ. Cumulative duration of "Triple Low" state of low blood pressure, low bispectral index, and low minimum alveolar concentration of volatile anesthesia is not associated with increased mortality. Anesthesiology 2015;59(1):44–5.
47. Onuigbo MAC, Agbasi N. Intraoperative hypotension - a neglected causative factor in hospital-acquired acute kidney injury; a Mayo Clinic Health System experience revisited. J Renal Inj Prev 2015;4(3):61–7.
48. Uthoff H, Breidthardt T, Klima T, et al. Central venous pressure and impaired renal function in patients with acute heart failure. Eur J Heart Fail 2011;13(4):432–9.
49. Ostermann M, Hall A, Crichton S. Low mean perfusion pressure is a risk factor for progression of acute kidney injury in critically ill patients - a retrospective analysis. BMC Nephrol 2017;18(1):151.
50. Alge JL, Arthur JM. Biomarkers of AKI: a review of mechanistic relevance and potential therapeutic implications. Clin J Am Soc Nephrol 2015;10(1):147–55.
51. Mishra J, Dent C, Tarabishi R, et al. Neutrophil gelatinase-associated lipocalin (NGAL) as a biomarker for acute renal injury after cardiac surgery. Lancet 2005;365(9466):1231–8.
52. Ho J, Tangri N, Komenda P, et al. Urinary, plasma, and serum biomarkers' utility for predicting acute kidney injury associated with cardiac surgery in adults: a meta-analysis. Am J Kidney Dis 2015;66(6):993–1005.
53. Kim S, Kim HJ, Ahn HS, et al. Is plasma neutrophil gelatinase-associated lipocalin a predictive biomarker for acute kidney injury in sepsis patients? A systematic review and meta-analysis. J Crit Care 2016;33:213–23.
54. Bonventre JV. Kidney injury molecule-1 (KIM-1): a urinary biomarker and much more. Nephrol Dial Transplant 2009;24(11):3265–8.
55. Bihorac A, Kellum JA. Acute kidney injury in 2014: a step towards understanding mechanisms of renal repair. Nat Rev Nephrol 2015;11(2):74–5.
56. Kashani K, Al-Khafaji A, Ardiles T, et al. Discovery and validation of cell cycle arrest biomarkers in human acute kidney injury. Crit Care 2013;17(1):R25.
57. Alge JL, Karakala N, Neely BA, et al. Association of elevated urinary concentration of renin-angiotensin system components and severe AKI. Clin J Am Soc Nephrol 2013;8(12):2043–52.
58. Kobori H, Alper AB, Shenava R, et al. Urinary angiotensinogen as a novel biomarker of the intrarenal renin-angiotensin system status in hypertensive patients. Hypertension 2009;53(2):344–50.

Hematologic Disorders

Germán Echeverry, MD[a],*, Allison Dalton, MD[b]

KEYWORDS

- Coagulopathies • Perioperative anemia • Hemoglobinopathies • Hemophilia

KEY POINTS

- Hematologic disorders are varied and require careful evaluation and management in the perioperative setting.
- Inherited coagulopathies and thrombophilias place affected patients at increased risk of bleeding and development of thromboembolic phenomena, leading to increased morbidity and mortality.
- Management may require careful coordination between numerous services, including pharmacy, blood bank, and hematology, to ensure appropriate treatment and monitoring of hematologic afflictions.

INTRODUCTION

The hematologic system is responsible for several of the body's most critical functions, including delivery of oxygen and nutrients to tissues, clearance of toxic metabolic byproducts, defense against offending pathogens, and maintenance of hemostasis in the setting of trauma. Its exquisite complexity is difficult to over-state and poses a great challenge to review in short form. Thus, this article pro-vides highlights and clinical pearls in managing patients suffering from some of the most common hematologic afflictions encountered in the perioperative setting.

ERYTHROCYTE DISORDERS

The World Health Organization defines anemia as hemoglobin (Hgb) less than 13 g/dL in adult men and less than 12 g/dL in adult nonpregnant women.[1] The prevalence of anemia is approximately 30% in adult nonpregnant women, 12% in adult men, and ap-proaches 24% in the elderly.[2] The prevalence of anemia in patients preparing for

Disclosure Statement: No disclosures.
[a] Department of Anesthesiology and Critical Care Medicine, Memorial Sloan Kettering Cancer Center, Cornell University, 1275 York Avenue, New York, NY 10065, USA; [b] Department of Anesthesia and Critical Care, University of Chicago, 5841 S. Maryland Avenue, MC 4028, Chicago, IL 60637, USA
* Corresponding author.
E-mail address: echeverg@mskcc.org

Anesthesiology Clin 36 (2018) 553–565
https://doi.org/10.1016/j.anclin.2018.07.006
1932-2275/18/© 2018 Elsevier Inc. All rights reserved.

surgery is even higher.[3] Iron deficiency is the most common type of anemia but multiple other causes may exist or coexist in preoperative patients.[2]

Along with history, components of the complete blood count may assist in elucidating the cause of anemia. Mean corpuscular Hgb (MCH) may provide information about conditions in which Hgb concentration may be decreased (ie, iron deficiency, thalassemia).[4] Low MCH concentration occurs in similar patients with low MCH, whereas elevated MCH concentration occurs in patients with spherocytosis and other congenital hemolytic anemias (ie, sickle cell anemia, Hgb C disease).[4] Mean corpuscular volume (MCV) is especially helpful in determining the cause of anemia based on the size of the individual red blood cell (RBC).[4]

Macrocytic Anemia

Normal MCV values range between 80 and 100 fL, although these norms do vary with age.[5] Megaloblastic anemias are associated with significantly higher MCV than non-megaloblastic anemias.[6] Folate and vitamin B12 deficiencies result in abnormal nucleic acid metabolism of erythrocyte precursors.[7] Megaloblastic anemias may occur in association with myelodysplastic syndrome and acute leukemia.[7] Use of multiple drugs may result in megaloblastic anemias and are detailed in **Table 1**. Non-megaloblastic anemias may be the result of alcoholism, liver disease, and hypothyroidism.[6] A first step in determining the cause of macrocytic anemia is to obtain levels of folate and vitamin B12. If levels are normal, the patient may require further workup, including hematology consultation and bone marrow evaluation.[6]

Microcytic Anemia

An MCV of less than 80 fL results in microcytic anemias. Microcytic anemias are the result of the inability to produce erythrocyte components due to altered iron availability, disorders of heme synthesis, or reduced globin production. The most common cause of microcytic anemia, and anemia in general, is iron deficiency anemia.[2] Iron acts as the oxygen carrier within the heme portion of the Hgb molecule. Iron deficiency may be the result of blood loss (ie, menstrual, gastrointestinal), lack of iron intake (ie, vegan or vegetarian diet), or inability to absorb adequate iron (ie, celiac disease, post-bariatric surgery). Iron deficiency anemia is characterized by low ferritin, low iron saturation, and increased transferrin total iron binding capacity levels.[8] Although oral iron supplementation can be effective long term in iron deficiency anemia, replacement of readily usable iron in the form of intravenous iron can lead to significant increases in Hgb over a shorter time course, which makes it more useful in the preoperative setting.[9] In addition to intravenous iron, the use of erythropoiesis-stimulating agents (ESAs) can increase the Hgb level by 1 g/dL per week.[9] ESAs are associated with increased risk of thromboembolism; however, this risk was noted with higher doses of ESAs over longer periods of time than is indicated for preoperative treatment of anemia.[9]

Disorders of Heme Synthesis

Sideroblastic anemia is a rare group of disorders that leads to microcytic anemia by decreased production of normal heme moieties.[10] Sideroblastic anemia is associated with elevated serum iron and transferrin levels due to decreased iron utilization and increased absorption.[10] Over time, serum ferritin may also increase. Iron may accumulate in hepatic and cardiac tissues. Mild liver and splenic enlargement may exist but clinically relevant hepatosplenomegaly is rare. Diagnosis of sideroblastic anemia is contingent on bone marrow assessment with findings of ringed sideroblasts.[10] Some forms of sideroblastic anemia respond to oral pyridoxine supplementation.

Table 1
Medications that may result in megaloblastic anemia

Drug Causes of Megaloblastic Anemia	
Interferes with nucleic acids	Azathioprine
	Mycophenolate mofetil
	Methotrexate
	Allopurinol
	Hydroxyurea
	Methotrexate
	Fluorouracil
	Trimethoprim
	Nitrous oxide
	Pentamidine
	Gadolinium
	Lamivudine
	Stavudine
	Zidovudine
Decreases folic acid	Alcohol
	Aminosalicylic acid
	Penicillins
	Estrogens
	Tetracycline
	Chloramphenicol
	Nitrofurantoin
	Erythromycin
	Phenobarbital
	Phenytoin
	Valproic acid
	Quinine
	Chloroquine
	Primaquine
Folate analogue activity	Methotrexate
	Trimethoprim
	Triamterene
Decreases vitamin B12	Isoniazid
	Metformin
	Aminosalicylic acid
	Colchicine
	H2 antagonists
	Proton pump inhibitors
	Sodium nitroprusside
	Nitric oxide
Causing hemolysis	Primaquine
	Dapsone
	Nitrofurantoin
	Rasburicase
	Methylene blue

Symptoms of iron overload may require phlebotomy to prevent associated morbidity (ie, diabetes, cirrhosis, and heart failure).[10]

Reduced Globin Production

Normal adult Hgb comprises 2 α-globin chains and 2 β-globin chains. This normal tetramer is recognized as Hgb A. Variations in the various globin chains lead to alternate

Hgb molecules. A single amino acid substitution (valine replaces glutamic acid) on the β-globin chain results in sickle Hgb (HbS).[11] If the mutation is carried on both β-chains, homozygous HbS (HbSS) develops.[11] If the autosomal recessive mutation is expressed on only 1 β-globin chain, sickle cell trait is present, which has significantly less clinical implications than HbSS. A separate single amino acid substitution (lysine replaces glutamic acid) on the β-globin chain results in HbC. Although HbC trait is relatively benign, producing mild hemolytic anemia and splenomegaly, a combination of HbC and HbS (HbSC) mimics a milder form of sickle cell disease associated with potentially severe morbidity.[12] When patients with HbSS and HbSC encounter hypothermia, dehydration, acidosis hypoxia, vasoconstriction, venous stasis, infection, and physiologic stress, abnormal HbS molecules polymerize and cause abnormal sickling of individual RBCs. The abnormally shaped cells adhere to each other and the vascular endothelium with resultant RBC sludging and vasoocclusive crises (VOC).[13,14]

Multiple organ systems are affected by sickling of red cells, leading to left ventricular hypertrophy, cardiomyopathy, pulmonary hypertension, restrictive or obstructive lung disease, stroke, neuropathy, renal insufficiency or failure, hepatic dysfunction, splenic infarction, hemolytic or aplastic anemia, osteomyelitis, and avascular necrosis.[14] Acute chest syndrome (ACS) is the result of vasoocclusive episodes in the pulmonary vasculature and is associated with increased mortality in sickle cell disease.[15]

Treatment of VOC requires reversal of triggering agents and pain control; however, treatment of ACS is additionally focused on optimization of oxygenation and ventilation as necessary, support of circulation, and restoration of normal RBC conformation.[14] Chronic treatment of sickle cell disease with hydroxyurea improves morbidity from VOC and ACS, and decreases mortality in patients with sickle cell disease.[14] Hydroxyurea stimulates the production of fetal Hgb and increases the release of endogenous nitric oxide. Perioperatively, there are multiple risk factors for the development of VOC and ACS, including anemia, hypothermia, dehydration, acidosis, hypoxia, and physiologic stress.[16] Patients with HbSS who are having surgery that is low to moderate risk and those with HbSC having surgery that is moderate to high risk should be transfused to Hgb of 10 g/dL or greater.[17] It is recommended that patients with HbSS disease who are scheduled for high-risk surgery should undergo exchange transfusion before surgery.[17]

Thalassemia syndromes are a group of inherited disorders that are characterized by the decreased presence or absence of the globin subunit. Alpha thalassemia is the

Table 2
Phenotypes of alpha-thalassemias and beta-thalassemias

	Thalassemia Phenotypes	
α-thalassemia	Deletion of 1 α-globin gene	Silent carrier state
	Deletion of 2 α-globin genes	Mild microcytic anemia without hemolysis
	Deletion of 3 α-globin genes (HbH)	Compensated hemolytic anemia
	Deletion of 4 α-globin genes (Hgb Barts)	Usually fatal in utero or shortly after birth
β-thalassemia	β-thalassemia minor	Mild to moderate microcytic anemia without hemolysis
	β-thalassemia intermedia	Moderate to severe partially compensated hemolytic anemia
	β-thalassemia major	Severe transfusion-dependent hemolytic anemia

Modified from Forget BG, Bunn HF. Classification of the disorders of hemoglobin. Cold Spring Harb Perspect Med 2013;3(2):a011684; with permission.

result of deletions of the α-globin gene and is distinguished by the number of deleted genes **(Table 2)**.[11] Beta-thalassemia usually results from point mutations on the β-globin genes, which leads to variable production of normal β-globin subunits.[11] For patients who have a heterozygous inheritance pattern (β-thalassemia minor), a mild hemolytic anemia will develop. For homozygote patients, a more severe transfusion-dependent hemolytic anemia will manifest. Due to the variety of molecular mutations found in β-thalassemia, there is an intermediate form that results in a more severe anemia than in β-thalassemia minor but does not require chronic transfusion, unlike β-thalassemia major.[11] Patients with β-thalassemia may additionally inherit the gene for sickle cell (HbS β-thalassemia), resulting in variable phenotypic expression depending on the amount of normal Hgb production by the β-thalassemia gene.[11]

Normocytic Anemia

Normocytic anemias are frequently a marker of underlying systemic disease. Anemia of inflammation is characterized by low serum iron, normal to elevated ferritin, and low TIBC. Whereas the laboratory findings in iron deficiency anemia highlight the lack of total body iron, the laboratory findings in anemia of inflammation demonstrate that iron stores cannot be appropriately used.[8] Even with normal ferritin levels in anemia of inflammation, intravenous iron may successfully increase Hgb due to low rates of mobilization of iron from ferritin stores.[18] Chronic kidney disease and renal disease as a result of heart failure result in normocytic anemia. Kidney disease–associated anemia should be treated with iron supplementation if transferrin saturation is less than or equal to 30% or ferritin is less than or equal to 500 ng/dL, and with ESAs when Hgb is less than or equal to 10 g/dL.[19] Many causes of hospital-acquired anemia result in normocytic anemia, including blood loss, hemodilution secondary to fluid administration, repeated or large-volume blood draws, and blunted erythropoiesis secondary to critical illness.

NORMAL COAGULATION

Clot formation is a crucial feature of the hematologic system, requiring a careful balance of a wide range of factors that help maintain hemostasis at sites of vascular injury but also prevent inappropriate clot formation that may lead to inadequate venous drainage, embolic events, and end-organ ischemia. This balance between the homeostatic and fibrinolytic mechanisms has been extensively studied over the centuries since Virchow first proposed a hypothesis for a cause of pulmonary emboli in which he identified 3 primary contributors, including stasis, vessel (endothelial) injury, and hypercoagulable states.

The coagulation and fibrinolytic systems consist of enzyme cascades that lead to the formation and degradation of a fibrin clot. Factors of the coagulation cascade are serine proteases that exist in plasma as zymogens, an inactive form that is proteolytically cleaved to release an active molecule.[20] Multiple positive and negative feedback loops ensure proper regulation of fibrin clot formation. The coagulation cascade is classically broken down into the extrinsic and intrinsic pathways, both ultimately culminating in a common pathway of thrombin formation. In vivo, the cascade is activated by tissue factor present at the surface of endothelial cells interacting with factor VIIa, leading to activation of factors IXa and Xa; together with Va they form a prothrombinase (so-called tenase) complex that converts prothrombin to thrombin. Thrombin then converts fibrinogen into fibrin; activates factor XIII, which crosslinks fibrin strands; and provides positive feedback to the cascade by activating Xa and IXa.[20] Fibrin forms an insoluble plug, activating platelets and forming an early clot, which is subsequently stabilized by undergoing covalent crosslinking in the presence of factor XIII. Fibrin also provides positive and negative feedback inhibition through activation of clotting factors, as well as exerting anticoagulant effects through its association with thrombomodulin, leading to activation of protein C.[20] Antithrombin (a serine protease inhibitor) and protein C (which as a complex with protein S proteolytically inactivate Va and VIIa) serve as the most important inhibitors of the coagulation cascade. Clot breakdown is, in part, carried out by plasmin, which degrades fibrin strands.[20] Plasmin exists in plasma as its inactive form, plasminogen, and is activated by the serine proteases tissue plasminogen activator and urokinase plasminogen activator. A careful balance between the thrombogenic and fibrinolytic systems exist, and any disruption of this equilibrium predisposes patients to inappropriate states of clotting or bleeding.[20]

Disorders of Coagulation

Disorders of coagulation, including bleeding diathesis and inherited thrombophilias, are rare but important clinical syndromes requiring a careful approach in the perioperative setting. Management of these patients often requires specialized consultation from a hematologist and, potentially, coordination with blood bank and pharmacy to ensure specific factor replacement or targeted pharmacotherapy is available should the patient necessitate acute treatment. Some of these blood products and medications are not readily available and come at significant financial cost.

Acquired dysregulation of the hemostatic system secondary to modifiable factors, such as effect of medications, immobility, pregnancy, and surgical intervention, are far more common. It is important for anesthesiologists and perioperative physicians to be familiar with this diverse group of clinical syndromes responsible for significant morbidity and mortality in this patient population.

INHERITED BLEEDING DIATHESIS

Given the complexity of the hemostatic system, inherited bleeding disorders are numerous and a comprehensive overview of each is beyond the scope of this article. Hematologic management of these patients in the perioperative period can be challenging and requires careful coordination of care. An expert should be consulted whenever possible. A brief overview of some of the most commonly occurring inherited bleeding disorders follows.

Hemophilia A

Hemophilia A is a bleeding disorder characterized by a deficiency of functional factor VIII. This occurs due to mutations in the factor VIII gene located on the X chromosome, leading to either low levels of circulating factor VIII (in severe cases <1%) or, rarely, normal levels but poorly reactive enzyme.[21,22] It is estimated the disease affects 1 in 5000 to 10,000 live births.[21,23,24] Severity of disease is variable, with most affected individuals presenting as children with spontaneous hemorrhage into joints, muscles, and soft tissues.[22] Patients with milder disease may only manifest after severe unexpected bleeding is observed in the setting of trauma or surgery.[23] Laboratory values are significant for a prolonged partial thromboplastin time and normal prothrombin time and bleeding time. Treatment varies depending on disease severity. In mild cases, preoperative desmopressin (DDAVP) may be sufficient because it increases baseline factor VIII levels by 3-fold to 6-fold.[21,25] Patients with severe disease who require surgery are treated prophylactically with recombinant factor VIII until normal levels (80%–100%) are achieved.[21,24] Repeated infusions are often necessary due to the short half-life of recombinant factor VIII to maintain adequate levels until wound healing is achieved.[23,26] Patients with mild disease or those receiving factor replacement for the first time should be screened for presence of inhibitors (see later discussion).[23]

Hemophilia B

Hemophilia B is another X-linked recessive inherited bleeding disorder characterized by decreased levels of functional factor IX.[22,23] Like hemophilia A, disease severity and clinical features exist on a spectrum with those most severely affected presenting as children with spontaneous hemorrhage.[21,22] Its incidence is much lower than hemophilia A, affecting 1 in 25,000 live births.[21,24] Patients are treated preoperatively with purified or recombinant factor IX until normal levels are reached.[23] As with hemophilia A, additional dosing in the postoperative period is needed until wound healing is achieved. DDAVP has no effect in circulating factor IX levels and, therefore, is not indicated in these patients.

Inhibitors to Factor VIII or IX

Patients with hemophilia A or B who have been treated with purified or recombinant factor VIII or IX, respectively, may develop inhibitors (antibodies) to these treatment modalities.[23,24,26] Genetically normal individuals may rarely develop autoantibodies.[26] Diagnosis is made via mixing studies revealing the presence of an inhibitor in the patient's plasma. It is important to identify this patient population in the preoperative period whenever possible to assure adequate factor replacement is available during surgery and wound healing. When surgery is indicated, agents bypassing the tenase complex, such as recombinant factor VII or prothrombin complex concentrate, have been used successfully to achieve hemostasis but no validated protocols exist for management of these patients.[26]

von Willebrand Disease

von Willebrand factor (vWF) facilitates platelet adhesion to sites of endothelial injury, activates platelets, and serves as a carrier protein for factor VIII. As such, it is a critical component of the hemostatic system. It is produced in vascular endothelium and in megakaryocytes, and is stored as multimers of varying molecular sizes.[27] von Willebrand disease is characterized by decreased vWF activity. It is the most common inherited bleeding disorder with a prevalence of 1% of the population.[21,27] Various types of the disease are differentiated by either low levels of plasma vWF (from either inadequate production or inadequate release from cellular stores) or qualitative defects leading to decreased protein activity.[27] Disease severity is variable, patients may be asymptomatic or present with spontaneous mucocutaneous bleeding. Type 1 disease is the most common form and is characterized by low levels of circulating vWF due to impaired release from Weibel-Palade bodies of endothelial cells. Type 2 disease is a qualitative defect resulting in lower or absent larger vWF multimers, resulting in decreased activity. Type 3 disease is characterized by a virtual absence of circulating vWF and often presents with most serious manifestations, including spontaneous internal hemorrhage. Treatment modalities in the perioperative setting include DDAVP (which stimulates release of vWF from endogenous stores) for patients with type 1 disease, exogenous vWF, antifibrinolytic therapy, tenase bypassing agents, and topical hemostatic agents.[21,27]

Dysfibrinogenemia

Dysfibrinogenemia is a genetic disorder leading to production of abnormal fibrinogen. Clinical presentation varies greatly, and most patients have no clinically significant disease, even in the setting of abnormal laboratory testing. Those with bleeding propensity may be treated with cryoprecipitate in the perioperative period.[21,26]

ACQUIRED COAGULOPATHIES

Coagulopathies may develop in response to various physiologic and pathophysiologic states, including trauma, major surgery, pregnancy, infection, and cardiopulmonary bypass, among others. Mechanisms vary, including relative platelet and factor deficiency from a consumptive process, such as DIC or HELLP syndrome; loss of vWF multimers from high sheer stress in acquired von Willebrand disease; development of autoantibodies and inhibitors, dilutional in the setting of major blood loss; or as a side effect of medications. Treatment is generally supportive and a hematology consultation is often useful in guiding diagnostic evaluation and treatment.

THROMBOPHILIAS

Thrombophilias are disorders of coagulation resulting in an increase propensity to pathologically form clot. They may be hereditary or acquired, and are a significant cause of morbidity and mortality in the perioperative setting.[24] They may be difficult to diagnose during a preoperative assessment unless the patient has already suffered sequelae such as recurrent spontaneous abortions or unprovoked thrombosis or thromboembolic phenomena. When and which patients should be screened, as well as adequate treatment of these patients, is a matter of ongoing debate in the literature.

Inherited Thrombophilias

Inherited thrombophilias include a group of inherited autosomal dominant genetic disorders that, as a net result, increase lifetime risk of developing venous thromboembolism (VTE). Most adult patients are heterozygotes who exhibit signs and symptoms later in life. Homozygote cases are more severe and may present as neonates with purpura fulminans.[28] A subset of these disorders follows in decreasing order of prevalence.

Factor V Leiden mutation: This is also known as activated protein C resistance, is a mutation in the factor V gene making factor Va less susceptible to inactivation by activated protein C (APC).[28,29] This leads to increased levels of factor Va, resulting in a hypercoagulable state. Additionally, factor V, together with protein S, has been identified as a potentiator of APC-mediated inhibition of factor VIIIa.[30] The name Leiden refers to the city in the Netherlands where it was first identified. Relative risk of any thrombosis is 2.2 compared with the normal population.

Prothrombin gene mutation: Results from a mutation at the prothrombin G20210 A gene, resulting in elevated circulating prothrombin and increased risk of thrombosis.[31] The relative risk of thrombosis is 8.1 compared with normal individuals.[32] This mutation is exceedingly rare in the nonwhite population.[28]

Protein C deficiency: As previously discussed, APC inactivates factors Va and VIIIa. Its effects are potentiated by the presence of protein S. This disorder is inherited in autosomal dominant manner. Prevalence in the white population is estimated to be 0.2% to 0.5%, and its relative risk of thrombus is 7.3 compared with the normal population.[32] Two major subtypes exist. Type I is more common, characterized by reduced plasma protein C concentration, whereas type II individuals have normal protein C levels but exhibit decreased activity. There is marked phenotypic variability in both types not explained by genetic factors alone.[28]

Protein S deficiency: protein S is cofactor for protein C. Three distinct phenotypes have been identified based on total and free protein S concentration and function. This disease is inherited in autosomal dominant pattern.[28] Relative risk of thrombosis is 8.5 compared with the normal population.[32]

Antithrombin deficiency: This is an autosomal dominant trait resulting in approximately 50% reduction in antithrombin levels. Of affected individuals, 70% develop a thromboembolic event before age 50 years. Like other thrombophilias, it rarely affects children.[28] The relative risk of thrombosis is 8.1 compared with the normal population.[32]

Other rarer causes of hereditary thrombophilia include elevated factor levels, severe homocystinemia, dysfibrinogenemia, and platelet glycoprotein gene polymorphisms, as well as deficiency of plasminogen or tissue plasminogen activator, among many others.

Thrombophilia Screening

Current expert opinion recommends selected screening, particularly in young patients with VTE, VTE during pregnancy, or before initiation of oral contraceptive therapy in patients with family history. Testing for inherited thrombophilias should not be performed in the acute state of VTE. Instead it should be deferred to 1 month following anticoagulation therapy or, otherwise, 3 months after VTE because there may be interference with test results.[33] To date, there are no controlled trials outlining a clear benefit for testing in reducing the recurrence of VTE but this information may be of clinical utility during pregnancy in the setting of recurrent pregnancy loss and for individuals from families with strong history of VTE.

Acquired Thrombophilias

Acquired thrombophilias result from modifiable and nonmodifiable factors predisposing the development of venous thrombosis and VTE. These include age; elevated body mass index; immobility; trauma; pregnancy (including mechanical venous compression by the gravid uterus, as well as upregulation of thrombogenic factors); recent major surgery (particularly orthopedic and cancer surgery); certain medications, including synthetic estrogens and some chemotherapeutic agents; antiphospholipid antibodies; lupus anticoagulant; myeloproliferative disorders; malignancy; nephrotic syndrome; and smoking, among others.[24]

Treatment

The mainstay of treatment includes early mobilization, modifiable risk factor reduction, and pharmacologic chemoprophylaxis for patients at risk for deep vein thrombosis (DVT), as well as systemic anticoagulation with heparin, low-molecular-weight heparin (LMWH), or coumadin as needed for treatment of DVT-VTE. Regardless of the mechanism, patients with inherited thrombophilias can be treated with prophylactic doses of heparin or LMWH, coumadin, or factor concentrate. Dose adjustments are not necessary because all these thrombophilias are sensitive to the effects of these medications. Duration of treatment may need to be extended given a higher propensity for clot formation in specific situations such as surgery and anticipated periods of prolonged immobility.

For specific factor deficiencies, replacement factors may be administered when indicated. A hematology consultation is valuable when managing these patients to guide medication or factor selection and duration of treatment. Patients presenting for high-risk surgery who have been identified as having a high risk for DVT-VTE may benefit from inferior vena cava filter placement in the preoperative period.[28]

PLATELET ABNORMALITIES

Immune Thrombocytopenia

Immune thrombocytopenia (ITP) is characterized by an acquired immune disorder leading to the destruction of platelets. This may occur via production of antiplatelet antibodies or impaired megakaryocytopoiesis, as well as T-cell–mediated mechanisms.[34,35] Its incidence is 3.3 per 100000 per year and may occur in children and adults.[36] A recent consensus report provided updated terminology that removed previous commonly used descriptors, including idiopathic and purpurea, to better characterize the disease process.[37] Secondary ITP is defined as ITP occurring in the setting of other underlying disorders and accounts for approximately 20% of cases.[35] Diagnosis of ITP is based on history and physical examination, results from routine laboratory work, and review of the peripheral blood smear. Specialized testing may be performed based on these findings to rule out secondary causes of ITP. Specialized testing for antiplatelet antibodies or routine screening for immunodeficiency or other autoimmune disease is not recommended. Treatment of ITP consists of immune suppression with steroids (methylprednisolone vs high-dose dexamethasone), rituximab, thrombopoietin receptor agonist, and splenectomy.[34,35] Treatment of secondary ITP is aimed at controlling the underlying condition.

Heparin-Induced Thrombocytopenia

Heparin-induced thrombocytopenia (HIT), including immune-mediated HIT or type II HIT, is a clinical syndrome characterized by the formation of antibodies to platelet factor 4 (PF4)-heparin complex.[38] In 1958, HIT was first reported by Weismann and Tobin[39] in a case series of 10 subjects who developed thrombi after heparin administration. Of note, this is a separate entity from thrombocytopenia caused by platelet aggregation following heparin administration, also known as type I HIT or heparin-associated thrombocytopenia, which is nonimmune-mediated and not clinically relevant.[40] These PF4-heparin complex antibodies are able to activate platelets via surface Fc receptors, leading to release of procoagulant microparticles and thrombi formation in a subset of patients.[41] Though heparin exposure classically precedes the development of HIT, infection and surgical inflammation have also led to its development in rare cases. Risk factors for HIT development include age (adults more than children), formulation (unfractionated heparin more than LMWH), and dose (treatment more than therapeutic).[42] Cardiac surgical patients receiving large doses of heparin for cardiopulmonary bypass have been shown to develop PF4-heparin complex antibodies up to 50% of the time, though few of these patients go on to develop persistent thrombocytopenia and thrombosis.[43] Clinical features include a moderate thrombocytopenia with 50% reduction of circulating platelets, typically 3 to 5 days following heparin exposure.[44] Severe thrombocytopenia (<20,000 platelets) is rarely seen. Thrombosis is the most severe complication and may affect any vascular bed, with predominance in the venous system and sites of vascular injury. Bleeding is seldom a complication of this clinical syndrome. Diagnosis involves screening and confirmatory antibody testing on patients suspected of having HIT. Heparin is discontinued in patients suspected of HIT based on clinical scoring tools, and a nonheparin anticoagulant is initiated to prevent thrombus formation while workup is ongoing. Vitamin K antagonists should be avoided until platelet counts have recovered because decreased protein C production in the setting of acute HIT can lead to limb-threatening and life-threatening thrombosis. A multidisciplinary approach, including expert consultation from a hematologist is warranted to help identify the most appropriate anticoagulant, guide subsequent diagnostic workup, and determine the appropriate duration of treatment. Current expert recommendation is to avoid heparin exposure in patients with history of HIT, except for seronegative patients presenting for cardiac surgery.

Essential Thrombocytosis

Essential thrombocytosis is a myeloproliferative disorder leading to inappropriate propagation of megakaryocytes and increased amounts of circulating platelets.[45] This disorder is associated with increased risk of thrombosis, as well as bleeding, in the perioperative setting.[46–49] The syndrome is characterized by dysplastic megakaryocyte and abnormal platelet morphology and function. Diagnosis involves a thorough clinical evaluation, as well as exclusion of other causes of thrombocytosis, such as malignancy and infection. Due to increased risk of VTE, perioperative treatment strategies focus on normalization of platelet count via cytoreductive medications or thrombocytapheresis, a strategy that has been used in the past for patients undergoing surgery.[45,50,51] No definitive guidelines exist in the optimal perioperative management of these patients.

Other causes of platelet number or function abnormalities include consumptive processes (TTP-HUS, HELLP syndrome, DIC), decreased production (bone marrow pathologic conditions, advanced liver disease), sequestration (splenomegaly), and recent exposure to antiplatelet agents such as aspirin and glycoprotein iib/iiia inhibitors. Treatment is variable, patients with platelet production disorders respond well to transfusions; however, those with consumptive processes should not be transfused except in the setting of life-threatening bleeding.

REFERENCES

1. McLean E, Cogswell M, Egli I, et al. Worldwide prevalence of anaemia, WHO vitamin and mineral nutrition information system, 1993-2005. Public Health Nutr 2009;12(4):444–54.
2. Bruno de Benoist EM, Egli I, Cogswell M. Worldwide prevalence of anaemia 1993-2005. WHO global database on anaemia. Geneva (Switzerland): World Health Organization; 2008.
3. Kansagra AJ, Stefan MS. Preoperative anemia: evaluation and treatment. Anesthesiol Clin 2016;34(1):127–41.
4. Yip R, Johnson C, Dallman PR. Age-related changes in laboratory values used in the diagnosis of anemia and iron deficiency. Am J Clin Nutr 1984;39(3):427–36.
5. Chanarin I, Metz J. Diagnosis of cobalamin deficiency: the old and the new. Br J Haematol 1997;97(4):695–700.
6. Takahashi N, Kameoka J, Takahashi N, et al. Causes of macrocytic anemia among 628 patients: mean corpuscular volumes of 114 and 130 fL as critical markers for categorization. Int J Hematol 2016;104(3):344–57.
7. Aslinia F, Mazza JJ, Yale SH. Megaloblastic anemia and other causes of macrocytosis. Clin Med Res 2006;4(3):236–41.
8. DeLoughery TG. Microcytic anemia. N Engl J Med 2014;371(14):1324–31.
9. Bou Monsef JB, Boettner F. Optimal management of perioperative anemia: current perspectives. Int J Clin Transfus Med 2015;3:65–73.
10. Camaschella C. Recent advances in the understanding of inherited sideroblastic anaemia. Br J Haematol 2008;143(1):27–38.
11. Forget BG, Bunn HF. Classification of the disorders of hemoglobin. Cold Spring Harb Perspect Med 2013;3(2):a011684.

12. Pecker LH, Schaefer BA, Luchtman-Jones L. Knowledge insufficient: the management of haemoglobin SC disease. Br J Haematol 2017;176(4):515–26.
13. Ware RE, de Montalembert M, Tshilolo L, et al. Sickle cell disease. Lancet 2017; 390(10091):311–23.
14. Khurmi N, Gorlin A, Misra L. Perioperative considerations for patients with sickle cell disease: a narrative review. Can J Anaesth 2017;64(8):860–9.
15. Vichinsky EP, Neumayr LD, Earles AN, et al. Causes and outcomes of the acute chest syndrome in sickle cell disease. National Acute Chest Syndrome Study Group. N Engl J Med 2000;342(25):1855–65.
16. Howard J, Malfroy M, Llewelyn C, et al. The Transfusion Alternatives Preoperatively in Sickle Cell Disease (TAPS) study: a randomised, controlled, multicentre clinical trial. Lancet 2013;381(9870):930–8.
17. Davis BA, Allard S, Qureshi A, et al. Guidelines on red cell transfusion in sickle cell disease Part II: indications for transfusion. Br J Haematol 2017;176(2): 192–209.
18. Auerbach M, Coyne D, Ballard H. Intravenous iron: from anathema to standard of care. Am J Hematol 2008;83(7):580–8.
19. KDIGO clinical practice guideline for anemia in chronic kidney disease. Kidney Int Suppl (2011) 2012;2(4):292–310.
20. Palta S, Saroa R, Palta A. Overview of the coagulation system. Indian J Anaesth 2014;58(5):515–23.
21. Mensah PK, Gooding R. Surgery in patients with inherited bleeding disorders. Anaesthesia 2015;70(Suppl 1):112–20.e39-40.
22. Blanchette VS, Key NS, Ljung LR, et al. Definitions in hemophilia: communication from the SSC of the ISTH. J Thromb Haemost 2014;12(11):1935–9.
23. Srivastava A, Brewer AK, Mauser-Bunschoten EP, et al. Guidelines for the management of hemophilia. Haemophilia 2013;19(1):e1–47.
24. Shah UJ, Narayanan M, Graham Smith J. Anaesthetic considerations in patients with inherited disorders of coagulation. Continuing Education in Anaesthesia Critical Care & Pain 2015;15(1):26–31.
25. Coppola A, Tagliaferri A, Franchini M. Old and new challenges in hemophilia management. Semin Thromb Hemost 2013;39(7):693–6.
26. Hines R, Marschall K. Anesthesia and co-existing disease. Philadelphia: Elsevier; 2008.
27. Stone ME, Mazzeffi M, Derham J, et al. Current management of von Willebrand disease and von Willebrand syndrome. Curr Opin Anaesthesiol 2014;27(3): 353–8.
28. Khan S, Dickerman JD. Hereditary thrombophilia. Thromb J 2006;4:15.
29. Kalafatis M, Bertina RM, Rand MD, et al. Characterization of the molecular defect in factor VR506Q. J Biol Chem 1995;270(8):4053–7.
30. Shen L, Dahlback B. Factor V and protein S as synergistic cofactors to activated protein C in degradation of factor VIIIa. J Biol Chem 1994;269(29):18735–8.
31. Poort SR, Rosendaal FR, Reitsma PH, et al. A common genetic variation in the 3'-untranslated region of the prothrombin gene is associated with elevated plasma prothrombin levels and an increase in venous thrombosis. Blood 1996;88(10): 3698–703.
32. Martinelli I, Mannucci PM, De Stefano V, et al. Different risks of thrombosis in four coagulation defects associated with inherited thrombophilia: a study of 150 families. Blood 1998;92(7):2353–8.
33. Colucci G, Tsakiris DA. Thrombophilia screening: universal, selected, or neither? Clin Appl Thromb Hemost 2017;23(8):893–9.

34. Lambert MP, Gernsheimer TB. Clinical updates in adult immune thrombocytopenia. Blood 2017;129(21):2829–35.

35. Cines DB, Bussel JB, Liebman HA, et al. The ITP syndrome: pathogenic and clinical diversity. Blood 2009;113(26):6511–21.

36. Moulis G, Palmaro A, Montastruc JL, et al. Epidemiology of incident immune thrombocytopenia: a nationwide population-based study in France. Blood 2014;124(22):3308–15.

37. Rodeghiero F, Stasi R, Gernsheimer T, et al. Standardization of terminology, definitions and outcome criteria in immune thrombocytopenic purpura of adults and children: report from an international working group. Blood 2009;113(11): 2386–93.

38. Amiral J, Bridey F, Dreyfus M, et al. Platelet factor 4 complexed to heparin is the target for antibodies generated in heparin-induced thrombocytopenia. Thromb Haemost 1992;68(1):95–6.

39. Weismann RE, Tobin RW. Arterial embolism occurring during systemic heparin therapy. AMA Arch Surg 1958;76(2):219–25 [discussion: 225–7].

40. Chong BH, Ismail F. The mechanism of heparin-induced platelet aggregation. Eur J Haematol 1989;43(3):245–51.

41. Chong BH, Fawaz I, Chesterman CN, et al. Heparin-induced thrombocytopenia: mechanism of interaction of the heparin-dependent antibody with platelets. Br J Haematol 1989;73(2):235–40.

42. Warkentin TE, Levine MN, Hirsh J, et al. Heparin-induced thrombocytopenia in patients treated with low-molecular-weight heparin or unfractionated heparin. N Engl J Med 1995;332(20):1330–5.

43. Bauer TL, Arepally G, Konkle BA, et al. Prevalence of heparin-associated antibodies without thrombosis in patients undergoing cardiopulmonary bypass surgery. Circulation 1997;95(5):1242–6.

44. Warkentin TE, Kelton JG. Temporal aspects of heparin-induced thrombocytopenia. N Engl J Med 2001;344(17):1286–92.

45. Ahmed K, Vohra HA, Milne A, et al. Aortic valve replacement in a young patient with essential thrombocytosis. J Cardiothorac Surg 2008;3:5.

46. Zhu Y, Jiang H, Chen Z, et al. Abdominal surgery in patients with essential thrombocythemia: a case report and systematic review of literature. Medicine (Baltimore) 2017;96(47):e8856.

47. Randi ML, Stocco F, Rossi C, et al. Thrombosis and hemorrhage in thrombocytosis: evaluation of a large cohort of patients (357 cases). J Med 1991;22(4–5):213–23.

48. Kessler CM. Propensity for hemorrhage and thrombosis in chronic myeloproliferative disorders. Semin Hematol 2004;41(2 Suppl 3):10–4.

49. Michiels JJ, Berneman Z, Schroyens W, et al. The paradox of platelet activation and impaired function: platelet-von Willebrand factor interactions, and the etiology of thrombotic and hemorrhagic manifestations in essential thrombocythemia and polycythemia vera. Semin Thromb Hemost 2006;32(6):589–604.

50. Edlich RF, Long WB 3rd, Cochran AA, et al. Management of femoral fracture in a patient with essential thrombocythemia treated with plateletpheresis and intramedullary rod fixation, followed by hydroxyurea: a case report. Am J Emerg Med 2008;26(5):636.e1-3.

51. Das SS, Bose S, Chatterjee S, et al. Thrombocytapheresis: managing essential thrombocythemia in a surgical patient. Ann Thorac Surg 2011;92(1):e5–6.

Surgical Prehabilitation
Nutrition and Exercise

John Whittle, MBBS, MD, FRCA, FFICM[a,b,*],
Paul E. Wischmeyer, MD, EDIC[c],
Michael P.W. Grocott, MBBS, MD, FRCP, FRCA, FFICM[d],
Timothy E. Miller, MB ChB, FRCA[e]

KEYWORDS

- Prehabilitation • Exercise • Preoptimization • Nutrition • Perioperative medicine

KEY POINTS

- Surgery is a significant physiologic challenge in an increasingly elderly and comorbid population.
- Malnutrition and impaired exercise tolerance are both associated with adverse perioperative outcomes.
- Exercise-based prehabilitation is associated with improved outcomes in many clinical settings, but its clinical utility in the perioperative period is yet to be confirmed.
- Nutritional interventions improve perioperative outcomes in both low-risk and high-risk patients.
- Combined exercise and nutritional strategies as part of an integrated approach to perioperative risk are most likely to yield positive results in terms of postoperative outcomes.

THE PHYSIOLOGIC CHALLENGE OF SURGERY

According to recent estimates, more than 300 million surgeries are undertaken worldwide each year.[1] In the developed world, the demographic of patients undergoing surgery is increasingly elderly, many of whom present with multiple comorbidities.

Mortality secondary to major surgery is around 4%,[2,3] and morbidity, more common than mortality, affects up to 18% of patients in the postoperative period.[3]

[a] Anesthesiology, Duke University School of Medicine, Duke University Health System, 5th Floor HAFS, DUMC 3094, 2301 Erwin Road, Durham, NC 27710, USA; [b] Perioperative Medicine, University College London, Gower Street, London, WC1E 6BT, UK; [c] Nutrition Support Service, Duke Clinical Research Institute, Duke University Hospital, Duke University School of Medicine, 2400 Pratt Street, Durham, NC 27705, USA; [d] Critical Care Research Group, NIHR Biomedical Research Centre, University Hospital Southampton NHS Foundation Trust, University Road, Southampton, SO17 1BJ, UK; [e] Duke University School of Medicine, Duke University Health System, 5th Floor HAFS, DUMC 3094, 2301 Erwin Road, Durham, NC 27710, USA
* Corresponding author. Anesthesiology, 5th Floor HAFS, DUMC 3094, 2301 Erwin Road, Durham, NC 27710.
E-mail address: john.whittle@duke.edu

Anesthesiology Clin 36 (2018) 567–580
https://doi.org/10.1016/j.anclin.2018.07.013
1932-2275/18/© 2018 Elsevier Inc. All rights reserved.
anesthesiology.theclinics.com

The development of even a single postoperative complication is not benign and may result in both short-term and long-term consequences,[3] resulting in reduced quality of life as well as decreases in functional capacity of up to 40%.[4] Persistent postoperative impairment is most apparent in the frail and is likely one of the major mechanisms linking the observed relationship between short-term morbidity and long-term adverse health outcomes. It is therefore of critical importance to address and attempt to modify risk of postoperative decline in function in the preoperative period through optimizing resilience to the stress of surgery.

Surgical trauma is associated with a variety of stressors. The ability of an individual to withstand these stressors in an adaptive manner depends on a multitude of interacting physiologic resilience factors, key among these being aerobic fitness and nutritional status.

These factors are strongly influenced by the physiologic age of the patient, chronic health status, and acute physiologic derangements consequent to any presenting illness. In addition, many long-term behavioral factors, including smoking, diet, alcohol usage, and amount of physical activity performed, influence physiologic resilience. Similarly, factors related to the treatment of disease, such as chemotherapy-induced skeletal and cardiac myopathy,[5] negatively affect physiologic reserve and hence the ability of an individual to tolerate major surgery.

The use of neoadjuvant chemotherapy is common in the preoperative period. Skeletal muscle wasting secondary to chemotherapy has been associated with declines in physical fitness[6] and mitochondrial dysfunction both in and ex vivo. It would seem, therefore, that therapies targeted at increasing cancer-free survival could influence long-term functional outcomes through impairments in physiologic reserve.

Fitness for surgery is a composite concept whereby a panoply of influences interacts in a given individual to modify physiologic resilience to perioperative stressors. Increasing interest is being generated in enhancing the functional capacity of individual patients through preemptive exercise and nutrition; this is the foundation of preoperative prehabilitation.

PREOPERATIVE PREHABILITATION: AN OPPORTUNITY THAT IS OFTEN MISSED

Many contemporary surgical pathways leave little leeway to offer comprehensive preoperative optimization, despite the potential benefits that could accrue.

Even given these constraints, opportunities to optimize modifiable risk factors are being missed.[7]

Surgery often seems routine to the doctors and allied health professionals engaged in delivering care but is a major life event for each individual patient. Surgical preassessment is in some patients the first time that a comprehensive health evaluation has been undertaken in many years. Patients may be particularly amenable to interventions that change behavior when faced with a major life event. In the preoperative period, patients are often anxious and have feelings of powerlessness and loss of control. Opportunities to engage in their own care may offer patients a means to achieve these goals and alleviate some of the emotional distress of the perioperative period.[8]

The perioperative period offers not just an opportunity to identify and optimize medical conditions but also a teachable moment for modifying behaviors such as physical inactivity. The perioperative health care team is therefore presented with an opportunity to influence not only perioperative outcomes but also wider health behavior.

AGING, HOMEOSTENOSIS, AND PHYSIOLOGIC RESERVE

The world population is aging,[9] and this is reflected in an aging surgical population.[10] Normal aging involves many complex biological changes that affect most organ systems and reduce the capacity of individuals to withstand physiologic stress.[11] Increased age is further variably associated with a variety of factors, including reduced exercise capacity, frailty, malnutrition, and a high chronic comorbidity burden.

Older patients are less likely to exercise regularly (in the United States, only 22% of individuals aged 65 years or older report regular activity)[12] and are more likely to present for surgery malnourished.[13] In combination, these factors result in a reduced physiologic reserve. This concept is also known as homeostenosis, a process in which, from maturity to senescence, diminishing physiologic reserves are available to buffer challenges to homeostasis,[11,14] so resilience to stress is reduced.

When an individual is subjected to stress, physiologic reserves are engaged to maintain homeostasis and to adapt to the new physiologic conditions. A physiologic limit may be conceptualized, beyond which the individual fails to adapt, resulting in organ injury or a disease state. With aging, physiologic reserves reduce, with a consequent decrease in this limit and reduced capacity to adapt to any given insult (**Fig. 1**). A stressor, easily tolerated by a young organ, may therefore exceed the physiologic limit in an older patient, resulting in injury.

Reduced exercise capacity in the elderly is a good example of this concept. With age, peak heart rate, peak oxygen consumption (Vo_2 peak), and cardiac output are reduced, limiting the ability to respond to exertional stress. This limitation is associated with a corresponding limitation in the capacity to respond to surgical stress, predisposing the heart and other organ systems to injury, and may contribute to the predisposition of elderly individuals to frailty.

Many predictors of poor operative outcome center on factors that impair physiologic resilience or reserve (**Fig. 2**), including:

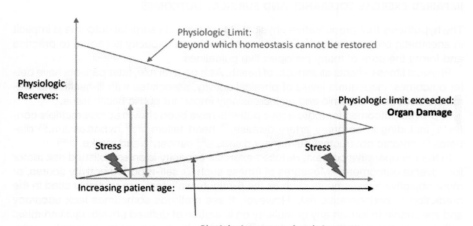

Fig. 1. Homeostenosis. Physiologic reserves maintain homeostasis and allow allostasis in the presence of environmental or physiologic stress. With increasing age, the physiologic limit that may be tolerated decreases, whereas physiologic reserves in use increase. A stressor (eg, surgery) may be tolerated at a young age that at an older age will exceed the physiologic limit, resulting in organ damage.

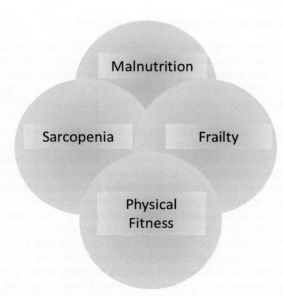

Fig. 2. The tetrad of preoperative fitness. All 4 of these factors independently and combined predict poor postoperative outcomes. The presence of one of these factors increases the likelihood of the development of another. All 4 are potentially modifiable with corresponding improvements in patient outcome.

- Impaired exercise tolerance
- Malnutrition
- Sarcopenia
- Frailty

IMPAIRED EXERCISE TOLERANCE AND SURGICAL OUTCOMES

The hypothesis that preoperative physical fitness predicts surgical outcome is implicit in anesthetic preassessment.[15] Evaluation of functional capacity is central to practice and forms the core of many perioperative guidelines.

Physical fitness affects all aspects of health. As a general rule, fitter patients have better outcomes. Inadequate levels of physical activity, associated with ill-health and premature death, are endemic and an increasingly important public health issue.[16,17]

Improved outcomes for more active patients have been shown across multiple contexts, including in coronary artery disease,[18] heart failure,[19,20] hypertension,[21] diabetes,[22] chronic obstructive pulmonary disease,[23] cancer,[24] and stroke.[15,25]

In the perioperative context, reduced exercise capacity is an established risk factor for adverse outcomes.[26] Measures of fitness such as self-reported activity scores, or more objective assessments such as the 6-minute walk test, are routinely used in the prediction of perioperative risk. However, these methods sometimes lack accuracy and are unable to furnish any granularity on limitation of defined physiologic variables.

Compounding the effects of endemic low activity levels among the surgical population are further modifiers of physical activity related to the medical conditions that underlie presentation for surgery. Osteoarthritis, malaise caused by chemotherapy, or reduced appetite, among others, meaningfully affect individual patient fitness. Given the rapidity with which bed rest and inactivity reduce physical fitness,[27] it is incumbent on treating physicians to promote ongoing physical activity throughout the perioperative period in order to overcome innate patient caution and years of accumulated medical practice.

Much of the current data on the consequences of reduced fitness on surgical outcome comes from preoperative cardiopulmonary exercise testing (CPET). CPET allows objective measurement of exercise capacity. Several systematic reviews to date have described a strong relationship between aerobic fitness and outcome.[28–30] Although several individual candidate variables have shown promise regarding prediction of perioperative risk, the strongest association with outcomes remains with a reduced anaerobic threshold, the threshold for increased risk of postoperative complications traditionally defined as being less than 11 $ml.O_2.kg$, although more recent studies suggest lower threshold levels.[28–30] Recently published clinical guidelines offer a clear framework for the perioperative use of CPET[31]

Data associating increased habitual activity and objective measures of aerobic fitness with improved perioperative outcome raise the question as to whether perioperative outcomes could be improved by intervening to improve physical fitness.

HOW DOES EXERCISE TRAINING BENEFIT HEALTH-RELATED OUTCOMES?

Exercise requires activation of multiple integrated physiologic processes, ultimately optimizing the delivery of oxygen to working muscles. The response to training results in increased efficiency of energy usage as well as delivery of substrate to respiring organs. Simply put, exercise training prepares the individual to compensate physiologically for other major systemic perturbations. Ultimately, the body becomes better adapted to tolerate stress over time.[32]

Cardiovascular, strength, and overall function improvements can occur within as little as 3 weeks after starting exercise training.[33,34] The limited time available for prehabilitation interventions before surgery may, therefore, still be sufficient for prehabilitation purposes to produce meaningful changes in outcome.

EXERCISE PREHABILITATION IN SURGERY

Prehabilitation has been defined as "the process of enhancing functional capacity of an individual to enable them to withstand an incoming stressor."[15]

Interest in exercise prehabilitation in the perioperative period has gained traction in recent years, although, to date, few clinical programs exist targeting systematic enhancement of physical performance in preparation for surgery.

The goal of exercise prehabilitation centers on the concept of enhancing physiologic reserve (**Fig. 3**).

In general, a dose-response relationship seems to exist between exercise and outcome. Underlying all exercise prescription is the necessity for a physiologic stress greater than normal for the individual patient in order to accrue a training effect.

Where preoperative exercise prehabilitation has been studied, there has been substantial variation in exercise interventions and outcome measures, making it challenging to draw clear conclusions as to the best approach.[35] In general, the greatest benefit has been seen in the least physically fit: the elderly, frail, and sedentary.

Early studies of prehabilitation[36–38] have shown feasibility, even in patients undergoing neoadjuvant chemotherapy, showing increases in physical fitness and reduced hospital stay as well as improved quality of life.

The first systematic review of exercise prehabilitation in noncardiac surgery was published in 2011. Twelve studies were reported, with great variety in the exercise intervention. Improvements in complication rates and hospital length of stay were seen in exercise cohorts.[38] A subsequent review of 15 studies reported improvements

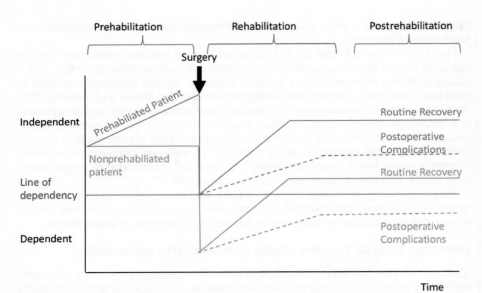

Fig. 3. The predicted impact of prehabilitation on outcomes in older patients after surgery. Surgery temporarily reduces physical independence in all patients. Under normal circumstances, a return to independence is expected in complication-free surgery, albeit with a reduced functional reserve. Postoperative complications may result in a failure to return to independent function. Prehabilitation improves preoperative function, thereby allowing return to independent function even if there is perioperative morbidity. (*Data from* Grocott M. Prehabilitation, fit-4-surgery: exercise interventions and outcome following surgery. The preoperative association. Available at: http://www.pre-op.org/useful-resources/prehabilitation. Accessed July 12, 2018.)

in pain, length of stay, and function but reported variable efficacy at improving health-related quality of life and aerobic fitness.[39] Another review of 10 studies reported physiologic improvement with exercise interventions but limited clinical benefits.[40]

Pooling of data from multiple studies has to date been limited by heterogeneity of interventions and outcome measures and inconsistent reporting of exercise interventions.

WHAT EXERCISE INTERVENTION?

The design of any exercise intervention is influenced by the type of exercise undertaken (eg, aerobic, strength), the time and frequency spent exercising, and the location (eg, home or supervised). This framework is summarized by the FITT (frequency, intensity, time, type) principle[41] (**Box 1**).

The perioperative period may be time poor. Patients may typically be engaged in a variety of other time-consuming preoperative activities. It is therefore incumbent on practitioners prescribing exercise programs in this period to ensure that they are not just cost-effective and efficacious at meaningfully increasing aerobic capacity but also that they are safe, time-efficient, and acceptable to patients. Supervised high-intensity interval training programs may fulfill these criteria.[18,43]

Although moderate exercise, such as walking at home, might be easier to achieve and even more effective in the long term for some conditions, such as the metabolic syndrome, the time constraints of surgery may not afford the physical improvements necessary for meaningful impact on clinical outcomes.

> **Box 1**
> **The FITT principle**
>
> The American College of Sports Medicine has released guidelines for and to describe exercise training. Frequency stands for the number of days a week, intensity reflects the work load while exercising, time refers to the duration of each exercise session, and type refers to the type of exercise undertaken. Moderate exercise has been defined as 80% of oxygen uptake at lactate threshold and severe exercise as 50% of the difference between oxygen uptake at lactate threshold and at peak Vo_2.[42]
>
> *From* National Heart, Lung, and Blood Institute. Clinical guidelines on the identification, evaluation, and treatment of overweight and obesity in adults: the evidence report. [Internet]. Rockville (MD): National Institutes of Health, National Heart, Lung, and Blood Institute; 1998. [cited 10/10/2010]. 228 p. Available at: http://www.nhlbi.nih.gov/guidelines/obesity/ob_gdlns.pdf.

A large portfolio of trials are in progress currently, aiming to answer questions around the optimum type of exercise (FITT), adherence to different types of exercise, feasibility when implemented at scale, and longer-term health impact (eg, WesFIt [Wessex Fit-4-Cancer surgery trial], PREHAB [Pre-operative Rehabilitation for Reduction of Hospitalization After Coronary Bypass and Valvular Surgery], PREPARE [prehabilitation, physical activity and exercise trial], CHALLENGE [Colon health and life long exercise trial]).

Exercise prescription alone in the preoperative period may not be sufficient to improve perioperative outcome. Care must also be taken to ensure compliance with exercise programs and, importantly, to optimize the nutritional status of the patient in order to maximize benefit seen from other interventions.

OPTIMIZATION OF PERIOPERATIVE NUTRITION

Malnutrition is endemic in the surgical population.[44] Malnutrition results in cachexia and sarcopenia and contributes to reduced physical fitness.

Malnutrition is particularly common in the elderly. In the community, up to 38% of older people either have or are at risk of malnutrition. In hospital, this may increase to up to 47% of patients being at risk of malnutrition and 39% being malnourished.

Malnourishment in surgical patients is particularly harmful: a malnourished patient is 3 times more likely to experience perioperative morbidity and 5 times more likely to die than a well-nourished patient. In addition, malnourished patients have increased hospital readmission rates and costs associated with their inpatient stays.[45,46]

Patients presenting for gastrointestinal and cancer surgeries seem to carry the highest risk of malnutrition, with up to 2 out of 3 individuals being malnourished.[47] Cancer cachexia is multifactorial and results from anorexia; tumor-related catabolism; altered nutrient metabolism; and, in some, physical gastrointestinal tract obstruction. Cancer cachexia has negative predictive value for survival, which was reduced to 8 months compared with 28 months in patients who had lost weight compared with those who had not in one study.[48]

Screening and management of malnutrition is generally inadequate in clinical practice. Only 1 in 5 hospitals have formal nutrition screening processes and a similar proportion of patients receive any preoperative nutritional intervention, despite an estimated $52 saving in hospital costs for every $1 spent on nutrition therapy.[49]

To be effective, nutritional prehabilitation before surgery therefore needs to be proactive and include nutritional assessments in addition to intervention. This approach has been emphasized in a recent Perioperative Quality Improvement initiative.[49]

NUTRITIONAL PREHABILITATION

Preoperative nutritional optimization aims to address the following goals:

- Optimize nutrient stores
- Optimize metabolic reserve
- Provide a buffer to trauma-induced catabolism
- Enhance immune response
- Provide a nutritional strategy for the entire perioperative period
- Target those at the highest risk

Perioperative nutritional interventions have been shown to improve postoperative outcomes across a variety of domains, including reducing surgical site infections[45] and other morbidity by 20% to 40%.[50,51]

Screening for and assessment of risk are central to the approach to nutritional prehabilitation.

Body mass index (BMI) is the most commonly used marker of nutritional status in clinical and research practice. In the research context, reduced BMI has been strongly associated with impaired survival in a variety of cancers and, with simple assessment of weight, remains a useful clinical prognostic tool in terms of grading the impact of weight loss on outcome.[52]

However, BMI and weight do not alone provide sufficient granularity in terms of assessment of nutritional deficit and sarcopenia. As a result, a variety[53] of nutritional screening tools incorporating biophysical measures and nutritional biomarkers have been developed in different clinical contexts. In hospitalized patients, the Malnutrition Universal Screening Tool (MUST), the Nutrition Risk Screening 2002 (NRS-2002), and the Short Nutrition Assessment Questionnaire (SNAQ) are commonly used. None of these tools have been specifically designed for use in the perioperative period.

The Perioperative Nutrition Screening (PONS) score has been proposed in an attempt to address this deficit (**Fig. 4**). It is an adaption of the MUST for perioperative use. If any question in the PONS tool results in a positive response, then a formal nutritional assessment and/or intervention is recommended.

Having screened for malnutrition, the appropriate nutritional intervention needs to be initiated (**Fig. 5**).

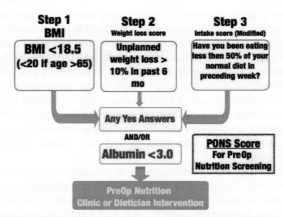

Fig. 4. The PONS score. Preop, preoperative. (*From* Wischmeyer PE, Carli F, Evans DC, et al. American Society for Enhanced Recovery and Perioperative Quality Initiative joint consensus statement on nutrition screening and therapy within a surgical enhanced recovery pathway. Anesth Analg 2018;126(6):1888; with permission.)

PREOPERATIVE NUTRITION CARE PATHWAY
Low Nutrition Risk

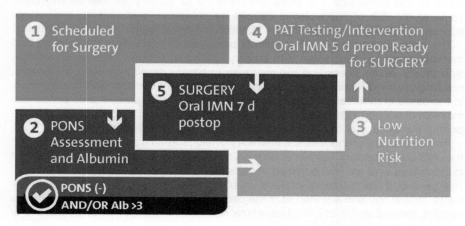

PREOPERATIVE NUTRITION CARE PATHWAY
High Nutrition Risk

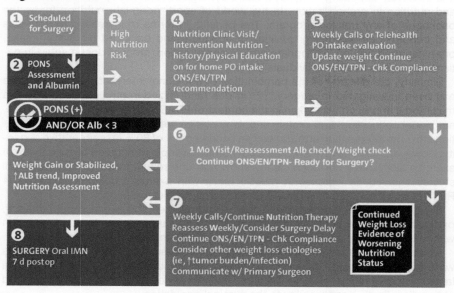

Fig. 5. Suggested low and high-risk nutrition pathways based on preoperative PONS scores. Alb, albumin; Chk, compliance; EN, enteral nutrition; IMN, immunonutrition; ONS, oral nutritional supplementation; PAT, preanesthesia testing clinic; PO, by mouth; PONS, preoperative nutrition score; TPN, total parenteral nutrition. (*From* Wischmeyer PE, Carli F, Evans DC, et al. American Society for enhanced recovery and perioperative quality initiative joint consensus statement on nutrition screening and therapy within a surgical enhanced recovery pathway. Anesth Analg 2018;126(6):1889; with permission.)

Enhanced recovery after surgery (ERAS) programs already recommend the use of carbohydrate-rich drinks in the 24 hours before surgery. Although this addresses some of the immediate metabolic requirements of surgery as well as mitigating some of the risk of hypovolemia caused by preoperative starvation, it does not address the chronic protein energy malnutrition present in higher risk surgical patients.

The content of preoperative nutritional packages should reflect the immune and metabolic demand associated with surgery, aiming to support physiologic reserve. Specifically, acute illness and the response to trauma result in protein catabolism, resulting in a need for protein supplementation beyond total energy deficits secondary to increases in metabolism. Protein supplementation in the preoperative period can maintain or support increases in lean body mass, ameliorating physical frailty and supporting the efficacy of other interventions such as exercise training.

As with exercise prehabilitation, in which training programs are most likely to benefit the unfit and sedentary, nutritional prehabilitation is likely to have the greatest impact in individuals who are malnourished at baseline.[54]

In general, if oral nutritional intake is unable to meet the needs of malnourished patients, enteral nutrition is preferred to the parenteral approach. If parenteral nutrition is needed, then a duration of 7 to 14 days is recommended, supplemented by oral and or enteral nutrition if possible.[55]

THE IMPACT OF NUTRITION AND EXERCISE PREHABILITATION COMBINED

It is intuitively appealing to hypothesize a synergistic relationship between exercise and nutrition in prehabilitation. In the world of sport, adequate nutrition forms the backbone of any training program. The benefits in terms of increased muscle size and performance-enhancing qualities of adequate and balanced nutritional intake, often centered around appropriate protein consumption, are well documented in patients as well as healthy individuals.[56,57]

Similarly, the efficacy of the combination of nutritional interventions and exercise has been investigated in surgery.[58,59] In one randomized controlled trial (RCT),[59] a multimodal approach was taken in the context of ERAS. Moderate physical exercise, nutritional counseling, and protein supplementation were prescribed to the intervention arm. The intervention arm showed an improvement of 80% in preoperative capacity. However, the relative, if any, merits of nutritional supplementation beyond those of exercise alone have not been clearly shown. In one recent systematic review,[60] all studies showed an increase in muscle mass with exercise, but only 8 out of 34 RCTs showed an additional benefit of nutritional supplementation.

Similarly, most reported studies showed improvements in exercise performance, particularly in otherwise healthy subjects aged 60 years or more, but an interaction with nutritional supplementation was found in less than 15% of reported results.

As with studies of exercise prehabilitation alone, a variety of nutritional approaches were taken, which may have confounded potential additional benefits. Similarly, a large number of reported studies included elderly individuals who were well nourished at baseline, limiting applicability to the surgical population.

SUMMARY

The concept of prehabilitation before surgery is attractive and underpinned by good explanatory mechanisms. Exercise and nutritional prehabilitation seem safe and effective, although, for exercise at least, meaningful clinical impact remains uncertain. Early data do support reduction in morbidity and improvements in quality of life for a combined approach.

Alongside nutritional and exercise-based approaches, efforts should be made to optimize other key modifiable risk factors. Any approach to prehabilitation should be multimodal and part of a global strategy for the perioperative period.

The key to the choice of any prehabilitation strategy is deciding on how to measure the success of the intervention. Length of stay may be confounded by a multitude of factors. Measurements of aerobic fitness and muscle size may be meaningless to individual patients. Therefore, the focus of preoptimization should be what is most important to the patient. Is it return to baseline activity? Or is it, for example, a return to social function and reintegration into the community? Ultimately, a paradigm shift is needed in terms of how success is measured in the perioperative period away from short-term economic and morbidity/mortality to longer-term patient-centered health outcomes.

REFERENCES

1. Weiser TG, Haynes AB, Molina G, et al. Estimate of the global volume of surgery in 2012: an assessment supporting improved health outcomes. Lancet 2015;385: S11.
2. Pearse RM, Moreno RP, Bauer P, et al. Mortality after surgery in Europe: a 7 day cohort study. Lancet 2012;380:1059–65.
3. Khuri SF, Henderson WG, DePalma RG, et al. Determinants of long-term survival after major surgery and the adverse effect of postoperative complications. Ann Surg 2005;123:326–41.
4. Christensen T, Kehlet H. Postoperative fatigue. World J Surg 1993;17:220–5.
5. West MA, Loughney L, Lythgoe D, et al. The effect of neoadjuvant chemoradiotherapy on whole-body physical fitness and skeletal muscle mitochondrial oxidative phosphorylation in vivo in locally advanced rectal cancer patients – an observational pilot study. PLoS One 2014;9(12):e111526.
6. West MA, Loughney L, Ambler G, et al. The effect of neoadjuvant chemotherapy and chemoradiotherapy on exercise capacity and outcome following upper gastrointestinal cancer surgery: an observational cohort study. BMC Cancer 2016;16:710.
7. Grocott MPW, Plumb JOM, Edwards M, et al. Re-designing the pathway to surgery: better care and added value. Perioper Med (Lond) 2017;6:9.
8. Spalding NJ. Reducing anxiety by pre-operative education: make the future familiar. Occup Ther Int 2003;10:278–93.
9. United Nations, Department of Economic and Social Affairs, P. D. World population ageing. United Nations. 2013. 114. doi:ST/ESA/SER.A/348.
10. Etzioni DA, Liu JH, Maggard MA, et al. The aging population and its impact on the surgery workforce. Ann Surg 2003;238:170–7.
11. Khan SS, Singer BD, Vaughan DE. Molecular and physiological manifestations and measurement of aging in humans. Aging Cell 2017;16(4):624–33.
12. Sun F, Norman IJ, While AE. Physical activity in older people: a systematic review. BMC Public Health 2013;13:449.
13. Dempsey D, Mullen J, Buzby G. The link between nutritional status and clinical outcome: can nutritional intervention modify it? Am J Clin Nutr 1988;47:352–6.
14. Kane RL, Shamliyan T, Talley K, et al. The association between geriatric syndromes and survival. J Am Geriatr Soc 2012;60:896–904.
15. Levett DZH, Grocott MPW. Cardiopulmonary exercise testing, prehabilitation, and enhanced recovery after surgery (ERAS). Can J Anaesth 2015;62:131–42.

16. Kohl HW, Craig CL, Lambert EV, et al. The pandemic of physical inactivity: global action for public health. Lancet 2012;380:294–305.
17. Lee IM, Shiroma EJ, Lobelo F, et al. Effect of physical inactivity on major non-communicable diseases worldwide: an analysis of burden of disease and life expectancy. Lancet 2012;380:219–29.
18. Elliott AD, Rajopadhyaya K, Bentley DJ, et al. Interval training versus continuous exercise in patients with coronary artery disease: a meta-analysis. Heart Lung Circ 2015;24:149–57.
19. Belardinelli R, Georgiou D, Cianci G, et al. Randomized, controlled trial of long-term moderate exercise training in chronic heart failure: effects on functional capacity, quality of life, and clinical outcome. Circulation 1999;99:1173–82.
20. O'Connor CM, Whellan DJ, Lee KL, et al. Efficacy and safety of exercise training in patients with chronic heart failure: HF-ACTION randomized controlled trial. JAMA 2009;301:1439–50.
21. Cornelissen VA, Smart NA. Exercise training for blood pressure: a systematic review and meta-analysis. J Am Heart Assoc 2013;2(1):e004473.
22. Weltman NY, Saliba SA, Barrett EJ, et al. The use of exercise in the management of type 1 and type 2 diabetes. Clin Sports Med 2009;28:423–39.
23. Watz H, Pitta F, Rochester CL, et al. An official European Respiratory Society statement on physical activity in COPD. Eur Respir J 2014;44:1521–37.
24. Brown JC, Winters-Stone K, Lee A, et al. Cancer, physical activity, and exercise. Compr Physiol 2012;2(4):2775–809.
25. Austin MW, Ploughman M, Glynn L, et al. Aerobic exercise effects on neuroprotection and brain repair following stroke: a systematic review and perspective. Neurosci Res 2014;87:8–15.
26. Levett DZH, Grocott MPW. Cardiopulmonary exercise testing for risk prediction in major abdominal surgery. Anesthesiol Clin 2015;33:1–16.
27. Coker RH, Hays NP, Williams RH, et al. Bed rest promotes reductions in walking speed, functional parameters, and aerobic fitness in older, healthy adults. J Gerontol A Biol Sci Med Sci 2015;70:91–6.
28. West M, Jack S, Grocott MPW. Perioperative cardiopulmonary exercise testing in the elderly. Best Pract Res Clin Anaesthesiol 2011;25:427–37.
29. Hennis PJ, Meale PM, Grocott MPW. Cardiopulmonary exercise testing for the evaluation of perioperative risk in non-cardiopulmonary surgery. Postgrad Med J 2011;87:550–7.
30. Smith TB, Stonell C, Purkayastha S, et al. Cardiopulmonary exercise testing as a risk assessment method in non cardio-pulmonary surgery: a systematic review. Anaesthesia 2009;64:883–93.
31. Levett DZH, Jack S, Swart M, et al. Preoperative cardiopulmonary exercise testing (PCPET): consensus clinical guidelines on indications, organisation, conduct and physiological interpretation. Br J Anaesth 2017;120:484–500.
32. Burton DA, Stokes K, Hall GM. Physiological effects of exercise. Continuing Education in Anaesthesia Critical Care & Pain 2004;4(6):185–8.
33. Murias JM, Kowalchuk JM, Paterson DH. Time course and mechanisms of adaptations in cardiorespiratory fitness with endurance training in older and young men. J Appl Physiol (1985) 2010;108:621–7.
34. Fielding RA. The role of progressive resistance training and nutrition in the preservation of lean body mass in the elderly. J Am Coll Nutr 1995;14:587–94.
35. O'Doherty AF, West M, Jack S, et al. Preoperative aerobic exercise training in elective intra-cavity surgery: a systematic review. Br J Anaesth 2013;110.

36. West MA, Loughney L, Lythgoe D, et al. Effect of prehabilitation on objectively measured physical fitness after neoadjuvant treatment in preoperative rectal cancer patients: a blinded interventional pilot study. Br J Anaesth 2015;114:244–51.

37. Mayo NE, Feldman L, Scott S, et al. Impact of preoperative change in physical function on postoperative recovery: argument supporting prehabilitation for colorectal surgery. Surgery 2011;150:505–14.

38. Valkenet K, van de Port IG, Dronkers JJ, et al. The effects of preoperative exercise therapy on postoperative outcome: a systematic review. Clin Rehabil 2011; 25:99–111.

39. Santa Mina D, Clarke H, Ritvo P, et al. Effect of total-body prehabilitation on postoperative outcomes: a systematic review and meta-analysis. Physiotherapy 2014; 100:196–207.

40. Lemanu DP, Singh PP, MacCormick AD, et al. Effect of preoperative exercise on cardiorespiratory function and recovery after surgery: a systematic review. World J Surg 2013;37:711–20.

41. Garber CE, Blissmer B, Deschenes MR, et al. Quantity and quality of exercise for developing and maintaining cardiorespiratory, musculoskeletal, and neuromotor fitness in apparently healthy adults: guidance for prescribing exercise. Med Sci Sports Exerc 2011;43:1334–59.

42. Loughney L, West MA, Kemp GJ, et al. The effects of neoadjuvant chemoradiotherapy and an in-hospital exercise training programme on physical fitness and quality of life in locally advanced rectal cancer patients (The EMPOWER Trial): study protocol for a randomised controlled trial. Trials 2016;17:24.

43. Weston M, Weston KL, Prentis JM, et al. High-intensity interval training (HIT) for effective and time-efficient pre-surgical exercise interventions. Perioper Med (Lond) 2016;5:2.

44. Williams JD, Wischmeyer PE. Assessment of perioperative nutrition practices and attitudes—a national survey of colorectal and GI surgical oncology programs. Am J Surg 2017;213:1010–8.

45. Weimann A, Braga M, Carli F, et al. ESPEN guideline: clinical nutrition in surgery. Clin Nutr 2017;36:623–50.

46. Correia MITD, Waitzberg DL. The impact of malnutrition on morbidity, mortality, length of hospital stay and costs evaluated through a multivariate model analysis. Clin Nutr 2003;22:235–9.

47. Thomas MN, Kufeldt J, Kisser U, et al. Effects of malnutrition on complication rates, length of hospital stay, and revenue in elective surgical patients in the G-DRG-system. Nutrition 2016;32:249–54.

48. Martin L, Birdsell L, Macdonald N, et al. Cancer cachexia in the age of obesity: skeletal muscle depletion is a powerful prognostic factor, independent of body mass index. J Clin Oncol 2013;31:1539–47.

49. Wischmeyer PE, Carli F, Evans DC, et al. American Society for Enhanced Recovery and Perioperative Quality Initiative joint consensus statement on nutrition screening and therapy within a surgical enhanced recovery pathway. Anesth Analg 2018;126(6):1883–95. Publish Ah, (9000).

50. Drover JW, Cahill NE, Kutsogiannis J, et al. Nutrition therapy for the critically ill surgical patient: we need to do better! JPEN J Parenter Enteral Nutr 2011;34: 644–52.

51. Drover JW, Dhaliwal R, Weitzel L, et al. Perioperative use of arginine-supplemented diets: a systematic review of the evidence. J Am Coll Surg 2011;212(3):385–99, 399.e1.

52. Elia M. THE 'MUST' REPORT nutritional screening of adults: a multidisciplinary responsibility Executive summary Section A: screening for malnutrition: a multidisciplinary responsibility. MAG, a Standing Comm. BAPEN. 2003.

53. Van Bokhorst-de van der Schueren MAE, Guaitoli PR, Jansma EP, et al. Nutrition screening tools: does one size fit all? A systematic review of screening tools for the hospital setting. Clin Nutr 2014;33:39–58.

54. Burden S, Todd C, Hill J, et al. Pre-operative nutrition support in patients undergoing gastrointestinal surgery. Cochrane Database Syst Rev 2012;(11):CD008879.

55. Miller KR, Wischmeyer PE, Taylor B, et al. An evidence-based approach to perioperative nutrition support in the elective surgery patient. JPEN J Parenter Enteral Nutr 2013;37:39S–50S.

56. Esmarck B, Andersen JL, Olsen S, et al. Timing of postexercise protein intake is important for muscle hypertrophy with resistance training in elderly humans. J Physiol 2001;535:301–11.

57. Burke LM, Hawley JA, Ross ML, et al. Preexercise aminoacidemia and muscle protein synthesis after resistance exercise. Med Sci Sports Exerc 2012;44: 1968–77.

58. Li C, Carli F, Lee L, et al. Impact of a trimodal prehabilitation program on functional recovery after colorectal cancer surgery: a pilot study. Surg Endosc 2013;27:1072–82.

59. Gillis C, Loiselle SE, Fiore JF Jr, et al. Prehabilitation with whey protein supplementation on perioperative functional exercise capacity in patients undergoing colorectal resection for cancer: a pilot double-blinded randomized placebo-controlled trial. J Acad Nutr Diet 2015;116:802–12.

60. Beaudart C, Dawson A, Shaw SC, et al. Nutrition and physical activity in the prevention and treatment of sarcopenia: systematic review. Osteoporos Int 2017;28: 1817–33.

Diabetes Mellitus
Preoperative Concerns and Evaluation

Roshni Sreedharan, MD[a], Basem Abdelmalak, MD, FASA[b,c],*

KEYWORDS

- Diabetes mellitus • Hyperglycemia • Preoperative • Anesthesia

KEY POINTS

- Diabetes is an important cause of morbidity in the adult population resulting in hypoglycemia, hyperglycemia, renal dysfunction, and cardiovascular complications. Such morbidities may have an impact on the perioperative anesthetic care and outcomes.
- In this review, the authors discuss the preoperative considerations in managing patients with diabetes as well as those without diabetes albeit hyperglycemic.
- The authors propose a plan for managing preoperative diabetes pharmacotherapy, including the use of a subcutaneous insulin pump with the goal to avoid both hypoglycemia and hyperglycemia.
- The authors discuss the decision whether to proceed or cancel surgery for a given hemoglobin A1c percentage or blood glucose concentration.

INTRODUCTION

Diabetes as a disease has a profound impact on the quality of the human life. Not only is it the most common endocrine disease in the United States but also widely prevalent Worldwide; in 2014, 8.5% of the world's population was diagnosed with diabetes. Hyperglycemia and diabetes were responsible for about 3.7 million deaths worldwide and was the seventh leading cause of death in the United States in 2012.[1] Risk factors for diabetes including obesity and inactivity have been steadily increasing. Diabetes has a significant impact on the economy as well. In the United States, the total estimated cost of diabetes (direct and indirect) in 2012 was about $245 billion. Individuals diagnosed with diabetes have 2.3 times higher health care expenditures than those without diabetes.[2]

Disclaimer: The authors have no relevant financial conflict of interest to disclose.
[a] Department of General Anesthesiology, Center for Critical Care, Anesthesiology Institute, Cleveland Clinic, E-31 9500 Euclid Avenue, Cleveland, OH 44195, USA; [b] Department of General Anesthesiology, Anesthesiology Institute, Cleveland Clinic, E-31 9500 Euclid Avenue, Cleveland, OH 44195, USA; [c] Department of Outcomes Research, Anesthesiology Institute, Cleveland Clinic, E-31 9500 Euclid Avenue, Cleveland, OH 44195, USA
* Corresponding author. Anesthesiology Institute, Cleveland Clinic, E-31 9500 Euclid Avenue, Cleveland, OH 44195.
E-mail address: abdelmb@ccf.org

Anesthesiology Clin 36 (2018) 581–597
https://doi.org/10.1016/j.anclin.2018.07.007
anesthesiology.theclinics.com
1932-2275/18/© 2018 Elsevier Inc. All rights reserved.

Diabetes is an important cause of morbidity in the adult population resulting in hypoglycemia, hyperglycemia, renal dysfunction, and cardiovascular complications; such morbidities have an impact on the perioperative anesthetic care of those who have them. Appropriate glycemic control is important in slowing the progression of diabetes. Consequent to the steady increase in the prevalence of diabetes over the past few decades, there is an increasing number of diabetic patients presenting for surgical procedures.

DISCUSSION
Classification of Diabetes

Diabetes is generally categorized as type 1 or type 2. Type 1 diabetes commonly is due to the autoimmune destruction of the beta cells. These patients usually are younger and present with an absolute insulin deficiency. Type 2 diabetes, on the other hand, is due to a progressive reduction in insulin secretion by the beta cells. This reduction is often coupled with insulin resistance.[3]

Other types of diabetes are attributed to specific causes like gestational diabetes, maturity-onset diabetes of the young, and drug-induced diabetes. Although the causes may vary, the anesthetic implications consequent to long-standing hyperglycemia and its treatment are fairly similar.

Diagnosis of Diabetes

The diagnostic criteria for diabetes as updated by the American Diabetes Association (ADA) in 2018 are as follows.[3] Meeting any one of the following criteria could confer a diagnosis of diabetes:

- Fasting plasma glucose of 126 mg/dL or greater
- 2-hour plasma glucose of 200 mg/dL or greater after an oral glucose tolerance test
- Hemoglobin A1c (HbA1c) of 6.5% or greater
- Random plasma glucose of 200 mg/dL or greater in patients with the classic symptoms of hyperglycemia or hyperglycemic crisis

Goals of preanesthetic evaluation in diabetic patients

- Document a diagnosis of diabetes: type, duration
- Document pharmacologic antihyperglycemic regimen and develop a plan for the perioperative period
- Document occurrence and frequency of hypoglycemia if present
- Document and evaluate microvascular and macrovascular complications from diabetes
- Document the current and chronic glycemic state
- Check patients' understanding of perioperative plan (pharmacologic and nonpharmacologic), especially for patients using insulin pumps, in which case, counseling and a thorough discussion of the care plan would be in order

Fig. 1 highlights an outline for the preoperative management of diabetic patients.

Undiagnosed Diabetic Patients

A global review of data across 74 countries found that 45.8% of all the cases of diabetes were undiagnosed. Undiagnosed diabetes is a significant concern in surgical patients.[4] A study looking at the prevalence of undiagnosed diabetes in patients undergoing noncardiac surgery found a prevalence of 10%.[5] Furthermore, they found that the mean preoperative blood glucose (BG) concentration in undiagnosed diabetic patients was higher than that in their diabetic counterparts. Another study examining the prevalence and outcomes from undiagnosed diabetes in patients undergoing

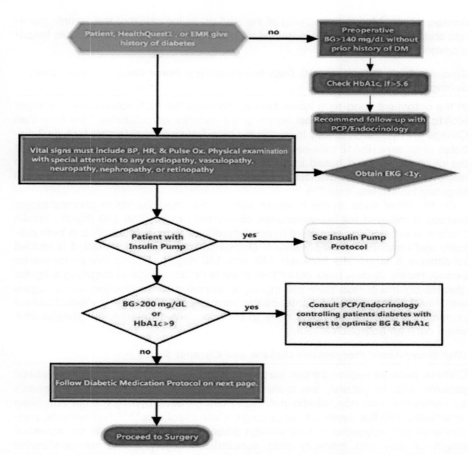

Fig. 1. Preoperative management algorithm for patients with diabetes. Diabetic patients (especially those taking insulin) are best done as first-round patients in the morning. BP, blood pressure; EKG, electrocardiogram; EMR, electronic medical record; HR, heart rate; Ox, oximeter; PCP, primary care physician. (*Courtesy of* Cleveland Clinic Center for Medical Art & Photography, Cleveland Clinic, Cleveland, Ohio © 2018. All Rights Reserved; with permission.)

cardiac surgery documented a prevalence of 5.2%.[6] Adverse outcomes, including reintubation, prolonged mechanical ventilation, and mortality, were more likely in patients with undiagnosed diabetes as compared with those without or diagnosed diabetes mellitus (DM) undergoing cardiac surgery.[6]

Abdelmalak and colleagues[7] reviewed the records of 62,000 relatively high-risk patients who underwent elective noncardiac surgery. They found an increased 1-year mortality with increasing levels of hyperglycemia among nondiabetic patients (many of whom were probably undiagnosed diabetic patients) versus patients with diabetes.

These outcomes are probably related to the lack of treatment, recognition of complications, and risk stratification. HbA1c would be useful to ascertain chronicity and to establish a diagnosis of DM in patients with elevated blood glucose values on preoperative laboratory work. The predicament in making a diagnosis of diabetes during preoperative evaluation is to help these patients on the long run, as early identification and management of diabetes helps reduce its burden and long term consequences. Moreover, learning of the HbA1c, as indicative of the chronic glycemic state of patients has the potential to impact the perioperative glycemic target/management plan.[8]

Glycemic Goals in Patients with Diabetes: Long-Term Home Versus Perioperative Setting

In the outpatient, long-term home setting, although the ADA recommends a target HbA1c of less than 7% in most nonpregnant patients with diabetes,[9] the American College of Physicians recently loosened the blood sugar control targets for type 2 diabetes to achieve HbA1c between 7% and 8%.[10] The thought behind the relaxation of the glycemic target is based on trials that showed minimal if any reduction in the microvascular and macrovascular complications from an intensive glycemic control targeting HbA1c less than 7%.[10]

On the other hand, in the inpatient setting, diet modification or pharmacologic therapy is initiated for hyperglycemia consistently more than 140 mg/dL. Insulin therapy is initiated for persistent hyperglycemia more than 180 mg/dL in both critically and noncritically ill inpatients.[11] Once insulin therapy is initiated, it is titrated to achieve a target BG between 140 and 180 mg/dL. During the perioperative period, recent studies have noted that there is no advantage in targeting a tighter glucose control of less than 140 mg/dL as opposed to maintaining blood sugars less than 180 mg/dL.[12,13] A tighter control may be appropriate in very select patient populations, and the providers have to be cognizant of the risk of hypoglycemia when such an approach is used.[8]

Why Worry About Preoperative Diabetic and Glycemic State?

Diabetic patients require certain surgical procedures more often than nondiabetic patients and, in general, are more likely to have adverse perioperative events as compared with nondiabetic patients. Postoperative hyperglycemia has been associated with the development of surgical site infections.[14,15] Furthermore, perioperative hyperglycemia with or without diabetes is associated with an increased length of stay and mortality after noncardiac surgery.[16] The neuroendocrine response during the perioperative period results in an increase in the level of catecholamines and stress hormones resulting in hyperglycemia.[17–19] This outcome, coupled with the difficulty managing oral hypoglycemic and other antihyperglycemic agents in the perioperative period, could result in the potential for uncontrolled hyperglycemia and its consequences, including diabetic ketoacidosis (DKA) or hyperosmolar hyperglycemic nonketotic syndrome (HHNS). More importantly, point-of-care blood sugar monitoring during the perioperative period is imperative, especially in diabetic patients and hyperglycemic nondiabetic patients, to monitor for and recognize both hyperglycemia and more importantly hypoglycemia. Hypoglycemia could be masked under general anesthesia, and its occurrence could result in irreversible neurologic damage and in adverse perioperative outcomes.[20,21]

When to Delay or Cancel a Procedure for Hyperglycemia, and/or Elevated Hemoglobin A1c

Patients who present to the preoperative clinic and have diabetes with either hyperglycemia or hypoglycemia outside of their target goal determined by their treating physician should be referred back to their physician to review their current treatment plan, compliance, and other contributing factors, as this is an opportunity to realign their health status with their treatment goals. Also, nondiabetic patients, who present with abnormally high glucose levels and/or high HbA1c should also be advised to seek specialized care to diagnose or rule out a diabetes diagnosis and get started on treatment of the same if indeed they have it, as early management of diabetes would have an impact on the disease progression and its impact on different organs. The impact of such interventions on surgical outcomes is not yet clearly delineated, but it is for the lifelong benefits of these patients.

The debate is still going regarding whether to proceed or not in elective surgeries when an abnormally high HbA1c concentration is encountered because of the lack of solid guidance on whether to proceed or not.[22] For example, the ADA does not recommend an HbA1c threshold above which elective surgery should be postponed. The Australian Diabetes Society recommends postponing elective procedures when the HbA1c is more than 9%.[23] The Association of Anesthetists of Great Britain and Ireland suggests more stringent criteria.[24] Many studies showed an association between poor outcomes and certain HbA1c percentages, like 7%, 8%, or 9%. It has been noted that the risk of adverse perioperative outcomes increases when the preoperative HbA1c is greater than 8 in this one study.[25] That said, association does not mean causation nor does it mean that normalization would result in reversal of that association or improve outcomes, as that has not been shown to date. Moreover, from a practical standpoint, it may be difficult to cancel elective procedures based on HbA1c criteria understanding that it would take about 3 months to show an improvement after pharmacologic and nonpharmacologic interventions to improve glycemic control are instituted. When joint arthroplasty was delayed for HbA1c greater than 7%, only 40% of the delayed patients were able to achieve such a target within a time range of 1 week to almost 3 years.[26]

When patients present in the morning of the surgery with abnormal BG concentrations, the decision becomes a bit more involved.

An emergency and potentially life-saving procedure will have to, and need to be, performed regardless; every effort should be done to maximize safety. In patients with complications of uncontrolled hyperglycemia like DKA or HHNS, it is prudent to delay surgery and treat the condition (obviously, unless it is an impending life-threatening emergency). Again as it is the case with HbA1c, many studies show an association between poor outcomes and certain glucose concentrations. Although, if the surgery gets delayed, there are no reliable data to support that if a specific optimal target glucose concentration and/or HbA1c are achieved and maintained for a given unknown optimal duration preoperatively, that it would in fact result in avoiding certain poor surgical outcomes.

Patients scheduled for surgery (as well as family and friends) have already planned their schedules, taken time off from their jobs, and psychologically prepared themselves for it. Delaying and/or canceling their surgery would constitute a major inconvenience with potential financial implications to the patients/family and the hospital to say the least. Therefore, the decision whether to reschedule surgery or not should be individualized, depending on the surgery, patient characteristics including chronic glycemic state and the clinician's experience with glucose management. In effect, many clinicians do not end up delaying elective surgery for mild to moderate hyperglycemia but rather treat it and the associated osmotic diuresis–induced hypovolemia. On the other hand, many think that it might be prudent to delay elective surgery when faced with glucose concentrations greater than 350 mg/dL and/or any concentration associated with DKA and/or a hyperosmolar state as stated earlier.[27,28] Some clinicians like the author (B.A.) of this article elect to use a higher cutoff value in certain patients in the absence of DKA. DKA can easily be diagnosed based on the clinical presentation and when certain laboratory criteria are met; the triad of hyperglycemia greater than 250 mg/dL, acidosis (arterial pH <7.3, serum bicarbonate <18 mEq/L, and anion gap of >10), and ketonemia (urine and serum ketones are positive).[29]

PHARMACOLOGIC THERAPY IN DIABETIC PATIENTS
Noninsulin Oral and Injectable Oral Hypoglycemic Therapy

In adults with type 2 diabetes, approximately 3 times as many patients have reported to be on the oral medications only as opposed to being on only injectable medications. In the absence of contraindications, metformin is chosen as the first-line oral therapy for type 2 diabetes.[30,31] Metformin has proven benefits in glycemic management, weight control, and cardiovascular outcomes. One concern, in the perioperative period with metformin, has been the risk of lactic acidosis. This risk has been proven not to be the case.[32] That said, in light of the fact that it is of long duration and because patients are expected to take nothing by mouth and to err on the safer side of hyperglycemia versus hypoglycemia, it might be prudent to hold metformin in the morning of the surgery. With most diabetic patients (70%) being on oral hypoglycemic therapy, the primary concern in these patients is the prevention of perioperative hypoglycemia. The risk of hypoglycemia is significant with oral hypoglycemic agents that can increase or stimulate insulin secretion like sulfonylureas and glinides. The common classes of oral hypoglycemic drugs, their physiologic effect, and their perioperative management are tabulated in **Table 1**.

Insulin Therapy

All patients with type 1 diabetes are on insulin because of its absolute deficiency. A smaller percentage of patients with type 2 diabetes are on insulin in addition to oral and injectable noninsulin antihyperglycemic agents to achieve adequate glycemic control. Because of insulin resistance, patients with type 2 diabetes may require a higher amount of insulin to achieve the same control as compared with patients with type 1 diabetes.

The insulin regimen in patients with type 1 covers the basal requirement, prandial and correctional insulin for anticipated nutritional intake or unanticipated accidental hyperglycemia, respectively.[11,31,33] It is of paramount importance to note that approximately 50% of the basal requirement of insulin is used to cover metabolic demands without inducing hypoglycemia.[33] These patients would need some insulin even while fasting to prevent ketosis.

Several different formulations of insulin are clinically used. They are classified according to their time of onset, peak, and duration of action into rapid-acting, short-, intermediate- and long-acting/basal insulins. In addition, there are premixed insulins as well, which could be a combination of intermediate- and short-acting or neutral protamine Hagedorn and regular insulins.

Long-acting insulin analogues (glargine, detemir, degludec) are less likely to result in hypoglycemia in the perioperative fasting state, as they do not peak, while maintaining a steady level of insulin. On the day before surgery, the usual dose of these medications could be administered. Although the risk of hypoglycemia is low with this formulation, some investigators suggest a 20% to 30% reduction in the dose either the night before or on the day of surgery because of a lack of consensus guidelines and to err on the side of safety.[24,31] Recently, Demma and colleagues[34] showed that administering 75% of the insulin dose the night before surgery was associated with more patients presenting to surgery with a BG concentration within the target range goal.

Table 1
Antihyperglycemic agents and their preoperative management

Class	Drug	Physiologic Effect	Risk of Hypoglycemia	Use on the Day Before Surgery	Use on the Day of Surgery
Biguanides	Metformin	Decrease hepatic glucose production	Low	Continue regular use	Skip dose
Sulfonylureas	Gliclazide, glipizide, glimepiride	Increase insulin secretion	Moderate to high	Continue regular use	Skip dose
Thiazolidinediones	Rosiglitazone, pioglitazone	Increase insulin sensitivity	Low	Continue regular use	Skip dose
Glinides	Nateglinide, repaglinide	Increase insulin secretion	Moderate	Continue regular use	Skip dose
Alpha glucosidase inhibitors	Acarbose	Slow intestinal carbohydrate absorption	Low	Continue regular use	Skip dose
Dipeptidyl peptidase-4 inhibitors	Sitagliptin, saxagliptin	Glucose-dependent increase in insulin section and decrease in glucagon secretion	Low	Continue regular use	Continue regular use
Glucagonlike peptide-1 analogues	Exenatide, liraglutide	Glucose-dependent increase in insulin secretion	Low	Continue regular use	Skip dose
Sodium glucose cotransporter-2 inhibitors	Dapaglifozina, canagliflozin	Decreases glucose reabsorption by the kidney	Low	Continue regular use	Skip dose
Long-acting basal insulin	Levemir, Lantus	Direct effect on reduction of serum glucose through multiple mechanisms	Low	Take 75% of dose	Take 50% of dose
Mixed insulin; combination of long- and short-acting (ie, 70/30 or 75/25)	NovoLog 70/30, Humalog 75/25	Direct effect on reduction of serum glucose through multiple mechanisms	Moderate to high	Take 75%–100% of dose	If morning BG is >200 mg/dL take 50% of dose, if ≤200 mg/dL skip dose

Courtesy of Cleveland Clinic Center for Medical Art & Photography, Cleveland Clinic, Cleveland, Ohio © 2017. All Rights Reserved; with permission.

With the intermediate-acting and premixed insulins, the risk of hypoglycemia could increase while fasting. With intermediate-acting insulins, both individually and as a component of premixed, the dose could be maintained the day before; but a 25% to 50% reduction in dose is recommended the night before and the day of surgery.[24,35,36] With premixed insulin, only the intermediate-acting component is given after dose reduction on the day of surgery; the short-acting component is best avoided (if feasible for patients to get separate prescriptions). Short-acting insulins are typically used to control prandial glucose elevation and, hence, are best avoided on the day of surgery and while patients are fasting.[24,31,35,36]However, in the absence of the ability to obtain separate components of premixed insulin, it is recommended to administer half the dose if the BG in the morning of surgery is greater than 200 mg/dL and hold it all together if the BG is 200 mg/dL or less.

Preoperative Management of Insulin Pumps

Insulin pumps are programmable devices that are capable of delivering a basal infusion and bolus doses of rapid-acting insulin analogues. Approximately 20% to 30% of patients with type 1 diabetes use insulin pumps. The preoperative visit is important in patients who use an insulin pump to establish the site of infusion, type of pump (**Table 2** shows some information on the most commonly used insulin pumps), formulation of insulin, and dosage regimen (basal and bolus) through the day. It would be useful to have an endocrinology consult to provide recommendations if changes are necessary preoperatively and to establish a relationship with patients and the caring team for inpatient management if patients are to be admitted to the hospital postoperatively.[37] Ideally this should be done a few days or weeks before an elective procedure. The basal dose of infusion is essential for maintenance of metabolic function in these patients. The recommendation is to maintain the basal dose during the preoperative fasting period, albeit reducing the dose by 10% to 20% in some situations, to reduce the risk of hypoglycemia.[38] For emergency procedures and for procedures lasting more than 3 hours, the insulin pump is disconnected and an external intravenous insulin infusion is run and titrated for target glycemic control.[37,38] **Fig. 2** shows a comprehensive plan for managing patients with an insulin pump starting with their preoperative visit to the preoperative preparation on the day of surgery and all the way through surgery.

COMPLICATIONS OF DIABETES AND THEIR ANESTHETIC IMPLICATIONS
The Airway and Musculoskeletal System in Diabetes Mellitus

Long-standing diabetes, especially type 1, when not well controlled, can lead to diabetic cheiroarthropathy. This condition is due to the accumulation of advanced glycation end products (AGE) and abnormal cross-linking of collagen in the joints.[39] Although joints of the hands and shoulders are commonly affected, the temporomandibular and cervical spine could be affected as well, leading to difficulty with laryngoscopy and intubation.[40] Approximately one-third of the patients with long-standing diabetes present with a difficult airway.[41] Stiff waxy hands and the presence of the prayer sign, wherein there is difficulty approximating the palms and bending fingers backwards, could indicate the presence of cheiroarthropathy and a potential difficult airway.[39] Advanced age, female sex, long duration of diabetes, poor glycemic control, and the presence of microvascular complications like neuropathy and retinopathy are associated with cheiroarthropathy.[39] A focused physical and airway examination in these patients would help identify a potential difficulty. Nonetheless, an encountered difficult airway is very rarely attributed to

Table 2
Insulin pumps

Manufacturer	Model	Reservoir	Basel Increment	Bolus Programming Methods	Battery Life	Battery Type
Animas (West Chester, PA)	OneTouch Ping Glucose Management System	200 plastic	0.025 unit	Menu, audio, vibrate, ezBolus	4–6 wk with lithium 2–4 wk with alkaline	1 AA lithium or 1 AA alkaline
Roche Insulin Delivery Systems, Inc (Ridgefield, CT)	ACCU-CHEK Spirit Insulin Pump System	315-unit Disposable plastic cartridge, system with integrated filling aid	0.1 unit	Menu, tactile Bolus (audible or vibrating)	appx 4 wk (alkaline), 1 wk (rechargeable)	One 1.5 v AA alkaline or NiMH AA rechargeable
Insulet Corporation (Billerica, MA)	OmniPod Insulin Management System	200-unit Reservoir integrated into Pod	0.05 unit	Menu	3 wk	2 AAA alkaline
Medtronic (Minneapolis, MN)	MiniMed Paradigm 522 MiniMed Paradigm 722	Disposable shock-resistant plastic	0.05 unit	Menu, remote and easy (audio) express	2–4 wk	One AAA alkaline; readily available
Nipro Diabetes Systems (Osaka, Japan)	Amigo	300-unit disposable plastic	0.05 unit	Audio, vibration or audio + vibration, via menu, or direct bolus	2–3 wk	1 Duracell, CR2

Abbreviations: appx, approximately; NiMH, nickel metal hydride.
Courtesy of Cleveland Clinic Center for Medical Art & Photography, Cleveland Clinic, Cleveland, Ohio © 2017. All Rights Reserved; with permission.

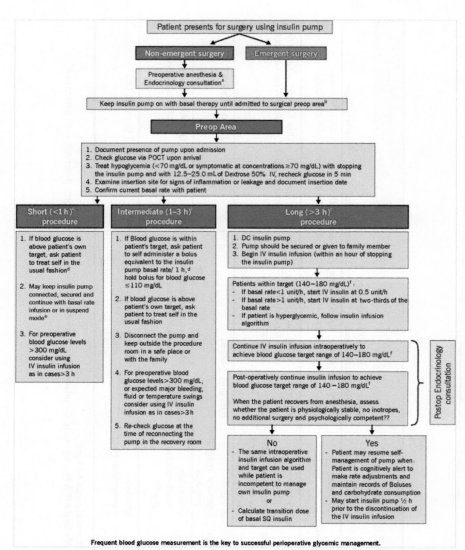

Fig. 2. Perioperative glycemic management in insulin pump patients undergoing noncardiac surgery. IV, intravenous; POCT, point-of-care testing; SQ, subcutaneous. [a] Patients scheduled for outpatient procedures may not require pre-operative endocrinology consult. [b] Do not withhold basal insulin if the patient is NPO. [c] The above stated duration, does not only include the procedure time, but spans the start of sedation/anesthesia till full recovery and patient judged competent to manage own pump. If patient's mental status is in question, disconnect the pump, and use an insulin infusion to manage blood glucose. [d] Before sedatives are administered. [e] Alternatively if there is expected X-ray, MRI, defibrillation shock exposure, disconnect the pump and keep outside the procedure room in a safe place or with the family. [f] Glucose target range may vary depending on the clinical situation and the Institution's policy. (*Courtesy of* Cleveland Clinic Center for Medical Art & Photography, Cleveland Clinic, Cleveland, Ohio © 2018. All Rights Reserved; with permission.)

diabetes, mostly because of other anatomic deformities, such as head and neck cancer.

MACROVASCULAR COMPLICATIONS
Coronary Artery Disease

Cardiovascular disease is a major contributor of mortality and morbidity in diabetic patients. Diabetes induces a proatherogenic procoagulant state by inhibiting nitric oxide, production of reactive oxygen species, increasing receptors for AGE, and impairing platelet function coupled with impaired fibrinolysis.[42] A combination of factors, including hypertension, hyperlipidemia, obesity, and uncontrolled BG, play a role in the accelerated atherosclerosis in these patients.[43,44] Heart failure, both systolic and diastolic, is more common in diabetic patients as compared with the nondiabetic population. Diabetes increases the risk of perioperative cardiac complications. Preoperative cardiac evaluation for noncardiac surgery in diabetic patients is done as per the AHA/ACC's 2014 guidelines. Diabetes mellitus requiring insulin has been recognized as one of the risk factors for the occurrence of a major adverse cardiac events in the perioperative period and is a component of the revised cardiac risk index for preoperative cardiac evaluation for noncardiac surgery.[45] Acute ischemic events could go unrecognized in these patients because of the existence of concomitant autonomic neuropathy, and increased vigilance to recognize them would serve well.

Peripheral Vascular Disease

Pathophysiologic factors that increase the risk of coronary artery disease also increase the risk of peripheral arterial disease (PAD) in diabetic patients. The prevalence of PAD in diabetic patients is about 20% with increasing age conferring a greater risk.[46] Presence of PAD in these patients might herald the presence of underlying coronary or cerebrovascular disease (CVD) with adverse cardiac and cerebrovascular events being more pronounced in diabetic patients with PAD than their counterparts.[46,47] Recognition of PAD in the preoperative period should alert the anesthesiologist of the potential for other cardiovascular manifestations and difficult invasive arterial access, due to increased arterial stiffness, should one be required.

Cerebrovascular Disease

The increased risk of atherosclerosis in diabetic patient translates to an increased risk of CVD as well. There is a high preponderance of all forms of stroke, especially ischemic stroke in young diabetic patients.[42] Depending on chronic glycemic control, diabetic patients could have impaired cerebrovascular reactivity under anesthesia.[48] Systemic inflammation, vascular smooth muscle dysfunction, and endothelial dysfunction play a pivotal role in the development of CVD in these patients.[49] Intraoperative hyperglycemia may worsen the sequelae of intraoperative neurologic insults. In the preoperative evaluation, looking for a history suggestive of CVD or carotid stenosis and maintaining adequate perfusion pressures may help minimize the risk of perioperative stroke.[50]

MICROVASCULAR COMPLICATIONS OF DIABETES
Diabetic Retinopathy

Diabetic retinopathy (DR) is the most common microvascular complication of diabetes. Retinopathy from diabetes could either be proliferative or nonproliferative. The presence of DR could signal the presence of long-term nephropathy.[51,52] Diabetic microangiopathy could result in capillary occlusion and retinal ischemia, which in turn increases the levels of vascular growth factors causing proliferative retinopathy. Vision loss from DR could result from maculopathy, vitreous hemorrhage, detachment, or neovascular glaucoma. Preoperative characterization of visual defects if any would be helpful, especially in cases whereby there is a potential for postoperative visual loss, such as spine surgery.

Diabetic Nephropathy

Diabetic nephropathy is characterized by albuminuria and progressive reduction of renal function. Diabetes is one of the primary causes for end-stage renal disease in the United States.[53] Preoperative evaluation of renal function might help strategize and develop a perioperative plan to reduce the risk of developing perioperative acute kidney injury (AKI). Nonsteroidal antiinflammatory drugs (NSAIDs) inhibit prostaglandins, impair renal blood flow, and worsen renal function.[54,55] It should be noted that selective cyclooxygenase-2 inhibitors could have a similar effect on renal function as well.[56] Patients with diabetes are commonly on medications that modulate the renin angiotensin aldosterone system (RAAS). A combination of hypovolemia, NSAIDs, and use of medications that modulate RAAS could have undesired consequences in these patients.[57] Efforts to maintain euvolemia, adequate renal perfusion, and avoidance of nephrotoxic medications should be considered to reduce the risk of AKI.

Autonomic Neuropathy

Diabetic autonomic neuropathy (DAN) primarily affects the cardiovascular and gastrointestinal systems. Although symptomatic autonomic neuropathy is rare in diabetic patients, recognition of its possibility is important so as to anticipate the adverse consequences in the perioperative period. Patients with DAN could be recognized from a history of inappropriate heart rate response to exercise and consequently poor exercise tolerance or from orthostatic blood pressure measurements. They could manifest with profound hypotension on induction due to poor vascular compensatory mechanisms. Sudden cardiac deaths due to dysrhythmias have been reported in these patients. During the preoperative visit, inquiring for symptoms of early satiety, bloating, and erectile dysfunction may help recognize underlying autonomic neuropathy. In patients in whom autonomic neuropathy is suspected, orthostatic blood pressure measurements might help corroborate the diagnosis. There are 5 tests that assess heart rate and blood pressure responses to various activities that have been validated to diagnose and quantify autonomic dysfunction, namely, heart rate response to Valsalva, standing and deep breathing to assess the parasympathetic system, and blood pressure response to standing and sustained hand grip to assess the sympathetic system. These are effective tests that are validated in preoperative clinic settings as well for screening patients for autonomic dysfunction, as long as the appropriate testing technique is used.[58] Typically in patients with DAN, parasympathetic dysfunction precedes sympathetic dysfunction.[58] The aforementioned tests could identify patients with DAN and, thus, assist the anesthesiologist in formulating an appropriate plan, such as considerations for invasive blood pressure monitoring and/or postoperative intensive care unit admission.

Gastrointestinal symptoms in patients with DAN affecting the gut present with nausea, vomiting, bloating, early satiety, and other symptoms suggestive of delayed gastric emptying.[33] Precautions to reduce the risk of aspiration on induction, including the use of prokinetic agents and H2 antagonists and/or proton pump inhibitors, may be prudent in patients who are symptomatic with long-standing or poorly controlled diabetes.[18] In severe cases of gastroparesis, the authors recommend awake intubation in a semisetting position versus intubation after induction of anesthesia (regardless of being conventional) or a rapid sequence induction with cricoid pressure. It seems that awake intubation may provide superior protection against aspiration through maintaining innate protective tracheal reflexes versus cricoid pressure that may or may not occlude the esophagus and, in some instances, make intubation more difficult.

Diabetic Peripheral Neuropathy

Distal symmetric polyneuropathy (DSPN) is the most common form accounting for about 75% of diabetic neuropathies. It occurs in 20% of patients with type 1 diabetes after 20 years of disease and 10% to 15% of patients with type 2 diabetes. Microvascular damage to the vasa nervosum and oxidative and inflammatory damage due to hyperglycemia are implicated in the pathogenesis of DSPN.[59,60] DSPN is the most important cause for diabetic foot ulceration and Charcot arthropathy. Initially small sensory fibers are involved, resulting in paresthesias and neuropathic pain. Later on, when larger fibers are involved, it could result in lack of painless paresthesias and loss of protective sensations.[59] Caution should be exercised while positioning patients with diabetic neuropathy, especially if they are insensate, to avoid causing pressure injuries or ulcerations to the extremities. Moreover, several factors need to be considered while performing regional anesthesia in patients with diabetic neuropathy. Common sense dictates that ultrasound-guided techniques may be favored in these patients, as the electric stimulation threshold is increased in diabetic neuropathy and there is an increased risk of stimulator needle trauma. Diabetic nerves are more sensitive to local anesthetics and result in prolonged block duration. There is an increase in the incidence of infection when nerve catheters are used for postoperative pain in patients with diabetes.[60]

SUMMARY

Diabetes is a systemic disease affecting several organ systems. There is a lack of consensus guidelines for the optimal perioperative management of these patients. It is prudent to use the preoperative visit as an opportunity to either diagnose undiagnosed diabetes or to check on and optimize the glycemic state of diagnosed diabetic patients. Diabetes-associated systemic complications should be investigated and optimized accordingly when needed. It is important to have an appropriate preoperative plan for management of pharmacotherapy, including subcutaneous insulin pump use to avoid both hypoglycemia and hyperglycemia on the day of surgery. Surgery for patients who present with DKA should be delayed (unless surgery is emergent), and patients should be treated and stabilized. Current evidence does not support canceling surgeries for a given abnormal HbA1c percentage. During the preoperative visit, a comprehensive perioperative plan for managing diabetes as outlined earlier and expectations should be formulated and shared with patients to assure them and alleviate their anxiety.

REFERENCES

1. for Disease Control C. National Diabetes Statistics Report, 2017 Estimates of Diabetes and Its Burden in the United States Background. 2017. Available at: https://www.cdc.gov/diabetes/pdfs/data/statistics/national-diabetes-statistics-report.pdf. Accessed March 6, 2018.
2. American Diabetes Association AD. Economic costs of diabetes in the U.S. in 2012. Diabetes Care 2013;36(4):1033–46.

3. American Diabetes Association AD. 2. Classification and diagnosis of diabetes: standards of medical care in diabetes-2018. Diabetes Care 2018;41(Suppl 1): S13–27.

4. Beagley J, Guariguata L, Weil C, et al. Global estimates of undiagnosed diabetes in adults. Diabetes Res Clin Pract 2014;103(2):150–60.

5. Abdelmalak B, Abdelmalak JB, Knittel J, et al. The prevalence of undiagnosed diabetes in non-cardiac surgery patients, an observational study. Can J Anesth 2010;57(12):1058–64.

6. Lauruschkat AH, Arnrich B, Albert AA, et al. Prevalence and risks of undiagnosed diabetes mellitus in patients undergoing coronary artery bypass grafting. Circulation 2005;112(16):2397–402.

7. Abdelmalak BB, Knittel J, Abdelmalak JB, et al. Preoperative blood glucose concentrations and postoperative outcomes after elective non-cardiac surgery: an observational study † †Preliminary results were presented at the American Society of Anesthesiologists Annual Meeting, October 18, 2010, in San Diego, CA, USA. Br J Anaesth 2014;112(1):79–88.

8. Abdelmalak BB, Lansang MC. Revisiting tight glycemic control in perioperative and critically ill patients: when one size may not fit all. J Clin Anesth 2013; 25(6):499–507.

9. American Diabetes Association AD. 6. Glycemic targets: standards of medical care in diabetes-2018. Diabetes Care 2018;41(Suppl 1):S55–64.

10. Qaseem A, Wilt TJ, Kansagara D, et al. Hemoglobin A $_{1c}$ targets for glycemic control with pharmacologic therapy for nonpregnant adults with type 2 diabetes mellitus: a guidance statement update from the American College of Physicians. Ann Intern Med 2018;168(8):569.

11. American Diabetes Association AD. 14. diabetes care in the hospital: standards of medical care in diabetes-2018. Diabetes Care 2018;41(Suppl 1):S144–51.

12. Umpierrez G, Cardona S, Pasquel F, et al. Randomized controlled trial of intensive versus conservative glucose control in patients undergoing coronary artery bypass graft surgery: GLUCO-CABG trial. Diabetes Care 2015;38(9):1665–72.

13. Sathya B, Davis R, Taveira T, et al. Intensity of peri-operative glycemic control and postoperative outcomes in patients with diabetes: a meta-analysis. Diabetes Res Clin Pract 2013;102(1):8–15.

14. Ata A, Lee J, Bestle SL, et al. Postoperative hyperglycemia and surgical site infection in general surgery patients. Arch Surg 2010;145(9):858.

15. Martin ET, Kaye KS, Knott C, et al. Diabetes and risk of surgical site infection: a systematic review and meta-analysis. Infect Control Hosp Epidemiol 2016;37(1): 88–99.

16. Frisch A, Chandra P, Smiley D, et al. Prevalence and clinical outcome of hyperglycemia in the perioperative period in noncardiac surgery. Diabetes Care 2010;33(8):1783–8.

17. Desborough JP. The stress response to trauma and surgery. Br J Anaesth 2000; 85(1):109–17.

18. Moitra VK, Meiler SE. The diabetic surgical patient. Curr Opin Anaesthesiol 2006; 19(3):339–45.

19. Abdelmalak BB, Bonilla AM, Yang D, et al. The hyperglycemic response to major noncardiac surgery and the added effect of steroid administration in patients with and without diabetes. Anesth Analg 2013;116(5):1116–22.

20. Cryer PE. Severe hypoglycemia predicts mortality in diabetes. Diabetes Care 2012;35(9):1814–6.

21. Kalra S, Bajwa SJS, Baruah M, et al. Hypoglycaemia in anesthesiology practice: diagnostic, preventive, and management strategies. Saudi J Anaesth 2013;7(4): 447–52.
22. Sebranek JJ, Lugli AK, Coursin DB. Glycaemic control in the perioperative period. Br J Anaesth 2013;111:i18–34.
23. Peri-operative diabetes management guidelines Australian diabetes society. 2012. Available at: http://diabetessociety.com.au/documents/Perioperative DiabetesManagementGuidelinesFINALCleanJuly2012.pdf. Accessed April 26, 2018.
24. Barker P, Creasey PE, Dhatariya K, et al. Peri-operative management of the surgical patient with diabetes 2015. Anaesthesia 2015;70(12):1427–40.
25. Underwood P, Askari R, Hurwitz S, et al. Preoperative A1C and clinical outcomes in patients with diabetes undergoing major noncardiac surgical procedures. Diabetes Care 2014;37(3):611–6.
26. Giori NJ, Ellerbe LS, Bowe T, et al. Many diabetic total joint arthroplasty candidates are unable to achieve a preoperative hemoglobin A1c goal of 7% or less. J Bone Joint Surg Am 2014;96(6):500–4.
27. Fasanmade OA, Odeniyi IA, Ogbera AO. Diabetic ketoacidosis: diagnosis and management. Afr J Med Med Sci 2008;37(2):99–105. Available at: http://www.ncbi.nlm.nih.gov/pubmed/18939392. Accessed April 30, 2018.
28. Akhtar S, Barash PG, Inzucchi SE. Scientific principles and clinical implications of perioperative glucose regulation and control. Anesth Analg 2010;110(2):478–97.
29. Kitabchi AE, Umpierrez GE, Murphy MB, et al. Management of hyperglycemic crises in patients with diabetes. Diabetes Care 2001;24(1):131–53. Available at: http://www.ncbi.nlm.nih.gov/pubmed/11194218. Accessed April 30, 2018.
30. American Diabetes Association AD. 8. Pharmacologic approaches to glycemic treatment: standards of medical care in diabetes-2018. Diabetes Care 2018; 41(Suppl 1):S73–85.
31. Vann MA. Management of diabetes medications for patients undergoing ambulatory surgery. Anesthesiol Clin 2014;32(2):329–39.
32. Nazer RI, Alburikan KA. Metformin is not associated with lactic acidosis in patients with diabetes undergoing coronary artery bypass graft surgery: a case control study. BMC Pharmacol Toxicol 2017;18(1):38.
33. Pontes JPJ, Mendes FF, Vasconcelos MM, et al. Avaliação e manejo perioperatório de pacientes com diabetes melito. Um desafio para o anestesiologista. Braz J Anesthesiol 2018;68(1):75–86.
34. Demma LJ, Carlson KT, Duggan EW, et al. Effect of basal insulin dosage on blood glucose concentration in ambulatory surgery patients with type 2 diabetes. J Clin Anesth 2017;36:184–8.
35. Joshi GP, Chung F, Vann MA, et al. Society for ambulatory anesthesia consensus statement on perioperative blood glucose management in diabetic patients undergoing ambulatory surgery. Anesth Analg 2010;111(6):1378–87.
36. Dhatariya K, Levy N, Kilvert A, et al. NHS Diabetes guideline for the perioperative management of the adult patient with diabetes. Diabet Med 2012;29(4):420–33.
37. Partridge H, Perkins B, Mathieu S, et al. Clinical recommendations in the management of the patient with type 1 diabetes on insulin pump therapy in the perioperative period: a primer for the anaesthetist. Br J Anaesth 2016;116(1):18–26.
38. Abdelmalak B, Ibrahim M, Yared J-P, et al. Perioperative glycemic management in insulin pump patients undergoing noncardiac surgery. Curr Pharm Des 2012; 18(38):6204–14. Available at: http://www.ncbi.nlm.nih.gov/pubmed/22762462. Accessed April 19, 2018.

39. Larkin ME, Barnie A, Braffett BH, et al. Musculoskeletal complications in type 1 diabetes. Diabetes Care 2014;37(7):1863–9.

40. Erden V, Basaranoglu G, Delatioglu H, et al. Relationship of difficult laryngoscopy to long-term non-insulin-dependent diabetes and hand abnormality detected using the "prayer sign. Br J Anaesth 2003;91(1):159–60.

41. Hogan K, Rusy D, Springman SR. Difficult laryngoscopy and diabetes mellitus. Anesth Analg 1988;67(12):1162–5. Available at: http://www.ncbi.nlm.nih.gov/pubmed/3057934. Accessed April 24, 2018.

42. Beckman JA, Creager MA, Libby P. Diabetes and atherosclerosis. JAMA 2002; 287(19):2570.

43. Kanter JE, Averill MM, Leboeuf RC, et al. Diabetes-accelerated atherosclerosis and inflammation. Circ Res 2008;103(8):e116–7.

44. Selvin E, Coresh J, Golden SH, et al. Glycemic control, atherosclerosis, and risk factors for cardiovascular disease in individuals with diabetes: the atherosclerosis risk in communities study. Diabetes Care 2005;28(8):1965–73. Available at: http://www.ncbi.nlm.nih.gov/pubmed/16043740. Accessed April 25, 2018.

45. Fleisher LA, Fleischmann KE, Auerbach AD, et al. 2014 ACC/AHA guideline on perioperative cardiovascular evaluation and management of patients undergoing noncardiac surgery: a report of the American College of Cardiology/American Heart Association Task Force on Practice Guidelines. Circulation 2014;130(24): e278–333.

46. Thiruvoipati T, Kielhorn CE, Armstrong EJ. Peripheral artery disease in patients with diabetes: epidemiology, mechanisms, and outcomes. World J Diabetes 2015;6(7):961–9.

47. American Diabetes Association. Peripheral arterial disease in people with diabetes. Diabetes Care 2003;26(12):3333–41. Available at: http://www.ncbi.nlm. nih.gov/pubmed/14633825. Accessed April 25, 2018.

48. Kadoi Y, Hinohara H, Kunimoto F, et al. Diabetic patients have an impaired cerebral vasodilatory response to hypercapnia under propofol anesthesia patients and methods. Stroke 2003;34:2399–403.

49. Chen R, Ovbiagele B, Feng W. Diabetes and stroke: epidemiology, pathophysiology, pharmaceuticals and outcomes. Am J Med Sci 2016;351(4):380–6.

50. Ng JLW, Chan MTV, Gelb AW. Perioperative stroke in noncardiac, nonneurosurgical surgery. Anesthesiology 2011;115(4):879–90.

51. Nentwich MM, Ulbig MW. Diabetic retinopathy - ocular complications of diabetes mellitus. World J Diabetes 2015;6(3):489–99.

52. Solomon SD, Chew E, Duh EJ, et al. Diabetic retinopathy: a position statement by the American Diabetes Association. Diabetes Care 2017;40(3):412–8.

53. Kazancioğlu R. Risk factors for chronic kidney disease: an update. Kidney Int Suppl 2013;3(4):368–71.

54. Clive DM, Stoff JS. Renal syndromes associated with nonsteroidal antiinflammatory drugs. N Engl J Med 1984;310(9):563–72.

55. Sivarajan M, Wasse L. Perioperative acute renal failure associated with preoperative intake of ibuprofen. Anesthesiology 1997;86(6):1390–2.

56. Perazella MA, Tray K. Selective cyclooxygenase-2 inhibitors: a pattern of nephrotoxicity similar to traditional nonsteroidal anti-inflammatory drugs. Am J Med 2001;111(1):64–7. Available at: http://www.ncbi.nlm.nih.gov/pubmed/11448662. Accessed April 25, 2018.

57. Lapi F, Azoulay L, Yin H, et al. Concurrent use of diuretics, angiotensin converting enzyme inhibitors, and angiotensin receptor blockers with non-steroidal anti-

inflammatory drugs and risk of acute kidney injury: nested case-control study. BMJ 2013;346:e8525.

58. Glick DB. The autonomic nervous system. In: Miller RD, Cohen NH, Eriksson LI, editors. Miller's Anesthesia. 8th edition. Philadelphia: Elsevier Saunders; 2015. p. 346–86.

59. Pop-Busui R, Boulton AJM, Feldman EL, et al. Diabetic neuropathy: a position statement by the American Diabetes Association. Diabetes Care 2017;40(1): 136–54.

60. ten Hoope W, Looije M, Lirk P. Regional anesthesia in diabetic peripheral neuropathy. Curr Opin Anaesthesiol 2017;30(5):627–31.

Preoperative Management of the Geriatric Patient
Frailty and Cognitive Impairment Assessment

Allison Dalton, MD[a],*, Zdravka Zafirova, MD[b]

KEYWORDS

• Frailty • Sarcopenia • Geriatric • Preoperative evaluation • Surgery

KEY POINTS

• Geriatric patients undergoing surgery benefit from age-specific preoperative evaluation, including evaluation for frailty, functional status, sarcopenia, and nutritional status.

• Geriatric patients are at increased risk for cardiovascular, pulmonary, renal, hepatic, and endocrine comorbidities.

• Identification of specific age-related comorbidities and geriatric syndromes allows for preoperative intervention, which can improve postoperative outcomes.

INTRODUCTION

In 2014, 15% of the US population was 65 years or older, and this percentage is expected to increase to more than 20% by 2030.[1] Geriatric patients, those 65 years or older, account for 43% of all hospital days, 35% of inpatient procedures, and 32% of outpatient procedures, resulting in a higher rate of surgical procedures than any other age group.[2–4] In addition to normal physiologic changes of aging, many pathologic conditions that contribute to elevated perioperative risk are more common in the geriatric patient, including neurocognitive disturbances, atherosclerosis, cancer, degenerative joint disease, cataracts, and prostatism.[5] Advanced age is a risk factor for prolonged postoperative length of stay, as well as postoperative morbidity and mortality.[6–8]

SURGICAL STRESS

Surgery results in activation of the sympathetic nervous system. After activation of the hypothalamus, epinephrine and norepinephrine are released from the adrenal medulla. Within the cardiovascular system, the increase in circulating catecholamines may result

Disclosure Statement: The authors have no disclosures.
[a] Department of Anesthesia and Critical Care, University of Chicago, 5041 South Maryland Avenue, MC 4028, Chicago, IL 60637, USA; [b] Section Critical Care, Department of Cardiovascular Surgery, Mount Sinai Hospital System, Icahn School of Medicine, Mount Sinai Medical Center, Box 1028, 1 Gustave L. Levy Place, New York, NY 10029, USA
* Corresponding author.
E-mail address: adalton@dacc.uchicago.edu

Anesthesiology Clin 36 (2018) 599–614
https://doi.org/10.1016/j.anclin.2018.07.008   anesthesiology.theclinics.com
1932-2275/18/© 2018 Elsevier Inc. All rights reserved.

in hypertension, tachycardia, and occasionally dysrhythmias.[9] For patients with known or covert cardiac comorbidities, these effects may predispose them to myocardial ischemia from demand-supply imbalance due to increased oxygen demand or coronary vasospasm and plaque disruption.[10] Activation of the hypothalamic-pituitary-adrenal axis leads to secretion of growth hormone, which results in decreases in protein breakdown and stimulates protein synthesis in addition to promoting lipolysis.[9] Growth hormone increases serum glucose levels by stimulating glycogenolysis and inhibits glucose uptake by cells. Adrenocorticotropic hormone (ACTH) is released by the anterior pituitary gland in response to stress. ACTH stimulates the release of cortisol from the adrenal cortex. Cortisol promotes protein breakdown and lipolysis.[9] In addition, surgical stress induces a relative insulin resistance (**Fig. 1**).

When tissue injury occurs, macrophages, fibroblasts, endothelial and glial cells release interleukins (ILs), interferons (IFNs), and tumor necrosis factor-alpha (TNF-α), inducing a proinflammatory state.[9] Increased cytokine production leads to increases in acute phase reactants, C-reactive protein, and complement and coagulation proteins.[9] Cytokines may also enhance the release of cortisol. Additional clinical effects include fever, hemostasis, and promotion of healing. Despite the depressed immune function related to aging, geriatric patients have been shown to have twofold to fourfold higher levels of proinflammatory cytokines present and prolonged effect after surgical stress.[10]

GERIATRIC SYNDROMES AND FUNCTIONAL ASSESSMENT

Specific geriatric conditions require unique consideration before elective surgery. A comprehensive geriatric assessment (CGA) has shown efficacy in improving mortality and prolonging independent living in nonsurgical geriatric patients.[11] The CGA is an evaluation of an elderly person's medical, psychosocial, functional, and environmental resources.[11] Following full assessment, a plan for management and follow-up is created and enacted. A full CGA is time-consuming and may not be practical for routine preoperative evaluation[12]; furthermore, the efficacy of its routine use in perioperative patients has not been fully established. However, focused evaluation of geriatric-specific domains should be performed. A geriatric assessment should include aspects of risk estimation, patient's decision-making capacity, preoperative optimization, anesthetic and surgical planning, perioperative surveillance, and postoperative and discharge planning.[12,13]

Frailty

Frailty is a geriatric syndrome that is characterized as decreased reserve and resistance to stressors as a result of physiologic decline.[14] There is no gold standard tool for the diagnosis of frailty. Multiple screening tools are available, including the Modified Frailty Index, Edmonton Frailty Scale, Rockwood-Robinson Frailty Index, and Fried Frailty Phenotype[10,12,15] (**Table 1**). Fried and colleagues[14] identified a standard phenotype of frailty that is characterized by shrinking, weakness, poor endurance, slow walking speed, and low physical activity levels. If 3 or more of the preceding criteria are present, the diagnosis of frailty may be made.[13] In geriatric patients, the prevalence of frailty is approximately 10%; it increases to 26% to 45% in patients 85 years and older and is as high as 46% in geriatric patients with cancer.[12] Frailty is associated with increased risk of postoperative complications, longer hospital stay, higher rate of discharge to a facility, and mortality.[15-17] Robinson and colleagues[18] suggested another set of criteria for the presence of frailty: Mini-Cog score, albumin, history of falls, hematocrit, assessment of activities of daily living

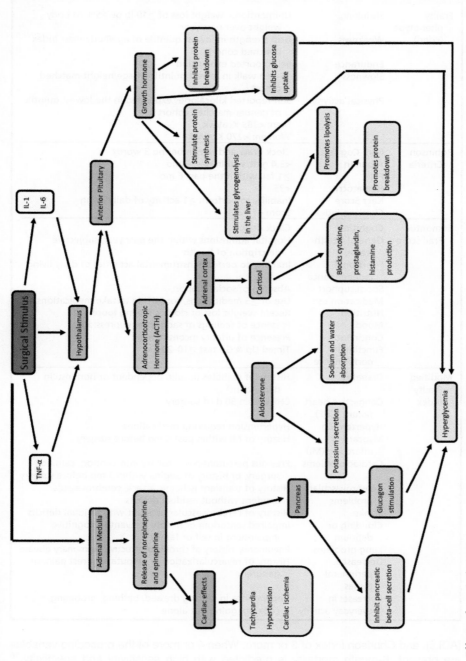

Fig. 1. Effects of surgical stress.

Table 1 Elements of various frailty screening tools		
Frailty phenotype (Fried)	Shrinking	Unintentional weight loss of ≥10 lb or ≥5% of body weight over past year
	Weakness	Grip strength in lowest quintile of age/body mass index matched cohort
	Endurance	Self-reported exhaustion
	Slowness	15-min walk in lowest quintile of age/height-matched cohort
	Physical activity	Self-reported kilocalories expended in the lowest quintile of gender-matched cohort Men: <383 Kcal/wk Women: <270 Kcal/wk
Robinson Criteria	Mini-Cog Test	Clock draw and remembering 3 words
	Albumin	<3.4 g/dL within past 3 mo
	Fall	≥1 fall within the past 6 mo
	Hematocrit	<35
	Katz Score	Inability to perform ≥1 activity of daily living
	Charlson Index	Score of ≥3
Edmonton Frail score	Cognition	Clock draw
	General health status	Hospital admissions within the past year, subjective description of health
	Functional independence	Inability to perform instrumental activities of daily living
	Social support	Absence of social support
	Medication use	Use of ≥5 medications, forgetting to take medications
	Nutrition	Recent weight loss or clothes feeling loose
	Mood	Presence of feelings of sadness or depression
	Continence	Presence of urinary incontinence
	Functional performance	Timed Up & Go test ≥10–20 s
Modified Frailty Index	Diabetes	History of diabetes (insulin dependent or non-insulin dependent)
	Congestive heart failure (CHF)	CHF within 30 d of surgery
	Hypertension	Hypertension requiring medications
	Myocardial infarction (MI)	History of MI within past 6 mo before surgery
	Cardiac problems	Previous percutaneous coronary intervention, cardiac surgery, or history of angina within 1 mo before surgery
	Cerebrovascular problems	History of transient ischemic attack, cerebrovascular accident without residual deficits
	Stroke	History of cerebrovascular accident with residual deficits
	Clouding or delirium	Impaired sensorium or history relevant to cognitive impairment in self or family
	Lung problems	Pneumonia, history of chronic obstructive pulmonary disease
	Decreased peripheral pulses	History of revascularization or amputation, rest pain, or gangrene
	Decreases in everyday activity	Dependence in getting dressed, bathing, grooming, cooking, going out alone

(ADLs), and Charlson index of 3 or more. When 4 or more of the preceding variables are present, 6-month mortality is predicted with high sensitivity and specificity.[18] Despite recognition of frailty as a common geriatric syndrome and improved ability to diagnose the condition, it is unclear whether the risks associated with preoperative frailty are modifiable.[13] The Society for Perioperative Assessment and Quality Improvement has published recommendations for the perioperative management of frailty, including preoperative assessment and perioperative interventions.[19]

Functional Status

Poor preoperative exercise tolerance is associated with postoperative surgical site infection, postoperative pulmonary complications, increased unanticipated hospital discharge to nursing home, and mortality.[10,18,20] Postoperative impaired mobility is associated with delirium, thromboembolism, and postoperative pulmonary and surgical site infections.[13,21] Evaluation of a geriatric patient's ability to perform the Katz ADL and Instrumental ADL (IADL) can determine his or her level of independent function.[13] Although not associated with increase in perioperative morbidity and mortality, patient dependence for ADLs and IADLs may contribute to overall risk assessment and prediction of mobility problems postoperatively.[12,13] The Timed Up and Go test identifies patients with deficits in strength, mobility, balance, and those at increased risk of fall.[13] In this examination, a patient is timed to determine how long it takes for him or her to rise from a seated position, walk 10 feet across a room, turn around, return to the chair, and sit back down. A score longer than 15 seconds is associated with increased perioperative mortality.[22] For patients with deficits in function status as determined by assessment of ADLs, IADLs, or the Timed Up and Go test, perioperative interventions to minimize fall risk and to coordinate hospital discharge to rehabilitation or nursing home can be instituted for appropriate patients.[13]

Prehabilitation

Prehabilitation is the process of initiating a preoperative exercise program including aspects of strength and/or endurance training. Although prehabilitation has mixed results in geriatric surgical patients, there is evidence that specific groups may benefit. In sarcopenic and frail patients, resistance exercise training may improve lean tissue mass, muscle strength, aerobic capacity, 6-minute walk, perceived quality of life, functional independence, gait balance, and may decrease risk of falls.[23] Patients with planned orthopedic surgery may have improved functional recovery after prehabilitation.[24] Prehabilitation is associated with decreased incidence of pneumonia and decreased length of stay in some patient populations.[25] However, association with improved survival postoperatively[13] has not been consistently demonstrated. In the geriatric patient, exercise programs designed to improve cardiovascular function may require 12 or more weeks to observe measurable benefit.[23] Given the lack of supportive studies regarding preoperative exercise programs, prehabilitation cannot be uniformly recommended for risk modification of geriatric-related sarcopenia, frailty, or decreased functional status.

Sarcopenia

Sarcopenia is a geriatric syndrome of progressive and generalized loss of skeletal muscle and strength[26] and in patients 80 years and older, it may be present in as many as half of the patients.[27] Sarcopenia is typically measured by taking an axial cross-section of the psoas muscle on computed tomography at the level of the L3 vertebral body. This syndrome is more specific to the diagnosis of frailty than is weight loss or nutritional status alone.[26] Sarcopenia is an independent predictor of morbidity (ie, infection, pressure ulcers, loss of autonomy, discharge to facility, and decreased quality of life) and mortality in hospitalized patients.[28]

Malnutrition

Surgery results in a hypermetabolic state. Elderly patients are at increased risk for malnutrition due to physiologic, social, and economic causes.[12] Malnutrition rates in the elderly can range from approximately 6% in the community to 14% in nursing home patients, and nearly 40% in hospitalized patients.[29] In addition to simple age-related malnutrition, patients with chronic illness may have coexisting cachexia. Cachexia is a metabolic syndrome associated with chronic illness that leads to weight loss.[15] In chronic illness, increases in inflammatory mediators (ie, IL-1, IL-6, TNF-α) result in lipolysis, muscle breakdown, and anorexia.[30] Malnourished patients are at increased risk of postoperative infections, poor wound healing, and increased hospital length of stay, and malnutrition may be an independent risk factor for postoperative mortality.[13,24] Multiple assessment tools including the Subjective Global Assessment, Nutritional Risk Screening, and Mini Nutritional Assessment instrument may assist in diagnosing geriatric patients with malnutrition.[13,24] Other markers of nutritional status may be valuable in efficient preoperative evaluation for nutrition including documentation of height, weight, and recent weight loss. Albumin and prealbumin are markers for nutritional status. Preoperative albumin levels predict postoperative outcomes including 30-day mortality.[10] Given its shorter half-life, prealbumin may be a better indicator of recent nutritional status.[10] In addition, prealbumin levels are less affected by changes in volume status, and, therefore, may be more reliable than serum albumin in patients on diuretics or dialysis.[10] Hypoprealbuminemia is predictive for postoperative morbidity (ie, infection, length of mechanical ventilation) and mortality.[10]

Patients with malnutrition on initial screening may benefit from evaluation by a dietician before elective surgery.[13] In malnourished surgical oncology patients, preoperative nutritional optimization may result in lower incidence of postoperative infection.[31] Klek and colleagues[32] have shown that despite aggressive preoperative nutritional replacement with enteral or parenteral nutrition, albumin levels will likely not improve, and the incidence of other complications may not decrease. The risk of malnutrition does not decrease following surgery. Sungurtekin and colleagues[33] showed that rates of malnutrition increased by approximately 20% during hospitalization after abdominal surgery. Therefore, postoperatively, adequate nutrition should be ensured. Malnourished patients should be assessed and aggressively treated for refeeding syndrome postoperatively.[13]

NEUROPHYSIOLOGY

As the brain ages, there is loss of both volume and weight of approximately 5% for every decade after age 40. At age 70, the rate of loss increases until approximately the age of 86.[34] There is a greater loss in gray matter than white.[35] Neuronal cell loss and changes in the blood-brain barrier account for at least a portion of the white matter death.[35,36] As the brain ages, neurotransmitter communication declines. Decreases in dopamine levels in the brain are associated with cognitive and motor deficits.[36] As serotonin levels decrease, there is evidence of decreased synaptic plasticity.[37] Neurogenesis decreases with aging and limits the ability to learn and may contribute to cognitive decline.[38] As patients age, multiple markers of brain function decline, including processing speed, reasoning ability, memory, and spatial cognitive abilities.[35,36] Physiologic changes in the neurologic system may predispose patients to postoperative cognitive complications.

Postoperative Delirium

Postoperative delirium (POD) is a disorder heralded by fluctuating course of impaired attention and disorganized thinking. Typically, delirium manifests early in the

Box 1
Risk factors for postoperative delirium

Patient Factors

Age $\geq$70 years

Poor nutrition

Polypharmacy

Lower education level

Poor functional status

Dehydration

Hearing or vision impairments

Hospital Environment

Sleep deprivation

Immobilization/physical restraints

Urinary catheter use

Inadequately controlled pain

Urinary retention/constipation

Hypoperfusion

Comorbidities

Cognitive impairment/dementia

Depression

Renal insufficiency

Sepsis

Critical illness

Cerebrovascular disease

Systemic vascular disease

Anemia

Alcohol use/withdrawal

Laboratory Findings

Hypoxia

Electrolyte abnormalities

Hypoglycemia

Medications

Penicillins

Sedatives/tranquilizers

Anticholinergic medications

Vasoactive agents

Histamine antagonists

postoperative course and may last days to weeks.[15] Delirium is a common postoperative complication with an incidence of 35% to 73%.[10,15,39] POD is thought to be caused by an absolute or relative decrease in acetylcholine or dopamine.[40] Elevated inflammation associated with major surgery may predispose to POD.[35] Galanakis and colleagues[41] found that higher age, depression, low educational level, and abnormal preoperative sodium, potassium, or glucose levels also correlated with increased incidence of POD.[42] There are multiple other risk factors for the development of delirium, as presented in **Box 1**. POD is associated with postoperative cognitive dysfunction (POCD), increased health care costs, increased hospital length of stay, increased likelihood of discharge to long-term care or rehabilitation facilities, and death.[39,42] Delirium likely is underreported, given the lack of standardized detection strategies especially for hypoactive delirium.[13] Despite its wide-reaching correlation with morbidity and mortality and its high prevalence in postoperative patients, there are few data supporting effective treatment for this disorder. Current clinical practices focus on avoidance of inciting factors, including minimizing sleep disturbances, encouraging use of hearing or vision assistance devices, avoidance of medications that result in cognitive depression, and ensuring adequate hydration.[13]

Postoperative Cognitive Dysfunction

POCD refers to impairment of memory, concentration, and social integration that first becomes evident days to weeks after surgery.[15] Symptoms of POCD tend to be milder than those of POD, but deficits may become permanent. Following noncardiac surgery, as many as 25% of geriatric patients demonstrate POCD.[43] At 3 months postoperatively, 10% of patients still were symptomatic.[43] Risk factors for POCD include multiple comorbidities and poor functional status.[15] POCD is associated with postoperative morbidity and mortality.[15] POCD is difficult to accurately diagnose and requires formal neurocognitive testing to evaluate for potentially subtle changes.[35] Even when the diagnosis is made, there is no standard treatment for POCD.[15]

Neurocognitive Assessment

It is estimated that approximately 14% of those older than 71 years have dementia, with an additional 22% of elderly patients with nondementia cognitive dysfunction.[44] Dementia in geriatric patients is associated with increased risk of morbidity and mortality.[44] This cognitive dysfunction may have perioperative effects, including reliability of medical history and diminished decision-making capabilities. The detection of preoperative cognitive dysfunction may assist in postoperative anticipation of delirium and function dependence.[10]

Preoperative Evaluation

Multiple evaluation methods exist for determining the presence of preoperative cognitive dysfunction. The Mini Mental Status Examination and the Montreal Cognitive Assessment test are 30-question validated tools to assess cognitive function. Given their length, they may be too time-consuming in a standard preoperative visit. The American College of Surgeons (ACS) and the American Geriatrics Society (AGS) recommend the implementation of The Mini-Cog assessment, a validated tool that allows for brief (3-minute) assessment of attention and executive function.[45,46]

CARDIOVASCULAR PHYSIOLOGY

Cardiovascular complications are the most common cause of perioperative death in the geriatric patient.[47] This may be a result of the physiologic changes in the cardiovascular system with aging, as well as the increased incidence of comorbid cardiovascular pathology.[15]

Vascular System

As a patient ages, arterial stiffness increases secondary to depleted elastin being replaced by collagen and calcium within the arterial walls.[48] The resulting systolic hypertension syndrome results in elevated systolic blood pressures with preserved or even diminished diastolic blood pressure in the geriatric patient.[49] In addition, with the decreased distensibility of arterial structures, there is a heightened nonlaminar and turbulent flow, leading to increased sheer force on the vascular walls,[50] which along with the widened pulse pressure leads to loss of the well-timed reflection of pulse waves resulting in decreased diastolic coronary artery filling. Aortic pulse wave velocity has been shown to be an important biomarker for arterial stiffness and an independent factor for cardiac risk.[48] With decreases in vascular relaxation, there is increased vascular permeability and vascular inflammation.[48] Age-related decline in vascular relaxation leads to elevated vascular expression of angiotensin II and aldosterone, which have been implicated in promoting vascular hypertrophy and fibrosis.[48,51] In addition to vascular remodeling, aging results in decreased production of nitric oxide (NO), increased generation of reactive oxygen species, stimulation of proinflammatory and profibrotic pathways, and extracellular matrix remodeling.[48] Diminished NO may be a result of deficiency in NO substrates and cofactors, presence of endogenous endothelial NO synthase (eNOS) inhibitors, and lower expression or activity of eNOS.[51] Decreased NO in the peripheral vessels may lead to additional organ dysfunction.[36] Increased oxidative stress in the sedentary geriatric patient results in decreased NO bioavailability, which can be counteracted by lifelong physical activity.[51]

Left Ventricular Function

In response to the decreased compliance of the arterial system, hypertrophy of the left ventricle (LV) develops. Resting diastolic filling of the LV decreases, but end-diastolic volume remains the same as in younger patients. The atrial contraction likely has a larger role in diastolic filling of the LV and atrial arrhythmias (ie, atrial fibrillation and flutter) may be more clinically significant in geriatric patients.[50] Although it is now believed that cardiac output and ejection fraction (EF) remain relatively constant as one ages, stroke volume decreases over time.[50] As cardiac muscle ages, some myocytes increase in size, whereas others are replaced with collagen, resulting in an overall increase in mass, albeit less functional. Due to fibrosis and myocardial hypertrophy, LV end-systolic volume (LVESV) and LV end-diastolic volume (LVEDV) both decrease with age. Because the LVEDV decreases more than the LVESV, the overall resting stroke volume decreases.[50] Despite previous assumptions that geriatric patients may respond similarly to surgical stress secondary to preserved EF, the increase in LV mass-to-volume ratio is associated with increased risk of cardiovascular complications.[50]

Right Ventricular Function

In the ideal system, right ventricle (RV) output would equal LV output. As the heart ages, the RV suffers from both systolic and diastolic dysfunction. Reduced systolic function is evident in echocardiographic evaluation of tricuspid annual plane systolic excursion (TAPSE), which is a marker for longitudinal contraction of the RV. With age, TAPSE decreases significantly as a result of increased pulmonary artery resistance.[50] Increases in pulmonary artery pressures may lead to diastolic dysfunction as evidenced by progressive decreases in early to late ventricular filling velocity (E/A) ratio on echocardiography.[52]

Sympathetic Nervous System and Cardiac Response

As a patient ages, there is an increase in sympathetic nervous system activity, resulting in higher circulating levels of norepinephrine.[36] Despite higher catecholamine levels, geriatric patients have a decreased response to them secondary to a decrease in adenylate cyclase coupling rather than due to decrease in the number of beta receptors.[53] Geriatric patients are most likely to exhibit lower intrinsic heart rate, maximal heart rate, and decreased chronotropic and inotropic response to endogenous and exogenous catecholamines.[53] The decreases in maximal heart rate to maintain cardiac output ensure that older patients will depend more heavily on increases in stroke volume than their younger counterparts.[50] When exposed to surgical stress, geriatric patients are shown to have significantly lower cardiac index, heart rate, and oxygen delivery.[54]

Preoperative Evaluation

The preoperative management of geriatric patients requires assessment of cardiovascular risk and risk reduction. ACS/AGS guidelines recommend evaluation of perioperative risk on the basis of the American College of Cardiology (ACC) and American Heart Association (AHA) guidelines for noncardiac surgery.[46,55] Risk calculators may be of additional assistance such as the National Surgical Quality Improvement Program (NSQIP) risk calculator: a validated tool using basic patient information, including age, sex, functional status, American Society of Anesthesiologists (ASA) class, body mass index, and patient comorbidities to determine individualized scores for risk.[56] Specific outcomes include pneumonia, cardiac complications, surgical site infection, urinary tract infection, renal failure, return to OR, death and other serious complications.[56]

Due to the increased incidence of cardiac comorbidities in the geriatric patient, thorough history and physical examination should be performed seeking signs and/or symptoms of coronary artery disease, systolic and diastolic heart failure, valvular abnormalities, and arrhythmias. Preoperative testing should take into account patient history, physical examination findings and the AHA/ACC guidelines for perioperative testing for noncardiac surgery.

RESPIRATORY PHYSIOLOGY

Among adults age 65 and older, lower respiratory tract disease is the third leading cause of death.[57] Approximately 15% of geriatric patients will experience postoperative pulmonary complications leading to increased morbidity and mortality.[58] Geriatric patients experience decreases in respiratory drive and diminished sensitivity to hypercapnia and hypoxia. Consequently, there is a higher incidence of central sleep apnea as compared with younger patients. Increased sensitivity to respiratory depressants further complicates this issue.[15]

Chest Wall

As patients age, the thoracic intervertebral disks spaces shorten resulting in kyphosis. Subsequently, intercostal spaces narrow, leading to altered intercostal muscle mechanics. As a consequence, fraction of exhaled volume over 1 second (FEV1) and forced vital capacity decrease as much as 30 mL per year.[59] In addition to structural changes, respiratory muscle mass and strength decrease with age leading to decreased ability to respond appropriately to increases in metabolic demand.[60]

Lung Parenchyma

With age, loss of parenchymal elasticity leads to increased lung compliance and decrease in lung elastic recoil.[60] Alterations in the organization of elastic fibers of the lung parenchyma result in enlargement of air spaces and reduction in alveolar surface area leading to decreases in diffusing lung capacity for carbon monoxide of up to 5% per decade.[60]

Airway

Geriatric patients tend to have shorter thyromental distance, smaller interincisor gaps, and higher Mallampati score that their younger counterparts.[60] Cervical degenerative disc disease and arthritis may lead to decreases in neck range of motion.[60] Poor dentition or presence of dentures may lead to difficulties with mask ventilation and airway management. Clearance of mucus and small particles is impaired due to sarcopenia-induced muscle loss and decreased mucociliary clearance processes in both the upper and lower airway.[60] Geriatric patients have an increased closing volume, which results in premature collapse of distal airways leading to ventilation/perfusion (V/Q) mismatch especially in the dependent portions of the lung.[60] This effect may be exaggerated in supine position. Loss of pharyngeal muscle tone, decreased cough and swallowing reflexes, and oropharyngeal colonization increase risk of aspiration in the geriatric patient.[15,36]

Preoperative Evaluation

Before elective surgery, geriatric patients should be screened for risk of postoperative pulmonary complications. The ACS/AGS recommendations cite age older than 60, presence of pulmonary comorbidities (ie, chronic obstructive pulmonary disease, obstructive sleep apnea, pulmonary hypertension), ASA class, functional dependence, current cigarette use, and other patient and procedural factors as risks for postoperative pulmonary complications.[61] For patients with underlying pulmonary comorbidities, preoperative optimization is paramount. Smoking cessation should be encouraged. Although routine preoperative chest radiography and/or pulmonary function testing are unnecessary in most geriatric patients, these studies may be appropriate in select patients to determine etiology of dyspnea or to ensure patients with pulmonary comorbidities are at their functional baseline.[61]

GASTROINTESTINAL PHYSIOLOGY

In addition to the airway changes predisposing a geriatric patient to aspiration, disorganized esophageal contractions and slowing of esophagogastric motility lead to delayed gastric emptying and increase the risk of gastric aspiration in the elderly.[36] Esophageal contractions decrease in amplitude and number as a patient ages, leading to increased incidence of dysphagia. Gastroesophageal reflux is present in approximately 30% of geriatric patients.[15] Gastric atrophy and gastritis predispose geriatric patients to gastrointestinal (GI) bleeding, which can carry a mortality rate of 10% to 25%.[15] Liver volume decreases by 20% to 40% over the course of a patient's life.[36] Hepatic blood flow decreases by 10% per decade.[62] The decline in the liver's ability to perform phase I reactions with aging leads to prolonged duration of action of medications like benzodiazepines, specific opioids, and neuromuscular blocking agents.[36,62] Phase II reactions are not affected by aging.[63] Geriatric patients are prone to constipation, especially when exposed to medications that slow GI transit time (ie, opioids).[15] Additional risk factors include immobility, decreased oral fluid intake, and dietary changes.[15]

Preoperative Evaluation

According to the ACS and AGS, albumin level is indicated in all preoperative geriatric patients.[46] In patients with coexisting liver disease, consideration may be given to obtaining liver function tests and coagulation studies.[46] Considering the depression in phase I reactions, medications undergoing metabolism in the liver should be used with caution with appropriate dosing adjustments. The increased risk for gastric aspiration should be considered and strict nil per os (NPO) guidelines should be discussed with patients.

RENAL PHYSIOLOGY

Renal senescence relates to the age-related irreversible structural and functional changes.[64] Total body water is decreased by 10% to 15% in geriatric patients.[65] Maintaining adequate fluid status is imperative in elderly patients, as dehydration secondary to even a 2% loss of total body water may result in cognitive and functional deficits.[66] In geriatric patients, volume overload is associated with increased development of acute kidney injury (AKI), progression to severe AKI, and increased mortality in patients with AKI.[67] Salt and fluid overload is associated with increased risk of infection, cardiopulmonary complications, impaired GI function, and prolonged hospital stay.[15]

Renal cortical mass decreases by 25% by the age of 80 years.[63] After the age of 30, glomerular filtration rate decreases by 1 mL per year. Renal blood flow deceases by 10% each decade after the age of 40.[36] Renal tubule dysfunction impairs the ability of the kidney to concentrate urine, leading to electrolyte disturbances. The renal tubules are less responsive to renin and aldosterone, leading to additional abnormalities in fluid and electrolyte balance.[15] Hyponatremia is common in the geriatric population.[21] Hypernatremia in the geriatric population is associated with increased mortality.[15] Secondary to the changes in the nephron, the excretion of multiple medications is decreased with aging, including benzodiazepines, certain opioids, and neuromuscular antagonists.[63]

Preoperative Evaluation

The ACS and AGS suggest obtaining baseline renal function and electrolytes in geriatric patients.[46] Medications should be dosed accordingly, considering the decreased clearance.

ENDOCRINE PHYSIOLOGY

As patients age, their endocrine function declines secondary to decreased tissue responsiveness and a decrease in hormone secretion.[68] Thyroid-stimulating hormone secretion and triiodothyronine levels are decreased.[68] Fifty percent of geriatric patients have impaired glucose tolerance by the age of 80 years secondary to decreased insulin production and increased tissue insulin resistance.[36] Poor diet, increases in intra-abdominal fat, and decreases in lean muscle mass may account for this glucose intolerance. After menopause, decreased estrogen levels, increase a geriatric woman's risk of cardiovascular events, decline in skeletal muscle mass, and vasomotor instability.[36]

Preoperative Evaluation

For patients with impaired glucose tolerance or diagnosed diabetes, preoperative glucose and assessment of renal function are indicated.[46] For patients with known or suspected thyroid dysfunction, consider thyroid function studies.

SUMMARY

Aging affects the physiology of every major organ system.[36] In addition to organ-specific comorbidities, particular geriatric syndromes exist and can impact clinical care. Geriatric patients are at unique risk for frailty, sarcopenia, malnutrition, and POCD and delirium. The focus of the preoperative evaluation of geriatric patients should include awareness of the age-specific physiology, identification of risk, and mitigation of perioperative risk of complications.

REFERENCES

1. Colby SL, Ortman JM. Projections of the size and composition of the U.S. population: 2014-2060. Curr Popul Rep 2014;1–13.
2. Hall MJ, DeFrances CJ, Williams SN. National hospital discharge survey: 2007 summary. Natl Health Stat Report 2010;29:1–20.
3. Cullen KA, Hall MJ, Golosinsky A. Ambulatory surgery in the United States, 2006. Natl Health Stat Rep 2009;11:1–25.
4. Etzioni DA, Liu JH, Maggard MA, et al. The aging population and its impact on the surgery workforce. Ann Surg 2003;238:170–7.
5. Wozniak SE, Coleman J, Katlic M. Optimal preoperative evaluation and perioperative care of the geriatric patient: a surgeon's perspective. Anesthesiol Clin 2015; 33:481–9.
6. Turrentine FE, Wang H, Simpson VB, et al. Surgical risk factors, morbidity, and mortality in elderly patients. J Am Coll Surg 2006;203:865–77.
7. Kiran RP, Attaluri V, Hammel J, et al. A novel nomogram accurately quantifies the risk of mortality in elderly patient undergoing colorectal surgery. Ann Surg 2013; 257:905–8.
8. Jarvinen O, Huhtala H, Laurikka J, et al. Higher age predicts adverse outcome and readmission after coronary artery bypass grafting. World J Surg 2003;27: 1317–22.
9. Burton D, Nicholson G, Hall G. Endocrine and metabolic response to surgery. Contin Educ Anaesth Crit Care Pain 2004;4:144–7.
10. Kim S, Brooks AK, Groban L. Preoperative assessment of the older surgical patient: honing in on geriatric syndromes. Clin Interv Aging 2015;10:13–27.
11. Stuck AE, Siu AL, Wieland GD, et al. Comprehensive geriatric assessment: a meta-analysis of controlled trials. Lancet 1993;342:1032–6.
12. Huisman MG, Kok M, de Bock GH, et al. Delivering tailored surgery to older cancer patients: preoperative geriatric assessment domains and screening tools–a systematic review of systematic reviews. Eur J Surg Oncol 2017;43:1–14.
13. Knittel JG, Wildes TS. Preoperative assessment of geriatric patients. Anesthesiol Clin 2016;34:171–83.
14. Fried LP, Tangen CM, Walston J, et al. Frailty in older adults: evidence for a phenotype. J Gerontol 2001;56:146–56.
15. Schlitzkus LL, Melin AA, Johanning JM, et al. Perioperative management of elderly patients. Surg Clin North Am 2015;95:391–415.
16. Makary MA, Segev DL, Pronovost PJ, et al. Frailty as a predictor of surgical outcomes in older patients. J Am Coll Surg 2010;210:901–8.
17. Feng MA, McMillan DT, Crowell K, et al. Geriatric assessment in surgical oncology: a systemic review. J Surg Res 2015;193:265–72.
18. Robinson TN, Eiseman B, Wallace JI, et al. Redefining geriatric preoperative assessment using frailty, disability and co-morbidity. Ann Surg 2009;250:449–55.

19. Alvarez-Nebreda ML, Bentov N, Urman RD, et al. Recommendations for Preoperative Management of Frailty from the Society for Perioperative Assessment and Quality Improvement (SPAQI). J Clin Anesth 2018;47:33–42.
20. Legner VG, Doerner D, Reilly DF, et al. Risk factors for nursing home placement following major nonemergent surgery. Am J Med 2004;117:82–6.
21. Sanguineti VA, Wild JR, Fain MJ. Management of postoperative complications: general approach. Clin Geriatr Med 2014;30:261–70.
22. Robinson TN, Wu DS, Sauaia A, et al. Slower walking speed forecasts increased postoperative morbidity and 1-year mortality across surgical specialties. Ann Surg 2013;258:582–8.
23. Vigorito C, Giallauria F. Effects of exercise on cardiovascular performance in the elderly. Front Physiol 2014;5:51–8.
24. Oresanya LB, Lyons WL, Finlayson E. Preoperative assessment of the older patient: a narrative review. J Am Med Assoc 2014;311:2110–20.
25. Hulzebos EHJ, van Meeteren NLU. Making the elderly fit for surgery. Br J Surg 2016;103:e12–5.
26. Wagner D, DeMarco MM, Amini N, et al. Role of frailty and sarcopenia in predicting outcomes among patients undergoing gastrointestinal surgery. World J Gastrointest Surg 2016;8:27–40.
27. Lindle RS, Metter EJ, Lynch NA, et al. Age and gender comparisons of muscle strength in 654 women and men aged 20-93 yr. J Appl Physiol (1985) 1997;83:1581–7.
28. Malafarina V, Úriz-Otano F, Iniesta R, et al. Sarcopenia in the elderly: diagnosis, physiopathology and treatment. Maturitas 2012;71:109–14.
29. Kaiser MJ, Bauer JM, Ramsch C, et al. Frequency of malnutrition in older adults: a multinational perspective using the mini nutritional assessment. J Am Geriatr Soc 2010;58:1734–8.
30. Evans WJ, Morley JE, Argilés J, et al. Cachexia: a new definition. Clin Nutr 2008; 27:793–9.
31. Sandrucci S, Beets G, Braga M, et al. Perioperative nutrition and enhanced recovery after surgery in gastrointestinal cancer patients. A position paper by the ESSO task force in collaboration with the ERA society (ERAS coalition). Eur J Surg Oncol 2018;44:509–14.
32. Klek S, Sierzega M, Szybinski P, et al. Perioperative nutrition in malnourished surgical cancer patients–a prospective, randomized, controlled clinical trial. Clin Nutr 2011;30:708–13.
33. Sungurtekin H, Sungurtekin U, Balci C, et al. The influence of nutritional status on complications after major intraabdominal surgery. J Am Coll Nutr 2004;23: 227–32.
34. Hedman AM, van Haren NE, Schnack HG, et al. Human brain changes across the life span: a review of 56 longitudinal magnetic resonance imaging studies. Hum Brain Mapp 2012;33:1987–2002.
35. Strøm C, Rasmussen LS, Sieber FE. Should general anaesthesia be avoided in the elderly? Anaesthesia 2014;69:35–44.
36. Alvis BD, Hughes CG. Physiology considerations in geriatric patients. Anesthesiol Clin 2015;33:447–56.
37. Mattson M, Maudsley S, Martin B. BDNF and 5-HT; a dynamic duo in age-related neuronal plasticity and neurodegenerative disorders. Trends Neurosci 2004;27: 89–94.
38. Couillard-Despres S, Igleseder B, Aifner L. Neurogenesis, cellular plasticity and cognition; the impact of stem cells in the adult and aging brain–a mini review. Gerontology 2011;57:559–64.

39. Inouye SK, Westendorp RGJ, Saczynski JS. Delirium in elderly people. Lancet 2014;383:911–22.

40. Trzepacz PT. Is there a final common pathway in delirium? Focus on acetylcholine and dopamine. Semin Clin Neuropsychiatry 2000;5:132–48.

41. Galanakis P, Bickel H, Gradinger R, et al. Acute confusional state in the elderly following hip surgery; incidence, risk factors and complications. Int J Geriatr Psychiatry 2001;16:349–55.

42. Marcantonio EF, Goldman L, Mangione CM, et al. A clinical prediction rule for delirium after elective noncardiac surgery. J Am Med Assoc 1994;271:134–9.

43. Moller JT, Cluitmans P, Rasmussen LS, et al. Long-term postoperative cognitive dysfunction in the elderly ISPOCD1 study. ISPOCD investigators. International Study of Post-Operative Cognitive Dysfunction. Lancet 1998;351:857–61.

44. Plassman BL, Langa KM, Fisher GG, et al. Prevalence of cognitive impairment without dementia in the United States. Ann Intern Med 2008;148:427–34.

45. Borson S, Scanlan JM, Chen P, et al. The Mini-Cog as a screen for dementia: validation in a population-based sample. J Am Geriatr Soc 2003;51:1451–4.

46. Chow WB, Rosenthal RA, Merkow RP, et al. Optimal preoperative assessment of the geriatric surgical patient: a best practices guideline from the American College of Surgeons National Surgical Quality Improvement Program and the American Geriatrics Society. J Am Coll Surg 2012;215:453–66.

47. Rosenthal RA, Perkal MF. Physiologic considerations in the elderly surgical patient. In: Miller TA, editor. Modern surgical care: physiologic foundations and clinical applications. 2nd edition. New York: Informa; 2006. p. 1129–48.

48. Harvey A, Montezano AC, Lopes RA, et al. Vascular fibrosis in aging and hypertension: molecular mechanisms and clinical implications. Can J Cardiol 2016;32:659–68.

49. Izzo JL. Arterial stiffness and the systolic hypertension syndrome. Curr Opin Cardiol 2004;19:341–52.

50. Martin RS, Farrah JP, Chang MC. Effect of aging on cardiac function plus monitor and support. Surg Clin North Am 2015;95:23–35.

51. Rubio-Ruiz ME, Peréz-Torres I, Soto ME, et al. Aging in blood vessels. Medicinal agents for systemic arterial hypertension in the elderly. Ageing Res Rev 2014;18:132–47.

52. Lindqvist P, Waldenstrom A, Henein M, et al. Regional and global right ventricular function in healthy individuals aged 20-90 years: a pulsed Doppler tissue imaging study: Umea General Population Heart Study. Echocardiography 2005;22:305–14.

53. Rooke GA. Cardiovascular aging and anesthetic implications. J Cardiothorac Vasc Anesth 2003;17:512–23.

54. Belzberg H, Wo CC, Demetriades D, et al. Effects of age and obesity on hemodynamics, tissue oxygenation a, and outcome after trauma. J Trauma 2007;62:1192–200.

55. Fleisher LA, Fleischmann KE, Auerbach AD, et al. 2014 ACC/AHA guideline on perioperative cardiovascular evaluation and management of patients undergoing noncardiac surgery: executive summary: a report of the American College of Cardiology/American Heart Association task force on practice guidelines. Circulation 2014;130:2215–45.

56. ACS NSQIP surgical risk calculator. Available at: http://riskcalculator.facs.org. Accessed February 23, 2018.

57. Minino AM. Death in the United States, 2011. NCHS Data Brief 2013;115:1–8.

58. Smetana GW, Lawrence VA, Cornell JE. Preoperative pulmonary risk stratification for noncardiothoracic surgery: systematic review for the American College of Physicians. Ann Intern Med 2006;144:581–95.

59. Knudson RJ, Slatin RC, Lebowitz MD, et al. The maximal expiratory flow-volume curve. Normal standards, variability, and effects of age. Am Rev Respir Dis 1976; 113:587–600.

60. Ramly E, Kaafarani HMA, Velmahos GC. The effect of aging on pulmonary function: implications for monitoring and support of the surgical and trauma patient. Surg Clin North Am 2015;95:53–69.

61. Roberts J, Lawrence VA, Esnoala NF. ACS NSQIP best practices guidelines: prevention of postoperative pulmonary complications. Chicago: American College of Surgeons; 2010.

62. Akhtar S, Ramani R. Geriatric pharmacology. Anesthesiol Clin 2015;33:457–69.

63. Rana MV, Bonasera LK, Bordelon GJ. Pharmacologic considerations of anesthetic agents in geriatric patients. Anesthesiol Clin 2017;35:259–71.

64. Melk A. Senescence of renal cells: molecular basis and clinical implications. Nephrol Dial Transplant 2003;18:2474–8.

65. Allison SP, Lobo DN. Fluid and electrolytes in the elderly. Curr Opin Clin Nutr Metab Care 2004;7:27–33.

66. Grandjean AC, Grandjean NR. Dehydration and cognitive performance. J Am Coll Nutr 2007;26:S549–54.

67. Mårtensson J, Bellomo R. Prevention of renal dysfunction in postoperative elderly patients. Curr Opin Crit Care 2014;20:451–9.

68. Chahal HS, Drake WM. The endocrine system and ageing. J Pathol 2007;211: 173–80.

Management of Challenging Pharmacologic Issues in Chronic Pain and Substance Abuse Disorders

Elyse M. Cornett, PhD[a],*, Rebecca Budish, MS[a],
Dustin Latimer, BS[a], Brendon Hart, DO[a],
Richard D. Urman, MD, MBA[b], Alan David Kaye, MD, PhD[c,d]

KEYWORDS

- Chronic pain • Substance abuse • Addiction • Pain management • Opioids
- Drug abuse

KEY POINTS

- Chronic pain is challenging to understand, as pain is subjective, personal, and has a vast number of causes.
- Over the past 10 years (2006–2016), the total US deaths due to drugs has doubled.
- There is a need for more psychological support in pain patients nationwide.

INTRODUCTION

Substance abuse has a major impact on health care services. These patients present challenges with regard to general management, pharmacologic treatment selections, and financial strain. According to the Substance Abuse and Mental Health Services Administration (SAMHSA), approximately 1 (8.1%) in 12 persons older than 12 had

The authors have no financial disclosures and no conflicts of interest. The article has been read and approved by all the authors, the requirements for authorship have been met, and each author believes that the article represents honest work. All authors contributed equally to the article.

[a] Department of Anesthesiology, LSU Health Shreveport, 1501 Kings Highway, Shreveport, LA 71103, USA; [b] Department of Anesthesiology, Perioperative and Pain Medicine, Brigham and Women's Hospital, 75 Francis street, Boston, MA 02115, USA; [c] Department of Anesthesiology, LSU Health Science Center, Room 656, 1542 Tulane Avenue, New Orleans, LA 70112, USA; [d] Department of Pharmacology, LSU Health Science Center, Room 656, 1542 Tulane Avenue, New Orleans, LA 70112, USA
* Corresponding author. Department of Anesthesiology, LSU Health Shreveport, 1501 Kings Highway, Shreveport, LA 71103.
E-mail address: ecorne@lsuhsc.edu

Anesthesiology Clin 36 (2018) 615–626
https://doi.org/10.1016/j.anclin.2018.07.009
1932-2275/18/Published by Elsevier Inc.

a substance use disorder (SUD) in 2014.[1] These disorders encompass both alcohol and illicit drugs, including marijuana, cocaine, heroin, and nonmedical use of prescription drugs. Within that 8.1%, 0.7% had a specific pain reliever use disorder.[1] The National Center on Addiction and Substance Abuse also notes that 1 in 6 people with a substance use problem will have multiple substance disorders.[2] Although they all require treatment, only 10.9% received treatment at a specialty facility in the prior year.[3] Substance abuse costs total more than $740 billion annually in crime, health care, and lost work productivity. Further, prescription opioid misuse has contributed $78.5 billion and this number is still on the rise.

Data from the National Health Interview Survey in 2012 demonstrated 10.3% of people 18 and older report "a lot" of pain, whereas 11.2% experience chronic pain, defined as pain every day for the past 3 months.[4] Chronic pain may be challenging to understand, as pain is subjective, personal, and has a vast number of causes.[5] There are no laboratory or imaging tests to evaluate pain, thus the physician relies heavily on patient history and clinical presentation.[6] Without proper treatment, patients may experience a decline in their daily function and quality of life. Generally, it is believed that chronic pain cannot be "cured"; however, the pain can be managed through a variety of treatment approaches, including pharmacologic, surgical, and behavioral therapies.[7] In 2016, the Centers for Disease Control and Prevention (CDC) published a guideline for prescribing opioids to patients with chronic pain.[8] This guide includes recommendations for when to initiate opioid use, proper dosing, associated risks, and screening questions to evaluate a patient who may be at high risk for abuse.

When considering how many patients are prescribed chronic opioid medication, only 8% to 12% of them become addicted[9]; however, we also must consider that many people are using opioid medication for nonmedical uses. More than 67% of these people state they have obtained opioids from a friend or family member.[3] This is a concern for many reasons, the most essential being the rising rate of overdose. Over the period between 2006 and 2016, the total US deaths related to drugs doubled.[10] Natural and semisynthetic opioids were the number 1 drug type involved in overdoses, until recently, when heroin and synthetic opioid overdoses began exceeding in 2015 to 2016. Critically reviewing the statistics available, deaths by opioid overdose have continued to escalate at alarming rates, with 64,000 people dying from drug overdoses in 2016, including more than 42,000 related to opioid deaths.[11,12] These data represent a 20% increase from the 52,000 total from 2015. Overdoses related to illegally manufactured fentanyl represent the greatest contribution to the increase, accounting for 20,000 deaths in total, heroin accounted for 15,000 deaths, and prescription drugs for fewer than 15,000.

Given these current statistics, physicians must be vigilant in monitoring the trends and providing appropriate support to their patients. This review discusses the present opioid crisis, mechanisms behind chronic pain and substance abuse, and management plans for patients with these disorders.

OPIOID CRISIS

In the mid-1990s, a campaign entitled "Pain as the Fifth Vital Sign" was launched. The campaign focused on increasing both awareness and treatments of this subjective vital sign. Shortly following, the American Pain Society and the American Academy for Pain Medicine began strongly encouraging the use of opioid medication for noncancer patients with chronic pain. Since this time, the use of opioids as pain relievers has been steadily increasing. This rise was supported by an article published in 1986, stating that opioids were safe for patients with chronic pain.[13] Reasons for the increasing need for chronic pain management included aging populations, increases in the prevalence of chronic conditions, expectations from patients for complete relief of symptoms, and increasing complexity of surgical procedures.[14] The use of opioids continued to rise, and this increase was facilitated by the 1995 development of Oxycontin, an extended-release (ER) oxycodone.[15] Addiction, tolerance, and other safety concerns were diminished to promote avid prescribing.

Overdose deaths involving opioids quadrupled from 1999 to 2010, with oxycodone being the most commonly distributed during this time.[16] The number of emergency room visits increased, as an attempt to obtain additional opioid prescriptions. Opioids became a gateway to street drugs, and patients began transitioning to heroin due to its lower price and ease of obtaining. Products containing fentanyl and other analogs were becoming increasingly more common in 2013, and the death rate continued to rise over the next few years.[14] The opioid crisis was officially declared a public health emergency.

Ending this epidemic and preventing further crises is a multistep process. Public health officials suggest a primary, secondary, and tertiary prevention method. This includes preventing new-onset opioid addictions, identifying addiction earlier, and providing adequate treatments to those in need.[15] Although the focus has been on preventing new addiction through means such as pharmacist involvement[17] and modification of opioid formulations,[15] the medical community is far from achieving success. Many health care providers have been unaware of the serious risks of opioids, which include physical (ie, chronic constipation, increased pain sensitivity, respiratory depression) as well as psychological (addiction, distrust) factors. Inconsistent patient monitoring via contracts, drug screens, or state programs can create a negative environment and a fragile patient-doctor relationship if the patient senses bias or deceit.[14] Some physicians are refusing to treat patients they believe are "drug seeking," instead of uncovering the truth and guiding treatment for possible abuse. To make the problem even more challenging, Medicaid in certain states does not cover methadone as a maintenance treatment, making access to care extremely difficult for many patients.[14] Reasons for increased chronic opioid management are summarized in **Box 1**.

Many policies thus far have been focused on reducing the nonmedical use of opioids, and we have seen a mild decline in their use from 2002 to 2012.[15] However, there is a continuous rise in both overdoses and admissions to treatment centers, suggesting that even patients receiving prescription opioids for chronic pain are in danger of addiction and death.[7]

SUBSTANCE ABUSE

Substance abuse is a maladaptive pattern of drug use that leads to clinically significant impairment or distress as manifested by one or more behaviorally based

---

Box 1
Reasons for increased chronic pain management

Pain is now considered an additional vital sign

Longer life expectancy leads to continued management of chronic conditions

Patients are dissatisfied with only partial relief of pain

Failure to control initial pain

criteria.[18] Substance misuse and abuse are critical to differentiate between in order to access potential for substance addiction to develop. Substance misuse is defined as the incorrect use of medication by patients who may use a drug for a purpose other than its original intended purpose, combining medications without the instruction of physician, taking too little or too much of a drug, taking a drug too often, or taking a drug in ways the physician did not intend the patient to do.[18] Substance addiction is a primary, chronic disease of the brain involving dysfunction of reward, motivation, and memory-related circuitry. This change can be manifested in biological changes, psychological and spiritual alterations, and social shifts in a person's life. Inappropriate emotional responses and an inability to maintain lasting interpersonal relationships are often significant problems a patient suffering from addiction will face.[18] Alcohol, tobacco, marijuana, and opioids are among the most common substances associated with addiction, costing the nation more the $740 billion annually in costs related to crime, lost work productivity, and health care. Marijuana leads the nation in illicit drug use; prescription drug misuse is the second most common type of illicit drug use. Being able to understand the reasons for misuse of prescription drugs and its prevalence makes for a major economic impact.[19] Substance abuse has long been seen as a social or criminal problem. In 1935, Alcoholics Anonymous was founded in response to mainstream psychiatric and general medicine providers not attending to SUDs, and the only other option being treated in an asylum away from the rest of health care.[18] In modern times, health care systems are becoming essential in addressing substance misuse and substance addiction.[19] Physicians are key in preventing a patient's substance addiction, treating patients who suffer from addiction, and implementing a safe and combative plan to correct for their addiction.[18] See **Fig. 1** created using information from DAWN, the Drug Abuse Warning Network public health surveillance system that monitored drug-related hospital emergency room department visits to elucidate drug use patterns in patients nationwide.

Physicians take the following steps to determine the most effective plan of action for someone suffering from addiction:

- Formulate diagnosis with differentials
- Psychological assessment including risk of addictive disorder
- Informed consent
- Treatment agreement
- Preintervention and postintervention assessment of pain level and function
- Trial of opioid therapy and/or adjunctive medication
- Routinely reassess pain score and function
- Regularly assess the "4 A's" (analgesia, activity, adverse effects, aberrant behaviors)
- Periodic review of pain diagnosis and the development of comorbid conditions, including addictive disorders
- Documentation

NEUROBIOLOGY OF PAIN AND REWARD

Pain is a subjective reporting by a patient that can be broken down into psychological and biological groupings. It is an individual's experience of sensory, affective, and cognitive dimensions.[20] The classification of pain can be accomplished by determining if the pain is linked to a medical etiology (eg, pain caused by ischemia, inflammation, tissue damage) or if the pain lacks measurable biological factors. Pain can be further classified based on acute or chronic, source, pathophysiology, nociceptive quality, location, distribution, or intensity.[21]

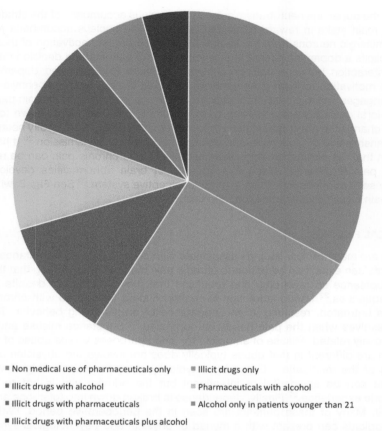

- ■ Non medical use of pharmaceuticals only
- ■ Illicit drugs only
- ■ Illicit drugs with alcohol
- ■ Pharmaceuticals with alcohol
- ■ Illicit drugs with pharmaceuticals
- ■ Alcohol only in patients younger than 21
- ■ Illicit drugs with pharmaceuticals plus alcohol

Fig. 1. Estimates of emergency department visits related to drug misuse or abuse. (*Data from* Drug abuse warning network (DAWN), Substance Abuse and Mental Health Services Administration (SAMHSA), 2008.)

The origins of pain trace back evolutionarily to elicit an amplified surge of motivation to escape or avoid the behavior that caused the pain. This allows for organisms to learn from experiences of pain and became a critical factor in future decision making.[20] The basal ganglia and associated limbic cortex became a cornerstone in the evolutionary process of vertebral brain function of selecting ideal behaviors to minimize consequences (ie, pain).[20] In modern humans, the thalamus, primary and secondary somatosensory cortex, insula, and the anterior cingulate cortex are the most commonly activated regions of the brain in response to acute pain. These regions of the brain receive direct nociceptive signaling from the spinal cord to determine the site and degree of pain to be perceived.[20] In addition to pain-receptive areas, the cortical and subcortical regions, are integrative in the reward/motivation circuit that encode for action selection and learning.[20] Scattered within the network of the subcortical region, opioid neurotransmission can be found.[21] Opioid neurotransmission activity is determined by the receptor that is activated on neurotransmission release. The μ and δ opioid receptors facilitate a dopamine release, whereas the κ receptors suppress dopamine being released.[21]

It is the dopamine neurotransmission in the nucleus accumbens of the striatum that is the main stake in reward-motivated behavior. The nucleus accumbens receives dopaminergic neurons from the ventral tegmental area, and activation of these neurons elicits a dopamine release that is important for learning and decision making.[20] The interaction between pain perceptive regions of the brain and dopaminergic-driven motivation to learn from behavior amplifies the pain-reward behavior. Acute pain engages an individual's motivational and emotional circuitry; chronic pain shifts behavioral goals toward achieving relief.[20] Chronic pain has been shown to extensively change the gray matter, alter white matter connectivity, and modify neurochemical transmission of glutamate, and opioid and dopamine transmission.[20] It has been shown that the cortical changes seen in patients with chronic pain can be reversed when pain is relieved, which it suggestive of brain abnormalities developing in response to continuous activation of the nociceptive system.[20] See **Fig. 2**, which details pain classifications, duration, and tissue type.

CLINICAL FINDINGS

There are many clinical findings associated with chronic pain and substance abuse. Patients can exhibit an addiction to chronic pain medication, meaning that they find the substance so rewarding and gratifying that they lose control despite harmful consequences.[22] Pseudoaddiction is another finding associated with chronic pain that is untreated, resulting in an appearance of drug-seeking behavior. Typically this resolves when the pain has been controlled.[23] Substance misuse and abuse are closely related. Misuse of an opioid for sleep purposes versus abuse of a medication are different in that abuse typically does not involve the physician or monitoring of the medication. Drug abuse typically gives the user a "high," whereas misuse can be accidental or intentional but the primary aim is not to have a euphoric experience.[22] Finally, dependence is broken down into tolerance and withdrawal. Many of these patients are seen in the perioperative period. Withdrawal from opioids can present with a myriad of physical and psychological symptoms. Physical symptoms include central nervous system hyperarousal responses, including diaphoresis, chills, myalgias, and diarrhea. Typically, the acute phase of withdrawal lasts 5 to 10 days, with a peak at day 2 to 3 depending on the half-life of the medication invovled.[22] Tolerance is the concept that patients require higher doses of the medication to achieve the same desired clinical effect over time. This is possibly due to the upregulation of receptors over time.[22] Other clinical symptoms from chronic opioid use are hyperalgesia and medication overuse headaches. Opioid-induced hyperalgesia is primarily mediated by N-methyl-D-aspartate and gamma-aminobutyric acid, and is defined as an increased sensitivity to an already painful stimulus, that is, surgery, in chronic opioid users. The difference between tolerance and hyperalgesia is that an increased or decreased dose of opioids will change the hyperalgesic response, whereas tolerance is gradual over time.[24] Overuse of nonsteroidal anti-inflammatory drugs (NSAIDs) in chronic pain can result in gastrointestinal, cerebrovascular, and renal adverse effects and must be monitored appropriately. Surgeons routinely prescribe opioids in the perioperative setting to help with acute pain control and, as such, can unknowingly contribute to the increasing risk of opioid abuse across the country.[25] There are a growing number of patients who receive opioids for postoperative pain control and then continue to receive them chronically thereafter. There is a risk of persistent opioid use even in opioid-naive patients who were exposed to opioids in the perioperative period.[25] Risk factors include a history of substance abuse, psychological

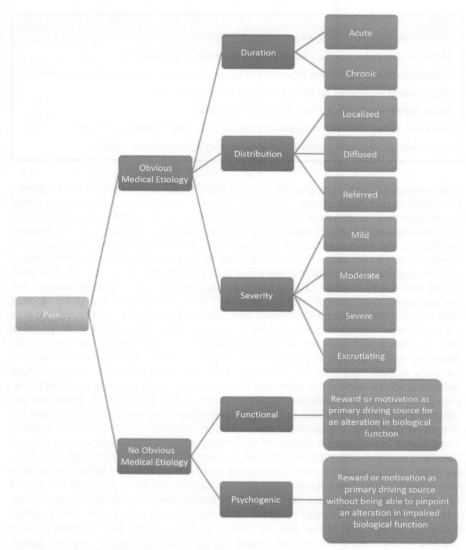

Fig. 2. Pain classification, duration, and tissue type.

conditions, female sex, and low socioeconomic class.[25–27] See **Box 2** for common drug abuse–associated terms and their definitions.

TREATMENT THERAPIES

The CDC recently came out with new guidelines regarding the prescribing and use of opioid prescriptions for primary care providers. This new approach focuses on limiting opioid use in chronic pain, using the lowest effective dose possible, and ensuring close monitoring of patients who use opioids.[28] The focus has shifted to a multimodal therapy of pain control with the focus on NSAIDs, anticonvulsants, and

---

Box 2
Common drug abuse–associated terms and definitions

Addiction: sense of euphoria, reward leading to misuse or overuse of medication

Pseudoaddiction: drug-seeking behavior due to untreated pain, resolves with treatment

Misuse: use of medication for other than what it was prescribed

Abuse: use of medication without physician monitoring

Tolerance: higher levels of medication needed for same effect, happens gradually

Withdrawal: physical and psychological symptoms after abrupt discontinuation

---

antidepressants, and treating acute pain quickly with opioids to prevent the long-term chronicity of potential abuse. There are various new and promising nonopioids currently in various stages of development to target novel receptors to treat chronic pain and decrease opioid consumption. An example is the endocannabinoid system; by blocking the molecules that degrade cannabinoids endogenously, thus increasing endogenous cannabinoids.[28] Other therapies targeted and the psychosocial aspect include cognitive behavioral therapy and mindful meditation practices. Studies have shown that the perception of pain has not changed with psychological therapy, but the perceived pain control is much greater.[28] The downside is that psychological care has a huge deficit in rural areas and even in some cities, and many patients may not have access or coverage for these therapies. Using the lowest possible dose of opioids and combing with another nonopioid novel therapy can significantly decrease tolerance and dependence.[28] There are many various novel therapies currently in trials right now, including peripherally restricted opioids, other selective therapies, and nonopioid therapies, but it will be many years until any potential therapies come to market. Finally, the close monitoring of those patients on opioid therapy will put a tremendous burden on primary care physicians, which may decrease the already limited time the provider has with each patient. To alleviate this burden, some states have set up a statewide monitoring system, but this has yet to show a decrease in opioid overdose and emergency room visits.[28] The CDC has given recommendations to possibly prevent a worsening opioid crisis, but what about the patients who already suffer from opioid dependence? Current evidence supports the use of opioid replacement therapy combined with psychosocial support. As mentioned, there is a need for more psychological support in patients nationwide. One possible future implementation of this may be related to digital health technologies through use of a smartphone or the Internet to meet the psychosocial needs.[28] Another potential therapy is the use of abuse deterrent opioid formulations. These formulations aim to reduce the extraction and bioavailability of the active substance.[29] A growing body of evidence has shown that the introduction of abuse deterrents results in a decrease in potential abuse and diversion, thereby benefiting the opioid epidemic.[29] Gabapentin, Gralise, for example, gastroretentive gabapentin, and pregabalin have been incorporated into multimodal pain regimens, but are those medications addictive as well? Bonnet and Scherbaum[30] report in a review that pregabalin appears to be more addictive than gabapentin but that gabapentinoids do not have substantial addictive effects. There is no evidence to suggest that gabapentinoids increase extracellular dopamine in the mesolimbic reward center. In those with substance abuse issues, the potential to abuse gabapentin and pregabalin is elevated but low. In this regard, it is generally recommended to avoid pregabalin in those with chronic opioid use and substance abuse disorders. See **Box 3** for current therapies aimed at reducing the opioid crisis.

Box 3
Current therapies aimed at reducing the opioid crisis
Limit opioid use for chronic pain
Use lowest adequate dose
Frequent monitoring
Multimodal approach
Cognitive behavioral therapy
Mindfulness and meditation

ABUSE DETERRENTS

Prescription opioids can be abused in their current state, or manipulated to be abused in another state. Possible routes of abuse include ingestion, inhalation, or intravenous. Medications can be manipulated by grinding them into a powder, dissolving them into a solvent like alcohol, or combining with other psychoactive substances.[31] The goal of any abuse deterrent is to give effective pain relief while reducing the rate of abuse by altering the formulation. Different routes include combining agonist/antagonist formulations together, extending the release of the drug, and novel routes of admission.[31] There are currently a number of Food and Drug Administration (FDA)-approved abuse deterrent formulations that have either aversive, for example, niacin, antagonistic, for example, naloxone, or physical barrier additives, for example, polyethylene oxide.

   Oxycontin is the original abuse deterrent and contains polyethylene oxide in its ER formulation. The tablet is difficult to crush and dissolve, becoming viscous, and when it came to market demonstrated an immediate reduction in overdoses in the United States.[31] This physical barrier and crush-resistant technology containing polyethylene oxide makes it hard to crush and turns into a plastic substance if dissolved.[32] Targiniq ER is a combined agonist/antagonist containing oxycodone and naloxone. The euphoric effect is blocked if attempts are made to crush the tablet. This has not yet been commercially available.[31] Embeda is a third abuse deterrent that is a combination of morphine and naloxone. The naloxone stays sequestered in the core if taken appropriately, but if crushed, then the antagonist effect blunts any euphoria from recreational use.[31] Hysingla is a fourth approved abuse deterrent and contains only hydrocodone. The formulation is difficult to crush and dissolve, making it a good abuse deterrent. It uses the same polyethylene oxide similar to Oxycontin.[32] Morphabond is a new abuse deterrent that is more resistant to crushing and cutting and becomes viscous if dissolved. This is the first morphine formulation without an antagonist serving as the deterrent.[31] Xtampza ER is another abuse deterrent and is oxycodone based. This drug is able to be opened and sprinkled on food, while still maintaining its ER potential. This makes it unattractive to drug seekers, because it maintains its ER activity even while crushed.[31] Suboxone is one of the more common agonist/antagonist formulations. It is a combination of buprenorphine and naloxone. Buprenorphine itself is a partial agonist at the mu receptor and antagonist at the kappa receptor.[33] The naloxone only takes affect if the drug is abused in ways other than sublingual absorption, for example, intravenous delivery.[32] There are other abuse deterrent drugs that are still being reviewed by the FDA. The potential to decrease opioid abuse with these formulations is great. One study even goes as far to say that it reduces overdose deaths by 87%.[34] The opioid epidemic is one that must be taken seriously in the medical community going forward. Abuse deterrents will play an increasingly important role going forward. **Box 4** lists common abuse deterrent drugs.

> **Box 4**
> **Common abuse deterrents**
>
> Targiniq; oxycodone/naloxone
>
> Embeda: morphine/naloxone
>
> Hysingla: hydrocodone
>
> Morphabond: morphine
>
> Xtampza: oxycodone
>
> Suboxone: buprenorphine/naloxone

SUMMARY

Chronic pain and opioid abuse is an ever increasing problem in the United States. It has been labeled a crisis by the federal government. This presents a number of challenges in the outpatient surgery setting for many patients with chronic pain issues and addiction because surgery typically requires the use of opioids and other pain medication. The most beneficial preoperative assessment is the establishment of realistic expectations.[35] The CDC recently came out with new guidelines regarding the prescribing and use of opioid prescriptions for primary care providers. This new approach focuses on limiting opioid use in chronic pain, using the lowest effective dose possible, and ensuring close monitoring of patients who use opioids. The CDC has also given recommendations to possibly prevent a worsening opioid crisis. However, the patients who already suffer from opioid dependence will likely need continued and longitudinal support in the form of opioid replacement therapy and psychosocial support.

REFERENCES

1. Hedden SL, Kennet J, Lipari R, et al. Behavioral health trends in the United States: results from the 2014 national survey on drug use and health.
2. Types of addiction | The National Center on Addiction and Substance Abuse.
3. Center for Behavioral Health Statistics. Results from the 2013 national survey on drug use and health: summary of national findings.
4. Nahin RL. Estimates of pain prevalence and severity in adults: United States, 2012. J Pain 2015;16(8):769–80.
5. Vadivelu N, Mitra S, Kaye AD, et al. Perioperative analgesia and challenges in the drug-addicted and drug-dependent patient. Best Pract Res Clin Anaesthesiol 2014;28(1):91–101.
6. Chronic pain: symptoms, diagnosis, & treatment | NIH MedlinePlus the Magazine.
7. Abrecht CR, Greenberg P, Song E, et al. A contemporary medicolegal analysis of implanted devices for chronic pain management. Anesth Analg 2017;124(4): 1304–10.
8. Dowell D, Haegerich TM, Chou R. CDC guideline for prescribing opioids for chronic pain—United States, 2016. MMWR Recomm Rep 2016;65(1):1–49.
9. Vowles KE, McEntee ML, Julnes PS, et al. Rates of opioid misuse, abuse, and addiction in chronic pain. Pain 2015;156(4):569–76.
10. Overdose death rates | National Institute on Drug Abuse (NIDA).
11. Dowell D, Noonan RK, Houry D. Underlying factors in drug overdose deaths. JAMA 2017;318(23):2295.

12. National Center for Health Statistics. Provisional counts of drug overdose deaths, as of 8/6/2017. 2016. Available at: https://www.cdc.gov/nchs/data/health_policy/monthly-drug-overdose-death-estimates.pdf. Accessed February 28, 2018.

13. Portenoy RK, Foley KM. Chronic use of opioid analgesics in non-malignant pain: report of 38 cases. Pain 1986;25(2):171–86.

14. Dasgupta N, Beletsky L, Ciccarone D. Opioid crisis: no easy fix to its social and economic determinants. Am J Public Health 2018;108(2):182–6.

15. Kolodny A, Courtwright DT, Hwang CS, et al. The prescription opioid and heroin crisis: a public health approach to an epidemic of addiction. Annu Rev Public Health 2015;36(1):559–74.

16. Jones CM. Trends in the distribution of selected Centers for Disease Control and Prevention.

17. Compton WM, Jones CM, Stein JB, et al. Promising roles for pharmacists in addressing the U.S. opioid crisis [published online ahead of print December 31, 2017]. Res Social Adm Pharm 2017. https://doi.org/10.1016/j.sapharm.2017.12.009.

18. Prater CD, Zylstra RG, Miller KE. Successful pain management for the recovering addicted patient. Prim Care Companion J Clin Psychiatry 2002;4(4):125–31.

19. (US). SA and MHSA (US); O of the SG. Health care systems and substance use disorders. In: Facing addiction in America: the surgeon general's report on alcohol, drugs, and health. 2016. Available at: https://addiction.surgeongeneral.gov/.

20. Navratilova E, Porreca F. Reward and motivation in pain and pain relief. Nat Neurosci 2014;17(10):1304–12.

21. Elman I, Borsook D. Common brain mechanisms of chronic pain and addiction. Neuron 2016;89(1):11–36.

22. Kahan M, Srivastava A, Wilson L, et al. Misuse of and dependence on opioids: study of chronic pain patients. Can Fam Physician 2006;52(9):1081–7.

23. Weaver M, Schnoll S. Abuse liability in opioid therapy for pain treatment in patients with an addiction history. Clin J Pain 2002;18(4 Suppl):S61–9.

24. Hsu ES. Medication overuse in chronic pain. Curr Pain Headache Rep 2017;21(1):2.

25. Demsey D, Carr NJ, Clarke H, et al. Managing opioid addiction risk in plastic surgery during the perioperative period. Plast Reconstr Surg 2017;140(4):613e–9e.

26. Kaye AD, Jones MR, Kaye AM, et al. Prescription opioid abuse in chronic pain: an updated review of opioid abuse predictors and strategies to curb opioid abuse (part 2). Pain Physician 2017;20(2S):S111–33. Available at: http://www.ncbi.nlm.nih.gov/pubmed/28226334. Accessed March 14, 2018.

27. Kaye AD, Jones MR, Kaye AM, et al. Prescription opioid abuse in chronic pain: an updated review of opioid abuse predictors and strategies to curb opioid abuse: part 1. Pain Physician 2017;20(2S):S93–109. Available at: http://www.ncbi.nlm.nih.gov/pubmed/28226333. Accessed March 14, 2018.

28. Wilson-Poe AR, Morón JA. The dynamic interaction between pain and opioid misuse. Br J Pharmacol 2018;175(14):2770–7.

29. Gasior M, Bond M, Malamut R. Routes of abuse of prescription opioid analgesics: a review and assessment of the potential impact of abuse-deterrent formulations. Postgrad Med 2016;128(1):85–96.

30. Bonnet U, Scherbaum N. How addictive are gabapentin and pregabalin? A systematic review. Eur Neuropsychopharmacol 2017;27(12):1185–215.

31. Hale ME, Moe D, Bond M, et al. Abuse-deterrent formulations of prescription opioid analgesics in the management of chronic noncancer pain. Pain Manag 2016;6(5):497–508.

32. Vadivelu N, Chang D, Lumermann L, et al. Management of patients on abuse-deterrent opioids in the ambulatory surgery setting. Curr Pain Headache Rep 2017;21(2):10.

33. Jonan AB, Kaye AD, Urman RD. Buprenorphine formulations: clinical best practice strategies recommendations for perioperative management of patients undergoing surgical or interventional pain procedures. Pain Physician 2018;21(1): E1–12. Available at: http://www.ncbi.nlm.nih.gov/pubmed/29357325. Accessed March 14, 2018.

34. Sessler NE, Downing JM, Kale H, et al. Reductions in reported deaths following the introduction of extended-release oxycodone (OxyContin) with an abuse-deterrent formulation. Pharmacoepidemiol Drug Saf 2014;23(12):1238–46.

35. Vadivelu N, Kai AM, Kodumudi V, et al. Pain management of patients with substance abuse in the ambulatory setting. Curr Pain Headache Rep 2017;21(2):9.

Preoperative Assessment of the Pregnant Patient Undergoing Nonobstetric Surgery

Michael P. Webb, MBChB, MSc[a], Erik M. Helander, MBBS[b],
Ashley R. Meyn, MD[c], Trevor Flynn, BS[b],
Richard D. Urman, MD, MBA[d], Alan David Kaye, MD, PhD[b],*

KEYWORDS

- Preoperative • Pregnant patient • Physiology • Airway • Pregnancy • Anesthesia
- Risk • Complications

KEY POINTS

- Risks and benefits for both the mother and the fetus should be discussed for any given procedure.
- The placental transfer of drugs varies by molecule size, lipid solubility, acidity, and protein-binding capacity.
- Hypoxemia, hypercapnia, stress, and hypotension can also produce teratogenic effects, and are common during general anesthesia.
- Women with preexisting cardiac disease are high-risk patients and should be counseled as such.

INTRODUCTION

In 2016 there were more than 3.9 million births in the United States, resulting in a birth rate of 12.2 per 1000 population, with 32% of these deliveries by way of cesarean.[1] Data show that up to 2% of pregnant women will undergo nonobstetric surgery per year.[2] With this in mind, it is highly likely that the anesthesiologist will have to perform a preoperative assessment of a pregnant patient before her subsequent encounter during childbirth. The anesthetic management of pregnant patients can present

Disclosure: Dr A.D. Kaye is a speaker for Depomed, Inc and Merck. Dr R.D. Urman has received research funding from Cara Pharmaceuticals, Mallinckrodt, Merck, and Medtronic. The other authors have no significant conflicts of interest to report.
[a] Department of Anesthesiology, North Shore Hospital, 124 Shakespeare Road, Takapuna, Auckland 0620, New Zealand; [b] Department of Anesthesiology, LSU School of Medicine, Room 656, 1542 Tulane Avenue, New Orleans, LA 70112, USA; [c] Department of Anesthesiology, Oschner Clinic, 1514 Jefferson Highway, Jefferson, LA 70121, USA; [d] Department of Anesthesiology, Perioperative and Pain Medicine, Brigham and Women's Hospital Main Campus, Harvard Medical School, 75 Francis Street, Boston, MA 02115, USA
* Corresponding author.
E-mail address: akaye@lsuhsc.edu

Anesthesiology Clin 36 (2018) 627–637
https://doi.org/10.1016/j.anclin.2018.07.010
1932-2275/18/Published by Elsevier Inc.
anesthesiology.theclinics.com

unique challenges; changes in airway anatomy, maternal-fetal physiology, specific risks, and potential crises all have to be considered during the assessment of the pregnant patient. Pregnant patients may require surgery for pregnancy-related issues (eg, cerclage placement, childbirth), fetal surgery, and nonobstetric-related issues, including abdominal, trauma, or orthopedic procedures.[3] All of these factors must be considered when cogitating a safe anesthetic for both the mother and the fetus.

HISTORY AND PHYSICAL

Every preoperative assessment of a pregnant patient starts with a history and physical examination. Thorough histories will include maternal health, anesthetic history, past obstetric history, allergies, family history, history of substance abuse, and baseline vital signs.[4] Major perioperative risk factors in these patients include hypertensive disorders of pregnancy, obesity, gestational diabetes or diabetes mellitus, thrombolytic syndromes, and coagulation disorders.[5–8] The physical should include an examination of the airway, heart, lungs, and lower back if considering a neuraxial anesthetic.[9]

Depending on the patient's individual history, The American Society of Anesthesiologists (ASA) additionally recommends an intrapartum platelet count, a blood type, and antibody screen.[9] Repeat screen with cross-matching results may be performed for high-risk patients. Platelet count will be specific to patients at risk of preeclampsia, with a history of coagulation disorders, or receiving anticoagulant therapies.[10] Blood type and antibody screen is indicated for those at risk of postpartum hemorrhage (PPH) or for those at risk of having blood antibodies (Rh).[9]

Informed Consent

Informed consent of the pregnant patient is complicated by the consideration of the "2 patients in one." The risks and benefits of a procedure, for both the mother and the fetus, have to be weighed by the practitioner and conveyed to the patient. An informed decision to consent on both her and her child's behalf can then be made. In addition to the standard issues of informed consent, pregnant women have several unique circumstances worth considering. These include capacity to consent during active labor, the maternal-fetal conflict, and the care of pregnant minors.[11]

Despite the anxiety and pain associated with active labor, women maintain the capacity to consent due to their ability to understand and recall information given to them while in labor. Giving the pregnant patient written information regarding the risks and benefits of anesthetics well before delivery or planned procedure may improve retention of information and maternal satisfaction.[12] A study by Jackson and colleagues[11] assessed postpartum patient satisfaction and awareness of the risks and complications associated with general anesthesia and also asked the participants what information they wish they had been given during the consent process. The study found that the risks were poorly conveyed. Knowledge of difficult intubation, dental damage, malignant hyperthermia, and medication-related apnea was known by less than 30% of the participants. The level of risk threshold varied; 50% of the participants wanted to know any risks that were known to occur up to 1 in 1000 cases, and 19% wanted to know about the risks greater than 1 in 1,000,000% and 30% of the participants responded that they wanted to know every known risk before consenting.[12]

ANESTHETIC RISKS

Along with standard surgical risks and patient-specific risks based on the pathology necessitating surgery and past medical history, a pregnant patient has numerous additional considerations. Of particular concern are risks resulting from physiologic changes of pregnancy, conditions compelling surgery during pregnancy, placental transfer of drugs, teratogenicity, preterm labor, and maternal factors leading to fetal compromise.

The placental transfer of drugs varies by molecule size, lipid solubility, acidity, and protein-binding capacity. Of the induction agents, ketamine is among the most completely transferred to the fetus. Thiopental and propofol are both highly lipid soluble and cross the placenta; however, thiopental is quickly cleared by the neonate, and the effects of propofol after delivery, including depression of the Apgar score and neurobehavioral effects, are rather transient.[13] Volatile anesthetics can have a more prolonged sedation effect if there is a longer time between induction and delivery of the infant. Nitrous oxide can produce a possible diffusion hypoxia in the neonate.[13] Fentanyl is more lipid soluble than morphine, and thus more readily crosses the placenta. Due to their size and polarity, neuromuscular blockers generally do not cross the placenta, and thus fetal uptake of neuromuscular blockers is negligible. The anticholinergic drug glycopyrrolate is fully ionized and does not cross the placenta as easily as atropine. Benzodiazepines are of moderate transferability and may result in neonatal depression; however, midazolam is shown to cross the placenta less compared with other drugs in its class. Neostigmine is a small molecule and rapidly transfers across the placenta and may cause fetal bradycardia. Atropine should be added to neostigmine to reduce this effect during nonobstetric surgery during pregnancy. Local anesthetics can accumulate in the fetus due to ion trapping if the fetus becomes acidotic during surgery.[13]

Teratogenicity of common anesthetic drugs is also of concern for surgery during pregnancy. This can be minimized by timing surgery to occur after organogenesis of the fetus, or after 18 weeks' gestation. The most teratogenic effects are seen between 2 weeks' and 2 months' gestation.[14] Hypoxemia, hypercapnia, stress, and hypotension also can produce teratogenic effects, and as these are common in the setting of general anesthesia, it is difficult to determine which abnormalities are drug induced, and which are due to a maternal physiologic response.

Despite the risk of preterm labor, current guidelines do not recommend routine prophylactic tocolytics, as there is no proven benefit. Minimizing uterine disruption and manipulation and avoidance of peritoneal irritation should be observed. Prophylactic glucocorticoids can be used for surgery between 24 and 34 weeks' gestation and administered 24 to 48 hours before surgery to reduce perinatal morbidity/mortality should preterm labor occur.[13]

The placenta is not autoregulated, and therefore maternal hypotension will result in decreased maternal-fetal exchange. This necessitates liberal use of intravascular fluids as well as ephedrine and phenylephrine, which are both currently considered effective vasopressors during pregnancy. Other factors that decrease uteroplacental blood flow are prolonged or significant maternal hypoxemia, maternal hypercapnia, and uterine hypertension, which can result from increased uterine irritability.[13]

As with any general anesthetic, there is a risk of death for both the mother and the fetus. The mother is at an increased risk of morbidity and mortality based on the previously described risks versus her nonpregnant counterpart, but these risks must be weighed against the risks of not having the procedure and the severity and acuity of her condition.

AIRWAY MANAGEMENT

Evaluation of the airway deserves special attention for pregnant populations due to increased risk for a difficult intubation associated with pregnancy-induced anatomic and physiologic changes in the airway. Weight gain and anatomic adaptations required for delivery can further complicate access to the airway.[15] Two studies found difficult intubations to occur in pregnant patients at a rate between 0.7% and 5.7%.[16,17] Tests used to predict difficult intubations include Mallampati scoring, thyromental distance, sternomental distance, mouth opening, and upper lip bite test.[17] The overall predictive value for screening methods of difficult intubations proved relatively limited; however a more recent study found high sensitivity (93.75%) and specificity (95.30%) for the combination of the upper lip bite test with thyromental distance when screening for difficult intubations.[18]

Increased levels of progesterone and prostaglandins result in maternal mucosal capillary engorgement. This predisposes the patient to a more friable airway, which together with increased blood volume, can result in a bloody, difficult-to-visualize glottis, particularly in the context of instrumentation. Nasal intubations should be avoided in a pregnant patient due to the increased risk of soft tissue trauma and bleeding.[19]

Decreased lower esophageal sphincter tone also predisposes the patient to reflux of gastric contents and aspiration during induction. Gastric emptying is not delayed until the onset of labor; however, pregnant patients should always be treated as not starved, regardless of time since last meal, although at least 6 to 8 hours of fasting is preferred.[20] Prophylaxis to prevent aspiration pneumonitis should be administered after 16 weeks' gestation. Prophylaxis of choice should be an H2-receptor antagonist and nonparticulate antacid. Rapid sequence induction also should be performed, with or without cricoid pressure, as recommendations vary on the efficacy of this maneuver.

During pregnancy, minute ventilation increases, but functional residual capacity decreases due to compression of the lungs by the gravid uterus resulting in rapid desaturation of the apneic pregnant patient. Preoxygenation should always be used whenever possible, using 100% oxygen for at least 5 minutes before induction.[13] Alternate methods include 4 deep breaths in 30 seconds, but its effectiveness is controversial.[21,22]

In 2015, the Obstetric Anesthetists' Association and Difficult Airway Society published algorithms to guide practitioners in their choices for airway management of obstetric patients. The first algorithm gives a framework on how to optimize a safe general anesthetic and emphasizes planning, multidisciplinary communication, preventing rapid oxygen desaturation by recommending nasal oxygenation and mask ventilation immediately after induction, limiting intubation attempts to 2, and early release of cricoid pressure if difficulties are encountered. The second algorithm discusses approaches after failed intubation, including the placement of a supraglottic airway device. The third algorithm covers the management of a "can't intubate, can't oxygenate" emergency, and includes emergency tracheotomy/cricothyrotomy and the necessity to perform a timely perimortem cesarean delivery if maternal oxygenation cannot be achieved. These guidelines also give practical considerations, such as waking the patient versus proceeding with surgery.[19]

In clinic, careful assessment of the airway must be made. Redundant airway tissue, increased breast mass, and vascular plethora of laryngeal structures conspire to make laryngoscopy more difficult.

MATERNAL-FETAL PHYSIOLOGY

During pregnancy there are significant physiologic alterations that occur in the parturient with the aim of maintaining a milieu conductive to supporting growth and development of the fetus. The central structure in the maternal-fetal relationship is the placenta. This is the interface of the 2 independent circulations and is a multifaceted organ, participating in gas and nutrient exchange, endocrine function, immunologic function, and acting as a reservoir. Clinically, the physiologic adaptation relevant to the anesthesiologist is very much related to the placenta and its functions.

Cardiovascular

The cardiovascular aims of pregnancy are to maintain a stable, uninterrupted blood flow to the placenta. The placenta is a low-resistance, non-autoregulated vascular bed that receives approximately 12% of cardiac output at term.[23] In pregnancy, the systemic vascular resistance is reduced and cardiac output is increased by increases in both stroke volume (SV) and heart rate. SV is increased primarily by increased end diastolic volume (~2000 mL increased blood volume), but also by increased ventricular mass and contractility. The blood volume is disproportionately increased by plasma rather than red cell mass, creating a physiologic anemia. This is due to progesterone-mediated and estrogen-mediated activation of the renin-angiotensin-aldosterone system.[23]

Pregnancy is a significant challenge to the cardiovascular system, but given the population of generally fit, young women, it is usually well tolerated. Clinical assessment and examination of cardiac history, functional status, volume status, and the precordium are routine. Of note, aortocaval compression by the gravid uterus can create a syndrome of syncope/near syncope in the supine mother, and may also produce fetal hypoxemia regardless of maternal symptoms.[23]

Women with preexisting cardiac disease are high-risk patients and should be counseled as such. A prospective study of pregnancy outcomes in women with heart disease noted that 13% of pregnancies in those with preexisting heart disease were complicated by a cardiac event, and approximately 20% had cardiac pharmacologic therapy started or augmented in pregnancy.[24] Complications were primarily acute pulmonary edema or tachydysrhythmia.[24] Where facilities exist, maternal cardiac disease should be managed in a multidisciplinary high-risk obstetric clinic.

Respiratory

To create a physiologic gradient for excretion of carbon dioxide and ingress of oxygen across the placenta, relative hyperventilation occurs owing to a hormonally mediated increased central sensitivity to carbon dioxide. The arterial blood gas demonstrates a renally compensated respiratory alkalosis.[23] The gravid uterus pushes the diaphragm cephalad, reducing the functional residual capacity (FRC). At term, closing volume can encroach into tidal volume, particularly in the supine patient. The maternal anterior-posterior and transverse diameter are increased to facilitate minute ventilation. The metabolic demand for oxygen is increased 60% at term.[23] Although breathlessness in pregnancy is common, and usually benign, a careful history must be taken to exclude cardiac causes. Breathlessness in pregnancy is associated with orthopnea, pain, and paroxysmal nocturnal dyspnea.[23]

Hematology and Rheology

Red cell mass increases in pregnancy due to hormone-induced excess of erythropoietin. White cell count increases progressively during pregnancy and peaks at term.[23] Platelet synthesis and function is increased, along with consumption, resulting in a relative thrombocytopenia. Pregnancy is a hypercoagulable state, with increased circulating coagulation factors. Venous thromboembolic (VTE) disease is a major risk in pregnancy. VTE has been shown to complicate 0.5 to 2.2 of every 1000 pregnancies, and this risk extends into the postpartum period. In fact, postpartum risk of

VTE is 15-fold to 35-fold that of the nonpregnant woman.[25,26] In clinic, VTE risk must be assessed, and a plan to mitigate risk postpartum must be made. Most obstetric societies advocate for early use of anticoagulant prophylaxis.[25] The 2012 American College of Chest Physicians clinical practice guideline on prevention and treatment of thrombosis recommends mechanical or pharmacologic thromboprophylaxis for all pregnant patients undergoing surgery.[27]

Renal, Gastrointestinal, and Endocrine

Glomerular filtration is increased, and plasma creatinine, urate, and bicarbonate are decreased. Glucose reabsorption falls, and a level of physiologic glycosuria may be present.[23] Progesterone-mediated smooth muscle relaxation leads to urinary stasis, and urinary tract infections may result. Dipstick analysis of urine may be helpful in clinic.

Liver function is typically maintained in pregnancy. Cholestasis may occur from low levels of cholecystokinin, and gallstones are relatively common. Biochemically, alkaline phosphatase produced from the placenta is raised, but other liver function assays are usually normal.[23] Plasma cholinesterase is quantitatively reduced in pregnancy, although this is usually not clinically relevant.[28]

Insulin resistance is physiologic in pregnancy. Diabetes in pregnancy is common, and can have effects on the developing fetus.[23]

Gastric reflux is also common in pregnancy, as the barrier pressure of the lower esophageal sphincter (LOS) is overcome by high intra-abdominal pressures.[23] The tone of the LOS is also reduced by progesterone. Antacid medications for the day of surgery are common practice and may be prescribed in clinic.

ANESTHETIC TYPES

There are 2 main techniques for achieving labor analgesia in the pregnant patient. The most effective and most commonly practiced technique is neuraxial analgesia, including epidural, combined spinal epidural (CSE), dural puncture epidural (DPE), single-shot spinal, and continuous spinal.[29] General anesthesia is less often used but can be an option when neuraxial is contraindicated or in emergency cesarean delivery.[30] Epidural and CSE are the most common and have been shown to be equally efficacious with some patient preference toward CSE over standard epidural technique.[31]

The ASA guidelines from 2016 recommend the lowest effective dose should be administered to achieve pain relief with the fewest adverse effects. The epidural local anesthetics most commonly used are bupivacaine and ropivacaine.[32] These drugs have an increased duration of action, reduced incidence of tachyphylaxis, and reduced incidence of lower limb motor block. Ropivacaine has fewer cardiotoxic effects and lower rates of motor block than bupivacaine.[33,34] Other local anesthetics used include lidocaine and chloroprocaine. Chloroprocaine has slightly faster onset of action than lidocaine, but otherwise both have been shown to be effective neuraxial anesthetics.[35]

Epidural opioids administered alone without local anesthetics do not provide complete analgesia. However, they may be used in conjunction with local anesthetics to provide a synergistic effect allowing for reduced dosing of both drugs. Lipophilic opioids, such as fentanyl or sufentanil, may be administered for induction of epidural anesthesia. Hydrophilic opioids such as morphine or hydromorphone are recommended for postoperative analgesia after delivery.[9] Meperidine has also been shown to be efficacious for increasing duration of postoperative analgesia in cesarean delivery.[36]

Adjuvant medications are often used to enhance the safety and efficacy of anesthetic solutions. Epinephrine has been widely used in epidural anesthesia and has been shown to produce a more intense block of both large-diameter and small-diameter sensory nerve fibers than lidocaine alone.[37] Additional studies have described how epinephrine as an epidural adjuvant is associated with fewer epidural vessel penetrations, fewer catheter insertion problems, and faster onset of surgical block and reduced incidence and severity of sedation.[38] Neostigmine has demonstrated significant reduction of local anesthetic consumption allowing for lower doses of anesthetic. A meta-analysis found that epidural administration of neostigmine did not cause the normal adverse effects associated with parenteral delivery when administered by intrathecal route.[39] Clonidine can improve duration and quality of analgesia, whereas sodium bicarbonate may be used to speed up the onset.[40]

It should be noted that cesarean delivery is associated with a greater risk of infection than vaginal delivery; one should consider prophylactic intravenous (IV) antibiotics, such as cefazolin or ampicillin before incision.[41] Clindamycin or gentamicin may be used in case of penicillin allergy.

CLINIC ASSESSMENT OF OBSTETRIC ANESTHETIC CRISES

Obstetric anesthesia has inherent risks. In the assessment of a pregnant woman, it is difficult to adjudicate who is at risk of major obstetric events. That said, planning and preparation starting in clinic may help mitigate consequences of major unanticipated events.

Rare Pharmacologic Anesthetic Crises

The pregnant woman's consultation with the anesthesiologist at preoperative assessment clinic may well be the patient's first-ever encounter with surgical services. The opportunity exists to screen those who may not have previously had anesthesia for rare but potentially fatal complications of anesthesia, outside of the emergency setting. Malignant hyperthermia and pseudocholinesterase deficiency are heritable conditions with low incident rates in the general population.[42] Malignant hyperthermia, an anesthetic drug-mediated hypermetabolic state, can result in a high mortality rate despite available treatment.[42] Pseudocholinesterase deficiency is a heritable defect in plasma cholinesterases, resulting in variable metabolism of some drugs, notably succinylcholine. Careful questioning of the patient and examination of the patient's history with particular reference to personal and family history of unexpected intensive care admissions, anesthetic "problems," or previous referral for additional tests related to anesthesia may unearth unforeseen issues.

Obstetric Hemorrhage

Bleeding in pregnancy is a major source of maternal morbidity and mortality worldwide. Major hemorrhage in pregnancy is the most common cause of maternal collapse and occurs in approximately 3.7 of 1000 maternities.[43] Bleeding can occur at any point in the pregnancy, and classification of bleeding is usually organized by the time at which it occurs. Antepartum hemorrhage is often from placental abruption, uterine rupture, ectopic pregnancy, or disorders of placental implantation (placenta previa and accreta). Postpartum hemorrhage (PPH) is commonly encountered, and its etiology can be usually traced to lack of uterine tone, trauma to the birth canal, retained tissue, or the presence of a disorder of coagulation.[43,44]

Disorders of placental implantation can be predicted by ultrasonography, and visualization of the placenta as it relates to the cervical os or to previous cesarean delivery scars. Uterine rupture occurs most commonly in women attempting vaginal birth after previous cesarean delivery, and particularly in those who have a short interval between pregnancies.[43–45]

The vast majority of PPH is due to uterine atony. Predictors of uterine atony are placenta previa, multiple pregnancy, polyhydramnios, previous PPH, Asian ethnicity, obesity, prolonged labor, and primiparae older than 40 years.[46] Traumatic PPH is predicted by cesarean delivery (with emergency more likely to result in bleeding rather than elective), episiotomy, operative vaginal delivery, and delivery of a large neonate (heavier than 4 kg).[46]

Coagulopathy can be predicted only by presence of an existing clotting disorder, be it acquired or congenital. It also occurs in those requiring massive transfusion. Previous episodes of bleeding may be a bellwether for future events.

Other events causing coagulopathy, such as fetal demise, are outside of the scope of this article.

Mitigation of the risk of obstetric hemorrhage in clinic can involve simple interventions, such as arranging for delivery at a tertiary center, provision for early large-bore IV access, cross-matching of blood, and organizing regular ultrasonography to elucidate placental position. Availability of adjuncts in bleeding, such as tranexamic acid and procoagulant blood products, cell salvage equipment, and access to prompt

Table 1
Considerations for assessment of the pregnant patient

Informed consent	"Two patients in one" Discussions should include information regarding risks to mother and fetus
Anesthetic risk	Placental transfer of drugs varies by molecular size, charge, and protein binding Teratogenicity minimized after 18 wk gestation Hypoxemia, hypercapnia, and hypotension can have teratogenic effects No routine use of tocolytics for prevention of preterm labor Increased morbidity and mortality compared with nonpregnant patients
Airway management	Increased risk for difficult intubation Mucosal capillary engorgement can lead to increased bleeding Avoidance of nasal intubations Rapid oxygen desaturation Aspiration prophylaxis should be given after 16 wk gestation
Maternal-fetal physiology	Patients with preexisting cardiac disease are considered high risk Decreased FRC and increased O2 consumption Hypercoagulable state: consider VTE prophylaxis Relative anemia
Anesthesia types	General vs regional (DPE, CSE)
Obstetric anesthetic crises	Bleeding is major source of morbidity and mortality Placental abruption Vast majority of PPH is from uterine atony Placenta previa, multiple gestations, obesity, primipare >40 y of age, prolonged labor, and previous PPHs are risk factors for atony Look for abnormal placental implantation Screen for coagulopathy

Abbreviations: CSE, combined spinal epidural; DPE, dural puncture epidural; FRC, functional residual capacity; PPH, postpartum hemorrhage; VTE, venous thromboembolism.

surgical intervention can all be organized preoperatively. Preoperative iron infusions may maximize iron stores for prophylactic production of endogenous hemoglobin.

SUMMARY

Considering the plethora of physiologic changes and potential risks to the mother and fetus, safe anesthesia can be provided for a wide variety of procedures. For nonobstetric surgery, timing can be important to fetal outcomes, with the second trimester being preferred for surgeries that cannot wait until the postpartum period.[47] The overall aims in assessing a pregnant patient are to identify potential issues that can lead to catastrophic complications, provide adequate information allowing the mother to make informed decisions, and to obtain knowledge for tailoring an anesthetic that maintains maternal and fetal homeostasis (**Table 1**). The anesthesia provider must have a well thought out anesthetic plan, but also must be ready to act swiftly, and not hesitate to call for help in the face of untoward events, as potential difficult airways, low oxygen reserve, and vigorous bleeding can quickly lead to true emergencies in this population.

REFERENCES

1. Centers for Disease Control and Prevention. Births—Method of Delivery. Available at: https://www.cdc.gov/nchs/fastats/delivery.htm. Accessed March 10, 2018.
2. Crowhurst JA. Anaesthesia for non-obstetric surgery during pregnancy. Acta Anaesthesiol Belg 2002;53(4):295-7.
3. Van De Velde M, De Buck F. Anesthesia for non-obstetric surgery in the pregnant patient. Minerva Anestesiol 2007;73(4):235-40.
4. Obenhaus T. Intraoperative anaphylaxis to latex in pregnancy. Anaesthesist 1995; 44(2):119-22 [in German].
5. Aya AG, Vialles N, Tanoubi I, et al. Spinal anesthesia-induced hypotension: a risk comparison between patients with severe preeclampsia and healthy women undergoing preterm cesarean delivery. Anesth Analg 2005;101(3):869-75. Table of contents.
6. Goodall PT, Ahn JT, Chapa JB, et al. Obesity as a risk factor for failed trial of labor in patients with previous cesarean delivery. Am J Obstet Gynecol 2005;192(5): 1423-6.
7. Leffert LR, Clancy CR, Bateman BT, et al. Hypertensive disorders and pregnancy-related stroke: frequency, trends, risk factors, and outcomes. Obstet Gynecol 2015;125(1):124-31.
8. Mhyre JM, Bateman BT, Leffert LR. Influence of patient comorbidities on the risk of near-miss maternal morbidity or mortality. Anesthesiology 2011;115(5):963-72.
9. Practice guidelines for obstetric anesthesia: an updated report by the American Society of Anesthesiologists task force on obstetric anesthesia and the Society for Obstetric Anesthesia and Perinatology. Anesthesiology 2016;124(2):270-300.
10. Horlocker TT, Wedel DJ, Rowlingson JC, et al. Regional anesthesia in the patient receiving antithrombotic or thrombolytic therapy: American Society of Regional Anesthesia and Pain Medicine Evidence-based Guidelines (third edition). Reg Anesth Pain Med 2010;35(1):64-101.
11. Jackson GN, Robinson PN, Lucas DN, et al. What mothers know, and want to know, about the complications of general anaesthesia. Acta Anaesthesiol Scand 2012;56(5):585-8.

12. Broaddus BM, Chandrasekhar S. Informed consent in obstetric anesthesia. Anesth Analg 2011;112(4):912–5.
13. Upadya M, Saneesh PJ. Anaesthesia for non-obstetric surgery during pregnancy. Indian J Anaesth 2016;60(4):234–41.
14. Tuchmann-Duplessis H. The teratogenic risk. Am J Ind Med 1983;4(1–2):245–58.
15. Djabatey EA, Barclay PM. Difficult and failed intubation in 3430 obstetric general anaesthetics. Anaesthesia 2009;64(11):1168–71.
16. Pilkington S, Carli F, Dakin MJ, et al. Increase in Mallampati score during pregnancy. Br J Anaesth 1995;74(6):638–42.
17. Shiga T, Wajima Z, Inoue T, et al. Predicting difficult intubation in apparently normal patients: a meta-analysis of bedside screening test performance. Anesthesiology 2005;103(2):429–37.
18. Yildirim I, Inal MT, Memis D, et al. Determining the efficiency of different preoperative difficult intubation tests on patients undergoing caesarean section. Balkan Med J 2017;34(5):436–43.
19. Mushambi MC, Kinsella SM, Popat M, et al. Obstetric Anaesthetists' Association and Difficult Airway Society guidelines for the management of difficult and failed tracheal intubation in obstetrics. Anaesthesia 2015;70(11):1286–306.
20. Macfie AG, Magides AD, Richmond MN, et al. Gastric emptying in pregnancy. Br J Anaesth 1991;67(1):54–7.
21. Baraka AS, Taha SK, Aouad MT, et al. Preoxygenation: comparison of maximal breathing and tidal volume breathing techniques. Anesthesiology 1999;91(3):612–6.
22. Benumof JL. Preoxygenation: best method for both efficacy and efficiency. Anesthesiology 1999;91(3):603–5.
23. Bedson R, Riccoboni A. Physiology of pregnancy: clinical anaesthetic implications. Cont Educ Anaesth Crit Care Pain 2014;14(2):69–72.
24. Siu SC, Sermer M, Colman JM, et al. Prospective multicenter study of pregnancy outcomes in women with heart disease. Circulation 2001;104(5):515–21.
25. Bates SM, Middeldorp S, Rodger M, et al. Guidance for the treatment and prevention of obstetric-associated venous thromboembolism. J Thromb Thrombolysis 2016;41(1):92–128.
26. Heit JA, Kobbervig CE, James AH, et al. Trends in the incidence of venous thromboembolism during pregnancy or postpartum: a 30-year population-based study. Ann Intern Med 2005;143(10):697–706.
27. Guyatt GH, Akl EA, Crowther M, et al. Executive summary: antithrombotic therapy and prevention of thrombosis, 9th ed: American College of Chest Physicians evidence-based clinical practice guidelines. Chest 2012;141(2 Suppl):7S–47S.
28. Whittaker M. Plasma cholinesterase variants and the anaesthetist. Anaesthesia 1980;35(2):174–97.
29. Silva M, Halpern SH. Epidural analgesia for labor: current techniques. Local Reg Anesth 2010;3:143–53.
30. Vincent RD Jr, Chestnut DH. Epidural analgesia during labor. Am Fam Physician 1998;58(8):1785–92.
31. Collis RE, Davies DW, Aveling W. Randomised comparison of combined spinal-epidural and standard epidural analgesia in labour. Lancet 1995;345(8962):1413–6.
32. Albright GA. Cardiac arrest following regional anesthesia with etidocaine or bupivacaine. Anesthesiology 1979;51(4):285–7.
33. Beilin Y, Halpern S. Focused review: ropivacaine versus bupivacaine for epidural labor analgesia. Anesth Analg 2010;111(2):482–7.

34. Halpern SH, Breen TW, Campbell DC, et al. A multicenter, randomized, controlled trial comparing bupivacaine with ropivacaine for labor analgesia. Anesthesiology 2003;98(6):1431–5.
35. Gaiser RR, Cheek TG, Adams HK, et al. Epidural lidocaine for cesarean delivery of the distressed fetus. Int J Obstet Anesth 1998;7(1):27–31.
36. Farzi F, Mirmansouri A, Forghanparast K, et al. Addition of intrathecal fentanyl or meperidine to lidocaine and epinephrine for spinal anesthesia in elective cesarean delivery. Anesth Pain Med 2014;4(1):e14081.
37. Sakura S, Sumi M, Morimoto N, et al. The addition of epinephrine increases intensity of sensory block during epidural anesthesia with lidocaine. Reg Anesth Pain Med 1999;24(6):541–6.
38. Denny JT, Cohen S, Stein MH, et al. Epinephrine adjuvant reduced epidural blood vessel penetration incidence in a randomized, double-blinded trial. Acta Anaesthesiol Scand 2015;59(10):1330–9.
39. Cossu AP, De Giudici LM, Piras D, et al. A systematic review of the effects of adding neostigmine to local anesthetics for neuraxial administration in obstetric anesthesia and analgesia. Int J Obstet Anesth 2015;24(3):237–46.
40. Bhatia U, Soni P, Khilji U, et al. Clonidine as an adjuvant to lignocaine infiltration for prolongation of analgesia after episiotomy. Anesth Essays Res 2017;11(3):651–5.
41. Smaill FM, Grivell RM. Antibiotic prophylaxis versus no prophylaxis for preventing infection after cesarean section. Cochrane Database Syst Rev 2014;(10):CD007482.
42. Hinova A, Fernando R. The preoperative assessment of obstetric patients. Best Pract Res Clin Obstet Gynaecol 2010;24(3):261–76.
43. Richardson AL, Wittenberg M, Lucas DN. An urgent call to the labour ward. Cont Educ Anaesth Crit Care Pain 2015;15(1):44–9.
44. Fitzpatrick KE, Kurinczuk JJ, Alfirevic Z, et al. Uterine rupture by intended mode of delivery in the UK: a national case-control study. PLoS Med 2012;9(3):e1001184.
45. Plaat F, Shonfeld A. Major obstetric haemorrhage. Cont Educ Anaesth Crit Care Pain 2015;15(4):190–3.
46. Royal College of Obstetricians and Gynaecologists Green Top 52. Postpartum haemorrhage, prevention and management. 2009. Available at: http://ww.rcog.org.uk/womens-health/clinical-guidance/prevention-and-managementpostpartum-haemorrhage-green-top-52. Accessed February 18, 2018.
47. Nejdlova M, Johnson T. Anesthesia for non-obstetric procedures during pregnancy. Cont Educ Anaesth Crit Care Pain 2012;12(4):203–6.

Genomics Testing and Personalized Medicine in the Preoperative Setting

Rodney A. Gabriel, MD, MAS[a,b,]*, Brittany N. Burton, MHS[c],
Richard D. Urman, MD, MBA[d], Ruth S. Waterman, MD, MSc[e]

KEYWORDS

- Pharmacogenomics • Preoperative • Genetics • Outcomes • Opioids

KEY POINTS

- The application of pharmacogenomics principles in perioperative medicine is fairly novel and only a limited number of studies have shown its potential benefit in this clinical setting.
- Many enzymes are involved with the metabolism of various analgesic medications, leading to genetic variability, and consequently play a role in drug toxicity and efficacy. It seems logical that having pharmacogenomics information on patients before surgery would be a valuable tool to anesthesiologists because it would allow tailored and effective analgesic use in each patient.
- Challenges in executing pharmacogenomics programs into health care systems include physician buy-in and integration into usual clinical workflow, including the electronic health record.
- The preoperative testing clinic, a facility usually run by anesthesiologists and designed to screen patients for appropriateness of surgery, is an ideal location to perform pharmacogenomics screening.

INTRODUCTION

Pharmacogenomics (PGx) is the study of how individuals' personal genotypes may affect their responses (phenotype) to various pharmacologic agents. The

Disclosure: R.A. Gabriel, R.S. Waterman, and R.D. Urman use CQuentia (Fort Worth, TX) for pharmacogenomics screening at their respective institutions.
[a] Division of Regional Anesthesia and Acute Pain, Department of Anesthesiology, University of California, San Diego, 200 W Arbor Dr, San Diego, CA 92103, USA; [b] Department of Medicine, Division of Biomedical Informatics, University of California, San Diego, 9500 Gilman Dr, La Jolla, CA 92093, USA; [c] School of Medicine, University of California, San Diego, 9500 Gilman Dr, La Jolla, CA 92093, USA; [d] Department of Anesthesiology, Perioperative and Pain Medicine, Harvard Medical School, Brigham and Women's Hospital, 75 Francis St, Boston, MA 02115, USA; [e] Department of Anesthesiology, University of California, San Diego, 200 W Arbor Dr, San Diego, CA 92103, USA
* Corresponding author. Department of Anesthesiology, University of California, San Diego, 9500 Gilman Drive, MC 0881, La Jolla, CA 92093-0881.
E-mail address: ragabriel@ucsd.edu

Anesthesiology Clin 36 (2018) 639–652
https://doi.org/10.1016/j.anclin.2018.07.014
1932-2275/18/© 2018 Elsevier Inc. All rights reserved.

application of PGx principles in perioperative medicine is fairly novel and only a limited number of studies have shown its potential benefit in this clinical setting.[1-3] During a patient's perioperative experience, anesthesiology providers are tasked with the management of multimodal pharmacotherapy; these involve medications that are used to manage pain, prevent nausea and vomiting, induce and maintain anesthesia, provide muscle relaxation, and manage hemodynamics. Although the mechanisms of action of the many medications anesthesiologists use are to some degree understood, the precise effect a given dose will have on an individual may not be known until it is given. These inherent variations in response to medications are partly caused by PGx, a profile that is unique to each individual. Thus, in theory, having this personalized information for every patient planned to undergo surgery may aid in fine-tuning precision medicine when it comes to optimizing perioperative care.

Enhanced recovery after surgery (ERAS) pathways and perioperative surgical home (PSH) models are being widely adopted in an effort to protocolize evidence-based medicine systematically.[4] The goal is therefore to improve outcomes. Integration of PGx into such pathways may provide a huge step in optimizing care even further by having available additional information on patient-specific response to medications. Enhanced recovery pathways involve integral steps at all stages in a patient's perioperative journey, including:

1. Preadmission (ie, surgery clinic and preoperative care clinic)
2. Preoperative (ie, day of surgery before operation)
3. Intraoperative
4. Immediate postoperative (ie, recovery, physical therapy, nutrition, pain management)
5. Long-term postoperative phase (**Fig. 1**)

There are a variety of pharmacologic agents that are used at each stage of this perioperative process. Integration of PGx early in this process (ie, preadmission) may help providers practice precision medicine at all subsequent stages.

This article discusses the current evidence highlighting the potential of PGx with various drug categories used in the perioperative process and the challenges of integrating PGx into a health care system and relevant workflows.

PHARMACOGENOMICS AND PERIOPERATIVE MEDICATIONS

It is important to discuss the current evidence of PGx as it applies to various drug classes relevant to surgical patients; these include opioids, nonopioids, antiemetics, anticoagulants, and β-blockers. Much of anesthesiologists' clinical practice involves the titration of various drugs individualized to each patient.[2,3] Many enzymes are involved with the metabolism of various analgesic medications, leading to genetic variability, and consequently playing a role in drug toxicity and efficacy. It seems logical that having PGx information on patients before surgery would be a valuable tool to anesthesiologists because it would allow tailored and effective analgesic use in each patient. More studies are still needed to assess the effects of personalized dosing of anesthetics and analgesics during the perioperative process for various major surgeries.

Opioids

An individual's metabolism of opioids is largely determined by variations of cytochrome P (CYP) enzymes, including CYP2D6[5] and CYP3A4.[6,7] Studies have shown variations in metabolism based on CYP2D6 for codeine,[8,9] tramadol,[10] and

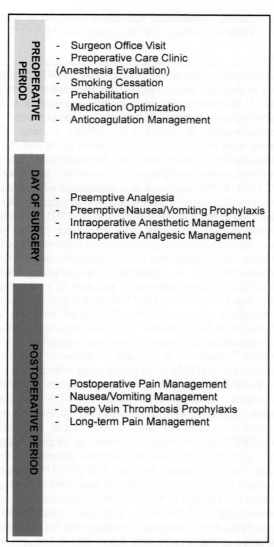

PREOPERATIVE PERIOD
- Surgeon Office Visit
- Preoperative Care Clinic (Anesthesia Evaluation)
- Smoking Cessation
- Prehabilitation
- Medication Optimization
- Anticoagulation Management

DAY OF SURGERY
- Preemptive Analgesia
- Preemptive Nausea/Vomiting Prophylaxis
- Intraoperative Anesthetic Management
- Intraoperative Analgesic Management

POSTOPERATIVE PERIOD
- Postoperative Pain Management
- Nausea/Vomiting Management
- Deep Vein Thrombosis Prophylaxis
- Long-term Pain Management

Fig. 1. Work flow of the perioperative process and how pharmacogenomics may be applied at each stage: preoperative, day of surgery, and postoperative phases.

hydrocodone.[11] Morphine metabolism has been shown to be affected by canalicular multispecific organic anion transporter 2 (ABCC3),[12] organic cation transporter,[12] CYP2D6,[5] and P-glycoprotein transporter (encoded by ABCB1).[13] Adverse events related to morphine may also be affected by mu-receptor genotype (OPRM1).[14] Fentanyl metabolism can be affected by the CYP3A4 enzyme.[6,7] Furthermore, postoperative requirements for fentanyl have been associated with genotypes for catechol-O-methyltransferase (COMT) enzymes.[15] Tramadol metabolism may be affected by variations in CYP3A4, CYP2B6, CYP2D6, and various other transporter and receptor genes.[10] Hydromorphone metabolism is related to several types of

CYP genes.[16] In addition, methadone has been associated with several genes, including ABCB1, CYP2B6, CYP3A4, OPRM1, and UGT1A.[8,17–20]

Nonopioid Analgesics

The World Health Organization developed the so-called pain ladder to guide treatment of mild to moderate acute pain, advocating for the administration of nonopioid analgesics as the first step.[21] Nonopioid analgesics comprise a diverse class of medications that have antiinflammatory properties. For example, animal studies have shown that metabolism of acetaminophen is mediated by CYP2E1 oxidation.[22] Acetaminophen overdose represents more than 50% of drug-related acute liver failure, and studies have identified polymorphisms associated with hepatotoxicity.[23] In their investigation of 15 adults with thalassemia/hemoglobin E, Tankanitlert and colleagues[24] showed that the UGT1A6*2/UGT1A1*28 haplotype was associated with increased paracetamol concentrations. Another study found decreased acetaminophen glucuronide concentrations in urine samples in patients expressing the UGT2B15*2 variant.[25] Acetaminophen glucuronidation partial clearance and increased plasma concentration of acetaminophen plasma protein complexes are largely determined by UGT2B15*2 polymorphism.[26] Moreover, sulfotransferase (SULT) enzymes are involved in the sulfate conjugation of acetaminophen. A systematic meta-analysis identified SULT1A1, SULT1A2, and SULT1A3 as determinants of sulfation of acetaminophen.[27] Several studies have shown that UGT1A6 and UGT1A9 are the primary human allele variants mediating acetaminophen glucuronidation. Compared with the UGT1A6*1 allele variant, UGT1A6*2 had 60% higher acetaminophen glucuronidation activity.[28] However, for select human populations, a reduction in glucuronidation activity is observed with the UGTA1*28 isoform.[28] Ibuprofen is primarily metabolized by cytochrome enzymes and excreted into the urine. CYP2C9 plays a major role in ibuprofen clearance. Studies have shown that concomitant administration of ibuprofen and CYP2C9 inhibitors leads to drug-drug interactions and toxic effects. CY2C8 and CYP3A4 are also involved in ibuprofen clearance. Although the contribution of UDP-glucuronosyltransferases (UGTs) in vivo remains unclear, in vitro studies show that UGT1A3, UGT1A9, UGT2B7, and UGT2B17 glucuronidate ibuprofen to ibuprofen-acyl glucuronide.[29] Most studies have suggested a decrease in ibuprofen clearance with CYP2C9*3 polymorphism compared with individuals with the CYP2C9*1/*1 genotype.[29] Naproxen metabolism is mediated by UGT2B7 and CYP2C9 and interindividual genetic variations that lead to decreased metabolism of naproxen have been linked to higher risk of acute gastrointestinal hemorrhage.[30–32] Celecoxib is primarily metabolized by CYP2C9 and CYP3A4.[33,34] Prieto-Pérez and colleagues[33] investigated the association of CYP polymorphisms and pharmacokinetics and they found that individuals with CYP2C9*1/*3 and CYP2C9*3/*3 had lower celecoxib clearance compared with individuals with CYP2C9*1/*1. Chan and colleagues[35] evaluated cytochrome polymorphisms on colorectal adenoma recurrence in 1660 adult patients with colorectal cancer receiving celecoxib and found that patients who expressed CYP2C9*3 genotypes and received high-dose celecoxib had a lower risk of recurrence; however, this association was not found for patients with CYP2C9*2.

Benzodiazepines

It is well established that benzodiazepines primarily act on the central nervous system and are clinically used as sedative-anxiolytics and antiepileptics. In nerve cells, benzodiazepines facilitate ionotropic γ-aminobutyric acid (GABA) action by increasing the frequency of chloride channel opening. Metabolism of benzodiazepines is determined largely by oxidative metabolizing cytochrome enzymes, such as CYP3A4 and

CYP3A5, which are expressed primarily in the liver and intestine.[36] One study showed that CYP3A activity reflected clearance of urinary ratios of endogenous steroids, which was positively correlated with midazolam clearance.[36] Several studies have shown interindividual variability in CYP3A expression and activity, which influences the adverse effect profile.[37] It has been shown that midazolam is largely metabolized by CY3A4 and CYP3B to its active metabolite, 1′-hydroxymidazolam.[38] Miao and colleagues[37] found that CYP3A5*3, the most prevalent variant, was expressed in 85% to 95% of white people, 27% to 50% of African Americans, and 60% to 73% in Asian people. Further studies have shown that CYP3A4 290 A>G and CYP3Ab 22893 A>G allelic variants lead to reduced drug clearance.[39] In European and African American adults, CYP3A*5 was associated with 50% increase in enzyme induction.[39] The average population clearance of midazolam was shown to be 22% lower in patients with cancer expressing CYP3A5*3.[40] Increased midazolam concentrations and decreased metabolite ratios were observed in patients with cancer expressing CYP3A4*22, which is associated with decreased CYP3A4 activity.[41] Studies have shown that UGT1A4, UGT2B4, and UGT2B7 isoforms are primarily involved in glucuronide conjugation of midazolam metabolites.[42] After midazolam undergoes oxidative phosphorylation to its metabolite (ie, hydroxymidazolam) by CYP3A4, glucuronidated metabolites are produced by UDP-glucuronosyltransferases (UGTs) and ultimately excreted into the urine.[42] Studies have shown that variation in the response to lorazepam is determined largely by UGT2B15. In in vitro studies, ketoconazole was associated with inhibition of UGT2B7 glucuronidation of lorazepam.[43] The UGT1A1*28 variant has been shown to be associated with reduced elimination and consequently increased toxicity of lorazepam.[44]

Antiemetics

Ondansetron is a 5-hydroxytryptamine (5-HT3) serotonin antagonist and is used to prevent postoperative and chemotherapy-induced nausea and vomiting. Ondansetron has been shown to be metabolized by CYP3A4, CYP2D6, and CYP1A2.[45] The most common CYP2D6 variants of ondansetron metabolism may be divided into groups such as normal function (ie, CYP2D6*1 and *2), decreased function (ie, CYP2D6*9, *10, and *41), and no function (eg, CYP2D6*3–*6).[46] Individuals who express CYP2D6*2 are ultrametabolizers who experience treatment failure and therefore have increased risk of nausea and vomiting.[47] ATP-binding cassette (ABC) proteins are important in transport of ondansetron across cellular membranes. He and colleagues[48] evaluated 215 patients with acute myeloid leukemia with clinical resistance to ondansetron and found that the ABC subfamily B member 1 (ABCB1) transporter C3435T polymorphisms were associated with grade 3/4 vomiting. Moreover, ondansetron metabolism has been shown to be associated with hepatic organic cation transporter 1 (OCT1).[49] Although metoclopramide is partially metabolized by cytochromes, CYP2D6 is the primary determinant of metoclopramide metabolism. Parkman and colleagues[50] investigated the metoclopramide adverse effect profile in 100 adult patients with gastroparesis and found that patients with polymorphisms in CYP2D6 (ie, rs1080985, rs16947, rs3892097) and potassium voltage-gated channel subfamily H member 2 (KCNH2; ie, rs3815459) were more likely to experience side effects, however KCNH2 (ie, rs1805123) and ADRA1D (ie, rs2236554) polymorphisms were associated with a favorable clinical response. Although the exact antiemetic mechanism of action of dexamethasone is unclear, studies show that dexamethasone is involved in reduction in prostaglandin synthesis in the nervous system.[51] Expression of CYP2D6*3/*4/*5/*6 results in poor metabolism of haloperidol. As such, these individuals are at risk of increased risk for QT prolongation and arrhythmias.[47] In their evaluation of novel loci associated with the response to antipsychotic medication, Yu and colleagues[52] found several polymorphisms associated with an increased risk of psychotic disorders and response to antipsychotic medications. CYP2D6 has been shown to be associated with metabolism of promethazine.[53] Moreover, CYP2D6 polymorphisms have been shown to be associated with H1 antihistamine–induced sedation.[54]

Anticoagulants

Anticoagulation is prescribed for a wide range of conditions, including, but not limited to, atrial fibrillation, acute coronary syndrome, pulmonary embolism, deep venous thrombosis, and cerebrovascular accident. It is well established that warfarin, which is most widely used in the prevention of venous thromboembolism and cerebrovascular accident in patients with atrial fibrillation, is metabolized by CYP2C9 and vitamin K epoxide reductase complex (VKORC1).[55] Studies have shown that CYP 2C9*2, CYP 2C9*3, and VKORC1 A haplotype warfarin polymorphisms are associated with slower metabolism.[55] The antiplatelet activity of clopidogrel has been shown to reduce the risk of vascular disease.[56] Roughly 25% of individuals treated with clopidogrel experience treatment failure, and studies have shown that CYP2C9 and CYP2C19 are involved in the metabolism of clopidogrel.[56] Polymorphism in ATP-Binding Cassette Subfamily B Member 1 (ABCB1), Paraoxonase-1 (PON1), Carboxyl Esterase 1 (CES1), and P2Y12 receptors are associated with clopidogrel metabolism.[56]

β-Blockers

Metoprolol is a β_1-adrenoreceptor antagonist and is often prescribed to manage myocardial infarction, supraventricular tachycardia, hypertension, and heart failure. Blocking adrenergic receptors reduces heart rate and contractility. Although there are more than 100 identified polymorphisms of CYP2D6, studies have shown that CYP2D6 is responsible for 70% to 80% of metoprolol metabolism. The wide genetic variation in CYP2D6 for metoprolol and carvedilol has been shown to lead to variation in clinical response. Individuals may be classified as poor, intermediate, extensive, and ultrarapid metoprolol or carvedilol metabolizers.[57,58] Studies have shown that CYP2D6 nonexpressors have roughly a 5-fold increase in plasma concentrations of metoprolol and consequently decreased cardioselectivity and increased risk of adverse effects.[59,60] As such, ultrarapid metabolizers are at risk of treatment failure, whereas poor metabolizers may experience toxic adverse effects. Gao and colleagues[59] evaluated 319 patients who received metoprolol succinate for heart rate control following percutaneous coronary intervention and found that CYP2D6*10 polymorphisms were associated with a lower heart rate. As such, metoprolol guidelines have been published to recommend dosing adjustments and requirements based on CYP2D6 polymorphisms.[47] Carvedilol is also commonly prescribed to treat hypertension and heart failure.[58] Luzum and colleagues[57] assessed the relationship of CYP2D6 polymorphisms and maintenance does of metoprolol and carvedilol. Patients with CY2D6*4 had lower and higher maintenance dose requirements for metoprolol and carvedilol, respectively.

Local Anesthetics

Common local anesthetics used in the perioperative period include lidocaine, bupivacaine, ropivacaine, and mepivacaine. Their primary site of action is neuronal sodium channels. Few studies have shown any clinical correlation between genomics and response to local anesthetics. Lidocaine and bupivacaine are metabolized by CYP3A4, whereas ropivacaine is metabolized by CYP1A2.[38] Furthermore, patients with MC1R variants have decreased response to lidocaine.[61]

Malignant Hyperthermia

Malignant hyperthermia (MH) is a rare and potentially life-threatening autosomal dominant inherited condition associated with inhaled anesthetics or succinylcholine. Roughly 50% of MH cases are associated with ryanodine receptors (RYRs) or calcium voltage-gated channels (CACNA1S).[62] RYR and CACNA1S polymorphisms have been identified in families with multiple cases of MH.[63] Genetics variations in RYR1 account for roughly 80% of all cases of MH, whereas polymorphisms of CACNA1S have been shown to account for less than 1% of MH cases.[64] Preoperative PGx information for RYRs would be useful in determining which patients should not receive succinylcholine or volatile anesthetics.

INTEGRATION INTO PERIOPERATIVE WORKFLOW

Although PGx is not new, its widespread implementation into perioperative care is still at its infancy. Challenges in executing such programs include physician buy-in and integration into usual clinical workflow, including the electronic health record (EHR).[1] To facilitate physician buy-in would require more published data reporting both the prevalence of genetic risk to various perioperative medications and definitive outcomes associated with tailoring medications based on PGx. Integration into clinical work flow is also key and would require a collaboration between health care providers and the informatics department to create useful and user-friendly interfaces and alerts that may lead to improved execution of PGx. In order to obtain more universal adoption of perioperative PGx, there needs to be:

1. More high-quality evidence that surgical outcomes improve with PGx
2. Easy-to-access and user-friendly interfaces integrated into electronic medical record systems
3. Protocols put into place that allow PGx to easily fit into regular clinical workflow

More High-Quality Evidence that Surgical Outcomes Improve with Pharmacogenomics

Integration of PGx-guided therapy for surgical patients has potential to improve outcomes; however, more large-scale definitive studies are required. To date, there have been some small-scale cohort studies reporting its impact.[2,3] In one cross-sectional study, approximately 150 patients with postoperative trauma were analyzed and genetic associations of OPRM1 and COMT and postoperative pain/opioid consumption were made. The investigators concluded that OPRM1 and COMT may contribute to the variability of opioid consumption.[65] Other studies have shown that there is no genetic association of various genes with fentanyl consumption in gynecologic patients[66] and obstetric patients.[67] Several studies, as described earlier, have shown associations between different genes and postoperative opioid use.[65-77] However, studies are now needed that focus on PGx interventions and postoperative outcomes. Senagore and colleagues[68] conducted a study whose methodology involved comparing results with historical controls in patients undergoing colorectal resections or ventral hernia repair and showed improvement in opioid consumption. The investigators produced a guided analgesic protocol based on the assessment of 6 CYP, COMT, OPRM1, and ABCB1 genes. Depending on the patients' genotypes, analgesics were dose adjusted or avoided as appropriate. Large-scale prospective randomized controlled trials are needed to prove its efficacy.

Easy-to-Access and Easy-to-Understand Interfaces Integrated into Electronic Medical Record Systems

Because there are several genes that have already been implicated in perioperative medication metabolism, a complete list of genetic interactions with pharmacologic agents may prove to be too long and complex for the average health care provider to review. Therefore, the interface presenting this information should be strategically designed. Specifically, integrating known PGx polymorphisms into ERAS protocols could prove to be the most useful for the health care provider.

Protocols Put into Place that Allow Pharmacogenomics to Easily Fit into Regular Clinical Workflow

The perioperative work flow needs to be an efficient process while maintaining patient safety. PGx screening results should be transferred directly into EHR systems and should contain some of these components: (1) customized report generation depending on provider and institution preferences; (2) data tracking and analytics; (3) easy-to-use provider-facing interface in the record explaining the key salient results for each patient as well as a separate section with more detailed information; and (4) EHR-integrated real-time alerts associated with genetic risks. On a daily operating room schedule integrated into the EHR, patients who have PGx screening available are identified by a unique icon next to their names. The presence of this icon alerts providers that results are available in the EHR. **Fig. 2**A is an example screenshot of 1 component of a patient's test results, listing each gene screened and the metabolism status of that gene. Based on the genes tested, providers are given information regarding potential drug responses to different pharmacologic categories, including anticoagulation, beta-blockade, sedatives, antiemetics, hypnotics, muscle relaxants, analgesics (opioid and nonopioids), and volatile anesthetics. **Fig. 2**B and C are example screenshots of a patient's thrombosis profile summary and response to analgesic medications, respectively.

WHEN TO PERFORM PHARMACOGENOMICS SCREENING

The time at which to perform PGx screening must take into consideration the time required to obtain the final results in relation to when the patient's surgery is scheduled. In addition, there must be an appropriate amount of allocated time to consent and educate the patient regarding PGx. The preoperative testing clinic (a facility usually run by anesthesiologists and designed to screen patients for appropriateness of surgery) is an ideal location to perform such tasks. At that time, health care providers can perform preoperative behavioral and medical risk assessments to determine appropriateness of PGx testing. Patients at risk for opioid dependence or pharmacologically associated adverse events can be recognized early and PGx may be used to potentially optimize perioperative care. Furthermore, genetics do not change and results may be used for multiple subsequent surgical encounters.

SUMMARY

The use of PGx to personalize perioperative care is promising, but there are several challenges that must be met before this becomes a widespread practice. This article discusses studies in the basic and clinical science showing the association of various genes and response to perioperative medications, both opioid and nonopioid medications. However, more evidence needs to be generated by high-quality large-scale randomized controlled trials to show efficacy and cost-effectiveness. Furthermore, protocols need to be developed that guide perioperative providers on how to

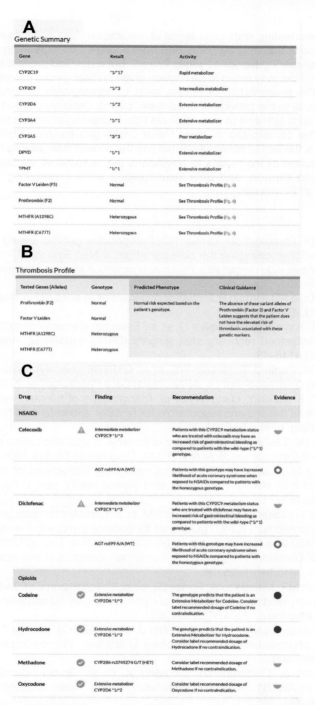

Fig. 2. Example screenshots of a pharmacogenomics tool integrated into the EHR. (*A*) A patients' metabolism status to various genes. (*B*) A patient's thrombosis profile based on pharmacogenomics. (*C*) A patient's response to various analgesics based on pharmacogenomics. (*Courtesy of* CQuentia, Fort Worth, TX.)

interpret genetic testing findings in terms of medication dose adjustment. There is a plethora of results that may be generated from a single PGx screening (especially if there are hundreds/thousands of genes tested), but a detailed presentation of these results to a provider may prove to be useless given the fast-paced nature of the operating room. The presentation of results must be strategically designed so that it proves functional to the providers. In addition, clinical decision support could be integrated into such systems to help improve PGx implementation into the perioperative space. The centerpiece to meet these challenges involves EHR integration, because this is the key to minimally disturbing the clinical flow, easing the visualization and execution of the results to physicians (eg, automated alerts/notifications, clinical decision support, and data visualization), while contributing to the cost-effectiveness of PGx testing.

REFERENCES

1. Gabriel RA, Ehrenfeld JM, Urman RD. Preoperative genetic testing and personalized medicine: changing the care paradigm. J Med Syst 2017;41(12):185.
2. Saba R, Kaye AD, Urman RD. Pharmacogenomics in pain management. Anesthesiol Clin 2017;35(2):295–304.
3. Saba R, Kaye AD, Urman RD. Pharmacogenomics in anesthesia. Anesthesiol Clin 2017;35(2):285–94.
4. Beverly A, Kaye AD, Ljungqvist O, et al. Essential elements of multimodal analgesia in enhanced recovery after surgery (ERAS) guidelines. Anesthesiol Clin 2017;35(2):e115–43.
5. Linares OA, Fudin J, Schiesser WE, et al. CYP2D6 phenotype-specific codeine population pharmacokinetics. J Pain Palliat Care Pharmacother 2015;29(1):4–15.
6. Tateishi T, Krivoruk Y, Ueng YF, et al. Identification of human liver cytochrome P-450 3A4 as the enzyme responsible for fentanyl and sufentanil N-dealkylation. Anesth Analg 1996;82(1):167–72.
7. Feierman DE, Lasker JM. Metabolism of fentanyl, a synthetic opioid analgesic, by human liver microsomes. Role of CYP3A4. Drug Metab Dispos 1996;24(9):932–9.
8. Armstrong SC, Cozza KL. Pharmacokinetic drug interactions of morphine, codeine, and their derivatives: theory and clinical reality, part I. Psychosomatics 2003;44(2):167–71.
9. Crews KR, Gaedigk A, Dunnenberger HM, et al. Clinical pharmacogenetics implementation consortium (CPIC) guidelines for codeine therapy in the context of cytochrome P450 2D6 (CYP2D6) genotype. Clin Pharmacol Ther 2012;91(2):321–6.
10. Lassen D, Damkier P, Brosen K. The pharmacogenetics of tramadol. Clin Pharmacokinet 2015;54(8):825–36.
11. Hutchinson MR, Menelaou A, Foster DJ, et al. CYP2D6 and CYP3A4 involvement in the primary oxidative metabolism of hydrocodone by human liver microsomes. Br J Clin Pharmacol 2004;57(3):287–97.
12. Venkatasubramanian R, Fukuda T, Niu J, et al. ABCC3 and OCT1 genotypes influence pharmacokinetics of morphine in children. Pharmacogenomics 2014;15(10):1297–309.
13. Sadhasivam S, Chidambaran V, Zhang X, et al. Opioid-induced respiratory depression: ABCB1 transporter pharmacogenetics. Pharmacogenomics J 2015;15(2):119–26.
14. Chidambaran V, Mavi J, Esslinger H, et al. Association of OPRM1 A118G variant with risk of morphine-induced respiratory depression following spine fusion in adolescents. Pharmacogenomics J 2015;15(3):255–62.

15. Zhang F, Tong J, Hu J, et al. COMT gene haplotypes are closely associated with postoperative fentanyl dose in patients. Anesth Analg 2015;120(4):933–40.
16. Benetton SA, Borges VM, Chang TK, et al. Role of individual human cytochrome P450 enzymes in the in vitro metabolism of hydromorphone. Xenobiotica 2004; 34(4):335–44.
17. Bunten H, Liang WJ, Pounder DJ, et al. OPRM1 and CYP2B6 gene variants as risk factors in methadone-related deaths. Clin Pharmacol Ther 2010;88(3):383–9.
18. Bunten H, Liang WJ, Pounder D, et al. CYP2B6 and OPRM1 gene variations predict methadone-related deaths. Addict Biol 2011;16(1):142–4.
19. Hodges LM, Markova SM, Chinn LW, et al. Very important pharmacogene summary: ABCB1 (MDR1, P-glycoprotein). Pharmacogenet Genomics 2011;21(3):152–61.
20. Kharasch ED, Hoffer C, Whittington D, et al. Role of hepatic and intestinal cytochrome P450 3A and 2B6 in the metabolism, disposition, and miotic effects of methadone. Clin Pharmacol Ther 2004;76(3):250–69.
21. Carlson CL. Effectiveness of the World Health Organization cancer pain relief guidelines: an integrative review. J Pain Res 2016;9:515–34.
22. Lee SS, Buters JT, Pineau T, et al. Role of CYP2E1 in the hepatotoxicity of acetaminophen. J Biol Chem 1996;271(20):12063–7.
23. Yoon E, Babar A, Choudhary M, et al. Acetaminophen-induced hepatotoxicity: a comprehensive update. J Clin Transl Hepatol 2016;4(2):131–42.
24. Tankanitlert J, Morales NP, Howard TA, et al. Effects of combined UDP-glucuronosyltransferase (UGT) 1A1*28 and 1A6*2 on paracetamol pharmacokinetics in beta-thalassemia/HbE. Pharmacology 2007;79(2):97–103.
25. Navarro SL, Chen Y, Li L, et al. UGT1A6 and UGT2B15 polymorphisms and acetaminophen conjugation in response to a randomized, controlled diet of select fruits and vegetables. Drug Metab Dispos 2011;39(9):1650–7.
26. Court MH, Zhu Z, Masse G, et al. Race, gender, and genetic polymorphism contribute to variability in acetaminophen pharmacokinetics, metabolism, and protein-adduct concentrations in healthy African-American and European-American volunteers. J Pharmacol Exp Ther 2017;362(3):431–40.
27. Yamamoto A, Liu MY, Kurogi K, et al. Sulphation of acetaminophen by the human cytosolic sulfotransferases: a systematic analysis. J Biochem 2015;158(6):497–504.
28. Mazaleuskaya LL, Sangkuhl K, Thorn CF, et al. PharmGKB summary: pathways of acetaminophen metabolism at the therapeutic versus toxic doses. Pharmacogenet Genomics 2015;25(8):416–26.
29. Mazaleuskaya LL, Theken KN, Gong L, et al. PharmGKB summary: ibuprofen pathways. Pharmacogenet Genomics 2015;25(2):96–106.
30. Sullivan-Klose TH, Ghanayem BI, Bell DA, et al. The role of the CYP2C9-Leu359 allelic variant in the tolbutamide polymorphism. Pharmacogenetics 1996;6(4):341–9.
31. Bowalgaha K, Elliot DJ, Mackenzie PI, et al. S-Naproxen and desmethylnaproxen glucuronidation by human liver microsomes and recombinant human UDP-glucuronosyltransferases (UGT): role of UGT2B7 in the elimination of naproxen. Br J Clin Pharmacol 2005;60(4):423–33.
32. Agundez JA, Garcia-Martin E, Martinez C. Genetically based impairment in CYP2C8- and CYP2C9-dependent NSAID metabolism as a risk factor for gastrointestinal bleeding: is a combination of pharmacogenomics and metabolomics required to improve personalized medicine? Expert Opin Drug Metab Toxicol 2009;5(6):607–20.
33. Prieto-Pérez R, Ochoa D, Cabaleiro T, et al. Evaluation of the relationship between polymorphisms in CYP2C8 and CYP2C9 and the pharmacokinetics of celecoxib. J Clin Pharmacol 2013;53(12):1261–7.

34. Wang B, Wang J, Huang SQ, et al. Genetic polymorphism of the human cytochrome P450 2C9 gene and its clinical significance. Curr Drug Metab 2009; 10(7):781–834.

35. Chan AT, Zauber AG, Hsu M, et al. Cytochrome P450 2C9 variants influence response to celecoxib for prevention of colorectal adenoma. Gastroenterology 2009;136(7):2127–36.e1.

36. Shin KH, Choi MH, Lim KS, et al. Evaluation of endogenous metabolic markers of hepatic CYP3A activity using metabolic profiling and midazolam clearance. Clin Pharmacol Ther 2013;94(5):601–9.

37. Miao J, Jin Y, Marunde RL, et al. Association of genotypes of the CYP3A cluster with midazolam disposition in vivo. Pharmacogenomics J 2009;9(5):319–26.

38. Cohen M, Sadhasivam S, Vinks AA. Pharmacogenetics in perioperative medicine. Curr Opin Anaesthesiol 2012;25(4):419–27.

39. Floyd MD, Gervasini G, Masica AL, et al. Genotype-phenotype associations for common CYP3A4 and CYP3A5 variants in the basal and induced metabolism of midazolam in European- and African-American men and women. Pharmacogenetics 2003;13(10):595–606.

40. Seng KY, Hee KH, Soon GH, et al. CYP3A5*3 and bilirubin predict midazolam population pharmacokinetics in Asian cancer patients. J Clin Pharmacol 2014; 54(2):215–24.

41. Elens L, Nieuweboer A, Clarke SJ, et al. CYP3A4 intron 6 C>T SNP (CYP3A4*22) encodes lower CYP3A4 activity in cancer patients, as measured with probes midazolam and erythromycin. Pharmacogenomics 2013;14(2):137–49.

42. Seo KA, Bae SK, Choi YK, et al. Metabolism of 1'- and 4-hydroxymidazolam by glucuronide conjugation is largely mediated by UDP-glucuronosyltransferases 1A4, 2B4, and 2B7. Drug Metab Dispos 2010;38(11):2007–13.

43. Sawamura R, Sato H, Kawakami J, et al. Inhibitory effect of azole antifungal agents on the glucuronidation of lorazepam using rabbit liver microsomes in vitro. Biol Pharm Bull 2000;23(5):669–71.

44. Herman RJ, Chaudhary A, Szakacs CB. Disposition of lorazepam in Gilbert's syndrome: effects of fasting, feeding, and enterohepatic circulation. J Clin Pharmacol 1994;34(10):978–84.

45. Dixon CM, Colthup PV, Serabjit-Singh CJ, et al. Multiple forms of cytochrome P450 are involved in the metabolism of ondansetron in humans. Drug Metab Dispos 1995;23(11):1225–30.

46. Bell GC, Caudle KE, Whirl-Carrillo M, et al. Clinical Pharmacogenetics Implementation Consortium (CPIC) guideline for CYP2D6 genotype and use of ondansetron and tropisetron. Clin Pharmacol Ther 2017;102(2):213–8.

47. MacKenzie M, Hall R. Pharmacogenomics and pharmacogenetics for the intensive care unit: a narrative review. Can J Anaesth 2017;64(1):45–64.

48. He H, Yin JY, Xu YJ, et al. Association of ABCB1 polymorphisms with the efficacy of ondansetron in chemotherapy-induced nausea and vomiting. Clin Ther 2014; 36(8):1242–52.e2.

49. Tzvetkov MV, Saadatmand AR, Bokelmann K, et al. Effects of OCT1 polymorphisms on the cellular uptake, plasma concentrations and efficacy of the 5-HT(3) antagonists tropisetron and ondansetron. Pharmacogenomics J 2012; 12(1):22–9.

50. Parkman HP, Mishra A, Jacobs M, et al. Clinical response and side effects of metoclopramide: associations with clinical, demographic, and pharmacogenetic parameters. J Clin Gastroenterol 2012;46(6):494–503.

51. Perwitasari DA, Gelderblom H, Atthobari J, et al. Anti-emetic drugs in oncology: pharmacology and individualization by pharmacogenetics. Int J Clin Pharm 2011; 33(1):33–43.
52. Yu H, Yan H, Wang L, et al. Five novel loci associated with antipsychotic treatment response in patients with schizophrenia: a genome-wide association study. Lancet Psychiatry 2018;5(4):327–38.
53. Nakamura K, Yokoi T, Inoue K, et al. CYP2D6 is the principal cytochrome P450 responsible for metabolism of the histamine H1 antagonist promethazine in human liver microsomes. Pharmacogenetics 1996;6(5):449–57.
54. Saruwatari J, Matsunaga M, Ikeda K, et al. Impact of CYP2D6*10 on H1-antihistamine-induced hypersomnia. Eur J Clin Pharmacol 2006;62(12): 995–1001.
55. Li J, Wang S, Barone J, et al. Warfarin pharmacogenomics. P T 2009;34(8):422–7.
56. Brown SA, Pereira N. Pharmacogenomic impact of CYP2C19 variation on clopidogrel therapy in precision cardiovascular medicine. J Pers Med 2018; 8(1) [pii:E8].
57. Luzum JA, Sweet KM, Binkley PF, et al. CYP2D6 genetic variation and beta-blocker maintenance dose in patients with heart failure. Pharm Res 2017;34(8): 1615–25.
58. Lymperopoulos A, McCrink KA, Brill A. Impact of CYP2D6 genetic variation on the response of the cardiovascular patient to carvedilol and metoprolol. Curr Drug Metab 2015;17(1):30–6.
59. Gao X, Wang H, Chen H. Impact of CYP2D6 and ADRB1 polymorphisms on heart rate of post-PCI patients treated with metoprolol. Pharmacogenomics 2017. https://doi.org/10.2217/pgs-2017-0203.
60. Dean L. Metoprolol therapy and CYP2D6 genotype. In: Pratt V, McLeod H, Dean L, et al, editors. Medical genetics summaries. Bethesda (MD): National Center for Biotechnology Information (US); 2012.
61. Liem EB, Joiner TV, Tsueda K, et al. Increased sensitivity to thermal pain and reduced subcutaneous lidocaine efficacy in redheads. Anesthesiology 2005; 102(3):509–14.
62. Kim JH, Jarvik GP, Browning BL, et al. Exome sequencing reveals novel rare variants in the ryanodine receptor and calcium channel genes in malignant hyperthermia families. Anesthesiology 2013;119(5):1054–65.
63. Muniz VP, Silva HC, Tsanaclis AM, et al. Screening for mutations in the RYR1 gene in families with malignant hyperthermia. J Mol Neurosci 2003;21(1):35–42.
64. Gonsalves SG, Ng D, Johnston JJ, et al. Using exome data to identify malignant hyperthermia susceptibility mutations. Anesthesiology 2013;119(5):1043–53.
65. Khalil H, Sereika SM, Dai F, et al. OPRM1 and COMT gene-gene interaction is associated with postoperative pain and opioid consumption after orthopedic trauma. Biol Res Nurs 2017;19(2):170–9.
66. Kim KM, Kim HS, Lim SH, et al. Effects of genetic polymorphisms of OPRM1, ABCB1, CYP3A4/5 on postoperative fentanyl consumption in Korean gynecologic patients. Int J Clin Pharmacol Ther 2013;51(5):383–92.
67. Landau R, Liu SK, Blouin JL, et al. The effect of OPRM1 and COMT genotypes on the analgesic response to intravenous fentanyl labor analgesia. Anesth Analg 2013;116(2):386–91.
68. Senagore AJ, Champagne BJ, Dosokey E, et al. Pharmacogenetics-guided analgesics in major abdominal surgery: further benefits within an enhanced recovery protocol. Am J Surg 2017;213(3):467–72.

69. De Gregori M, Diatchenko L, Ingelmo PM, et al. Human genetic variability contributes to postoperative morphine consumption. J Pain 2016;17(5):628–36.
70. Ren ZY, Xu XQ, Bao YP, et al. The impact of genetic variation on sensitivity to opioid analgesics in patients with postoperative pain: a systematic review and meta-analysis. Pain Physician 2015;18(2):131–52.
71. Henker RA, Lewis A, Dai F, et al. The associations between OPRM 1 and COMT genotypes and postoperative pain, opioid use, and opioid-induced sedation. Biol Res Nurs 2013;15(3):309–17.
72. Boswell MV, Stauble ME, Loyd GE, et al. The role of hydromorphone and OPRM1 in postoperative pain relief with hydrocodone. Pain Physician 2013; 16(3):E227–35.
73. Ochroch EA, Vachani A, Gottschalk A, et al. Natural variation in the mu-opioid gene OPRM1 predicts increased pain on third day after thoracotomy. Clin J Pain 2012;28(9):747–54.
74. De Gregori M, Garbin G, De Gregori S, et al. Genetic variability at COMT but not at OPRM1 and UGT2B7 loci modulates morphine analgesic response in acute postoperative pain. Eur J Clin Pharmacol 2013;69(9):1651–8.
75. Bartosova O, Polanecky O, Perlik F, et al. OPRM1 and ABCB1 polymorphisms and their effect on postoperative pain relief with piritramide. Physiol Res 2015; 64(Suppl 4):S521–7.
76. Hayashida M, Nagashima M, Satoh Y, et al. Analgesic requirements after major abdominal surgery are associated with OPRM1 gene polymorphism genotype and haplotype. Pharmacogenomics 2008;9(11):1605–16.
77. Zwisler ST, Enggaard TP, Mikkelsen S, et al. Lack of association of OPRM1 and ABCB1 single-nucleotide polymorphisms to oxycodone response in postoperative pain. J Clin Pharmacol 2012;52(2):234–42.

Creating a Pathway for Multidisciplinary Shared Decision-Making to Improve Communication During Preoperative Assessment

Timothy D. Quinn, MD[a,b],*, Piotr Wolczynski, MD[c],
Raymond Sroka, PharmD, MD[a,b], Richard D. Urman, MD, MBA[d]

KEYWORDS

- Perioperative medicine • Shared decision-making
- Preoperative anesthesia evaluation • Appropriateness • Multidisciplinary team
- High-risk • Anesthesiology • Quality improvement

KEY POINTS

- Shared decision-making (SDM) is vital for high-quality surgical decision-making.
- Lack of adequate time is a perceived barrier to effective SDM.
- Patients may seem to have an understanding of the risks and benefits of an intervention but may actually have deficits in decision-making.
- Multidisciplinary decision-making (MDM) before surgery is an opportunity for anesthesiologists to enhance communication through the preoperative anesthesia evaluation.
- The authors have developed a pathway for MDM and implemented it at their institution.

The authors have no disclosures to report.
[a] Department of Anesthesiology, Jacobs School of Medicine and Biomedical Sciences, State University of New York at Buffalo, 77 Goodell Street, Suite 550, Buffalo, NY 14203, USA; [b] Department of Anesthesiology, Critical Care and Pain Medicine, Roswell Park Comprehensive Cancer Center, Elm and Carlton Streets, Buffalo, NY 14263, USA; [c] Department of Internal Medicine, Jacobs School of Medicine and Biomedical Sciences, State University of New York at Buffalo, 462 Grider Street, Buffalo, NY 14215, USA; [d] Department of Anesthesiology, Perioperative and Pain Medicine, Center for Perioperative Research, Brigham and Women's Hospital, Harvard Medical School, 75 Francis Street, Boston, MA 02115, USA
* Corresponding author. Department of Anesthesiology, Critical Care and Pain Medicine, Roswell Park Comprehensive Cancer Center, 3rd Floor, Clinical Sciences Building, Elm & Carlton Streets, Buffalo, NY 14263.
E-mail address: Timothy.Quinn@roswellpark.org

Anesthesiology Clin 36 (2018) 653–662
https://doi.org/10.1016/j.anclin.2018.07.011
1932-2275/18/© 2018 Elsevier Inc. All rights reserved.

anesthesiology.theclinics.com

INTRODUCTION

Effective communication in the perioperative period is vital for safe surgical care.[1] Communication breakdowns have been cited in the preoperative, intraoperative, and postoperative periods.[2–4] There are 2 main forms of preoperative communication. The first is communication between clinicians and the patient, which is described in the literature as shared decision-making (SDM).[5] The preoperative anesthesia evaluation (PAE) provides an opportunity for anesthesiologists to engage in SDM before the day of surgery.[6] The second form of communication in the preoperative period is multidisciplinary decision-making (MDM) between different members of the health care team to optimize patient care and minimize risk. Anesthesiologists may play a pivotal role in this communication. Both types of communication involve consistent effort from all groups and systematic support to be effective. The end goal is to provide appropriate surgical care that is high-quality and patient-centered.[7–10]

This review discusses the fundamentals of SDM and MDM and proposes a pathway for anesthesiology-led SDM and MDM in the preoperative period.

APPROPRIATENESS IN SURGICAL CARE

Appropriate surgical care is not simply the surgeon choosing for the patient the correct surgery for the patient's disease. Appropriate surgical care is more complex and aims to do more good than harm and align with the patient's goals for treatment.[11] A conceptual framework to better understand the different facets of high-quality surgical decision-making has been previously developed.[7] It consists of 4 parts. The first component is choosing the right surgery for the disease based on current evidence-based practices. Second, the surgery should be performed at the right place to ensure compliance with standards and regulations, and availability of proper resources, to not only perform the surgery but also to manage any potential complications of the surgery to the patient. Third, the right provider should be chosen who has the proper training and expertise to perform the surgery. Finally, and potentially most important, is the patient must be right for the proposed surgery. Effective 2-way communication between the patient and the clinicians should be sought. Does the patient fully understand all that the surgery will entail from preoperative optimization, the risks and benefits of the surgery, and the anesthesia and rehabilitation required?

For example, a highly invasive procedure requiring substantial recovery time in an elderly patient near the end of life may be medically indicated but may not fulfill the patient's desire to maximize time with family away from medical institutions. This may seem intuitive, yet there are data demonstrating the high incidence of surgery in the last year of a patient's life and surgeries performed during a terminal admission.[12–14] The question for clinicians caring for surgical patients is how to ensure that health care decisions, at every stage of life or disease process, match the preferences and wishes of the patient.

SDM is vital to achieving the fourth component of high-quality decision-making for surgical care. The PAE may serve as a pause point to foster communication between members of the health care team and the patient.[6]

SHARED DECISION-MAKING
Background

A key component of patient autonomy is SDM. In 1982, describing patient and medical provider interactions that should form the basis of SDM, the Presidents' Commission for the Study of Ethical Problems in Medicine and Biomedical and Behavioral Research defined the interaction as follows[15,16]:

> It will usually consist of discussions between professional and patient that bring the knowledge, concerns, and perspective of each to the process of seeking agreement on a course of treatment. Simply put, this means that the physician or other health professional invites the patient to participate in a dialogue in which the professional seeks to help the patient understand the medical situation and available courses of action, and the patient conveys his or her concerns and wishes.

There has been a massive expansion in medical technology and surgical interventions available to patients over the past 40 years since the Commission convened. How do clinicians ensure there is adequate communication and engagement so that patients are making medical decisions with an informed understanding of the risks, benefits, and other potential treatment options?

Definition of Shared Decision-Making

SDM occurs when the clinician and the patient engage in an open dialogue about health care choices.[17] Each clinical scenario between the clinician and the patient may illicit different levels of interaction. Some health care decisions are straightforward because the best option is either clearly defined or the risks to the patient are relatively minor.[18] Other health care decisions are more complicated and may require more intensive back and forth communication and clarification, especially ones that involve how aggressively to treat a disease that is diagnosed in the early stages or that will require chronic and sustained exposure to treatments such as chemotherapy.

The 3 main components of SDM for the patient include[19]
- The patient must be given information about the treatment options available and the risks and benefits of each
- The patient should be given opportunity to weigh the risks and benefits against their own values and preferences for treatment and quality of life
- The patient should be able to discuss these issues with the clinician.

The clinician should possess the following competencies for SDM[20]:
- Develop a partnership with the patient
- Establish the patient's preferences for information (how much and how it is presented)
- Establish the patient's preferences for his or her role in decision-making
- Ascertain and respond to the patient's ideas, concerns, and expectations
- Identify choices and evaluate the evidence with respect to the patient
- Present the evidence to the patient in a way that maximizes the patient's understanding and processing of the information
- Resolve any conflict with the patient in a collaborative manner
- Agree on an action plan and follow-through.

The clinician should explain the risks and benefits of each treatment option and invite the patient to offer her or his opinions and wishes. The ultimate decision may not be what the clinician thinks is optimal. Rather, it might be the decision that best reflects the patient's values and preferences.

Clinicians should be wary about recommending any treatment option over another without engaging in SDM first. One study showed that patients were more involved in decision-making for a proposed surgery (lumpectomy vs mastectomy) if the provider did not make an initial recommendation either way.[21] The providers were less likely to present a balanced representation of both options if they recommended a specific surgery over another. In general, SDM principles have evolved from nonsurgical specialties, and there have been limited studies evaluating SDM practices in surgical and perioperative environments.

Deficits in Shared Decision-Making

Even when the clinician engages in open dialogue regarding all therapeutic options and the risks and benefits associated with each option, patients may not fully comprehend what is being told to them. In 1 study, 882 preoperative subjects seen at a preoperative anesthesia clinic at a tertiary academic medical center completed a survey with demographic, clinical, and psychosocial questions.[22] Questions were designed to gauge the subject's understanding of the proposed surgery, postoperative disposition (ie, admission to the intensive care unit), and discharge from the hospital. About 15% of subjects had deficits in knowledge of the diagnosis and/or procedure. Subjects with deficits in surgical decision-making were more likely to be older, black, or Asian, or those who used denial as a coping mechanism. A similar study surveyed 1034 subjects after the informed surgical consent was signed.[23] Non-English speaking subjects and subjects with a lower education level were more likely to demonstrate deficits in decision-making. The study also showed deficits in advanced care planning, including approximately 66% of respondents who had not completed an advance directive and nearly half who lacked a designated health care proxy. A recent pilot study by Urman and colleagues[24] showed poor compliance by perioperative providers in documenting code status limitations in surgical patients, even though there are established professional society guidelines from both surgery and anesthesiology societies for preprocedural reconsideration of code status limitations.

Studies such as these raise important ethical concerns regarding how well patients not only understand the risks and benefits associated with the proposed surgery but also the availability and efficacy of other treatment options. Patients may not reveal their deficits. Special attention should be paid to patient groups at high risk for deficits in surgical decision-making. Patients with preoperative deficits in surgical decision-making may encounter more challenges in the postoperative period, especially if the patient has a complicated hospital course and end-of-life decisions become a reality.[25]

Understanding which patient populations are most at risk is important; however, it is also important to determine which groups are most receptive to SDM. One cross-sectional study of 364 subjects undergoing anesthesia in Singapore aimed to identify demographic factors that can predict patient preferences in SDM. Subjects who preferred greater participation in medical decisions were in a younger age group, had a higher level of education, and were employed. Most subjects (52.2%) wished to make a joint decision with the anesthesiologist and the preferred method of communication was a discussion with the provider, as opposed to reading a pamphlet or watching a video.[26]

Barriers to Shared Decision-Making

A systemic review of 38 studies showed that the most common barrier to SDM was perceived time constraints by clinicians.[27] Patient characteristics and the clinical situation were also prevalent barriers. In other words, clinicians made assumptions about which patients would be interested in engaging in SDM. There is the possibility that clinicians will fail to engage in SDM in certain patient populations or understand how to approach SDM with different patient populations. For SDM to work in the preoperative setting, anesthesiologists need to invite patients to express their opinions and values and not defer to the opinion of the clinician. Patients consider a good patient–doctor relationship (eg, trust, honesty, equity) as essential in the implementation of SDM.[28]

The patient is at a decided disadvantage for effective SDM secondary to uncertainty about the prognosis and treatment course.[29] In a systemic review of 39 studies that measured SDM and evaluated the relationship between SDM and at least 1 subject outcome, researchers found it is critical to develop a better understanding of what actually makes decision-making shared because patient-reported measures of SDM tend to be higher than observer ratings of effective SDM.[30] The researchers point out that the problem may lie in the actual instruments used to measure SDM or in differences in understanding the conceptual definition of SDM. These observations are supported by recent work looking at responses of 80 preoperative patients who visited an outpatient preoperative anesthesiology clinic.[31] Patients and clinicians scored themselves better in achieving SDM than did observers who used validated questionnaires to measure SDM. Again, these findings beg the question of why such differences are observed. The investigators suggest that anesthesiologists may still be unaware of what truly defines SDM. Although they discuss the different options available and respective risks and benefits, they often do not wholeheartedly invite the patients to participate in the actual decision-making process. One of the causes in the difference between subjective and objective appreciations of the level of SDM is that clinicians and patients express their degree of satisfaction with the consultation rather than the perceived level of SDM.

Shared Decision-Making Aids

When multiple treatment or screening options exist, decision aids can be instrumental in educating patients. Decision aids can take many forms, including visual aids, flowcharts, printed material, videos, or online tutorials. It has been shown that when patients use decision aids, they believe it improves their knowledge of the options, consider themselves better informed and clearer about what matters most to them, have more accurate expectations of risks and benefits, and are more likely to engage in decision-making.[32] By conducting a prospective cohort study, Sepucha and colleagues[33] found that patient decision aids, when used as part of routine orthopedic care, were associated with increased knowledge, more SDM, higher patient experience ratings, and lower surgical rates.

The International Patient Decision Aid Standards (IPDAS) was founded in 2003 to enhance the quality and effectiveness of patient decision aids. A compilation of 13 articles within the first 10 years of the development of IPDAS offers valuable insight into the creation, evaluation, and implementation of patient decision aids.[34] The use of mobile health applications has emerged as another option to support SDM.[35] Research in this field has shown that the mobile apps can increase patient satisfaction and engagement in SDM. On the other hand, the apps may increase patient anxiety. There are also access issues for patients who lack the technological resources to support the apps. Clinicians interested in using these apps in their practice should ensure they conform to IPDAS standards and are accessible to the patient population they serve.

Has Shared Decision-Making Actually Taken Place?

It is difficult to assess if adequate SDM has been achieved. One study has looked at this topic in-depth and cited reasons why measuring SDM can be challenging.[36] Tools continue to be developed to better gauge, objectively from third-party observers and subjectively from patient feedback, whether SDM has taken place to a satisfactory level. Developing validated tools to measure the quality of SDM in the perioperative setting is an important topic for ongoing research.

Potential Benefits of Shared Decision-Making to the Clinician

Physician burnout, caused by stress and exhaustion with clinical responsibilities, can negatively affect patient care.[37,38] Burnout involves emotional exhaustion or loss of enjoyment for work, cynicism and loss of empathy for patients, and the feeling that work does not have meaning or worth.[39] Greater emphasis is being placed on developing ways to address and alleviate physician burnout.[40] Some investigators have proposed effective SDM with patients as an opportunity to reduce burnout.[41] The hypothesis is that by improving the interactions between physicians and patients, more meaningful interactions will occur and improve satisfaction and sense of personal worth for the provider. Improvement in physician burnout would not instantly improve with this single intervention. SDM would need to be part of a more comprehensive approach to reducing physician burnout, with attention to how the intervention is affecting physician attitudes.

MULTIDISCIPLINARY DECISION-MAKING BEFORE SURGERY

The concept of MDM to assess and manage disease is well-represented in the literature.[42] An example of the multidisciplinary team approach is a tumor board in cancer care that accurately stages disease and guides surgical and nonsurgical treatment options.[43,44] Anesthesiologists, especially those involved in perioperative medicine, are uniquely positioned to facilitate collaboration for appropriate surgical care through multidisciplinary communication. Anesthesiologists may be able to offer insight and expertise on how the patient's comorbidities may compound surgical stress, outcomes, and quality of life after surgery. There is increasing interest in fostering more collaboration in surgical care, especially for high-risk patients, although it is conceded that this approach will require a cultural shift and a commitment by all team members to share accountability for outcomes of surgical or nonsurgical care.[45] The Royal College of Anesthetists has proposed a multidisciplinary approach to surgical care in the perioperative period whereby the meetings should be used to make a collaborative decision about whether to operate, to optimize the patient preoperatively, and to outline the multidisciplinary care needed intraoperatively and postoperatively.[46]

A novel approach to better use the PAE would be to use the preoperative period as an opportunity to optimize patients before surgery while increasing the quality of SDM and MDM. At the authors' institution, Roswell Park Comprehensive Cancer Center, we have developed an anesthesiology-led model to identify the high-risk patients most vulnerable to complications. **Fig. 1** demonstrates a preoperative clinical pathway we have implemented in which enhanced MDM is conducted between members of the health care team.[47] The aim is to determine whether the proposed surgery is appropriate for the high-risk patient from a holistic standpoint of health status and patient values, not just the surgical indication. Ensuring the presence of an advance directive and designated health care proxy are part of the process.

As a center, Roswell Park gains several advantages from using this pathway to enhance MDM. A robust Anesthesia Preoperative Evaluation Clinic is maintained with administrative support and staffed with an anesthesiologist, as well as midlevel providers and nurses. The anesthesiologists are motivated and dedicated to the mission of advancing perioperative care and communication. Roswell Park is focused solely on the diagnosis and treatment of cancer; therefore, anesthesiologists have a close working relationship with their surgical colleagues. This likely promotes communication and collegiality when discussing challenging clinical situations.

The authors have modified this pathway to reflect points in the process in which SDM may be emphasized. We continue to adopt strategies to improve direct SDM in addition to MDM.

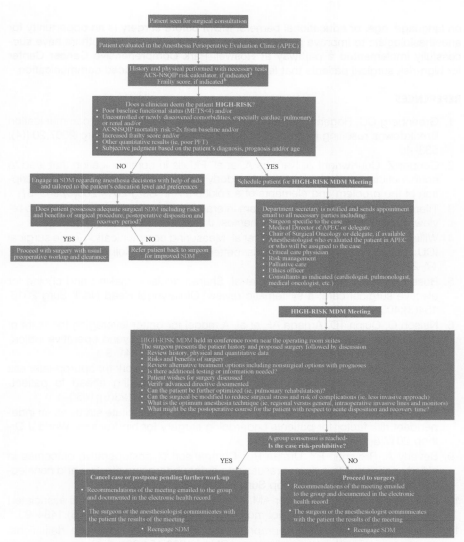

Fig. 1. Anesthesiology-led pathway development for SDM and MDM in the preoperative period for high-risk patients. ACS-NSQIP, American College of Surgeons National Surgical Quality Improvement Program; METS, measurement of exercise tolerance before surgery. [a] Consider for invasive procedures. Defer for American Society of Anesthesiologists Physical Status I or II. [b] Consider for invasive procedure. Hold for age younger than 65 years or METS greater than 7. PFT, pulmonary function test. (*Modified from* Sroka R, Gabriel EM, Al-Hadidi D, et al. A novel anesthesiologist-led multidisciplinary model for evaluating high-risk surgical patients at a comprehensive cancer center. J Healthc Risk Manag 2018; with permission.)

SUMMARY

SDM is essential for high-quality surgical care. Barriers to SDM exist in clinical practice but there is evidence these obstacles can be overcome with organizational support and committed clinicians.[17] SDM requires clinician and patient engagement. Though patients may indicate understanding, deficits in decision-making may persist based on language, age, or educational barriers. MDM before surgery is an opportunity for anesthesiologists to improve perioperative and surgical care. The authors have successfully implemented a pathway at Roswell Park Comprehensive Cancer Center for high-risk surgical patients that leverages the PAE for enhanced communication.

REFERENCES

1. Greenberg CC, Regenbogen SE, Studdert DM, et al. Patterns of communication Breakdowns resulting in injury to surgical patients. J Am Coll Surg 2007;204(4): 533–40.
2. Cooper Z, Courtwright A, Karlage A, et al. Pitfalls in communication that lead to nonbeneficial emergency surgery in elderly patients with serious illness: description of the problem and elements of a solution. Ann Surg 2014;260(6):949–57.
3. Tiferes J, Bisantz AM, Guru KA. Team interaction during surgery: a systematic review of communication coding schemes. J Surg Res 2015;195(2):422–32.
4. Williams M, Hevelone N, Alban RF, et al. Measuring communication in the surgical ICU: better communication equals better care. J Am Coll Surg 2010;210(1): 17–22.
5. Boss EF, Mehta N, Nagarajan N, et al. Shared decision making and choice for elective surgical care: a systematic review. Otolaryngol Head Neck Surg 2016; 154(3):405–20.
6. Nelson O, Quinn TD, Arriaga AF, et al. A model for better leveraging the point of preoperative assessment: patients and providers look beyond operative indications when making decisions. A A Case Rep 2016;6(8):241–8.
7. Cooper Z, Sayal P, Abbett SK, et al. A conceptual framework for appropriateness in surgical care: reviewing past approaches and looking ahead to patient-centered shared decision making. Anesthesiology 2015;123(6):1450–4.
8. Brovman EY, Pisansky AJ, Beverly A, et al. Do-Not-Resuscitate status as an independent risk factor for patients undergoing surgery for hip fracture. World J Orthop 2017;8(12):902–12.
9. Beverly A, Brovman EY, Urman RD. Comparison of postoperative outcomes in elderly patients with a do-not-resuscitate order undergoing elective and nonelective hip surgery. Geriatr Orthop Surg Rehabil 2017;8(2):78–86.
10. Walsh EC, Brovman EY, Bader AM, et al. Do-not-resuscitate status is associated with increased mortality but not morbidity. Anesth Analg 2017;125(5):1484–93.
11. Lavis JN, Anderson GM. Appropriateness in health care delivery: definitions, measurement and policy implications. CMAJ 1996;154:321–8.
12. Kwok AC, Semel ME, Lipsitz SR, et al. The intensity and variation of surgical care at the end of life: A retrospective cohort study. Lancet 2011;378:1409–13.
13. Barnet CS, Arriga AF, Hepner DL, et al. Surgery at the end of life: a pilot study comparing decedents and survivors at a tertiary care center. Anesthesiology 2013;119(4):796–801.
14. Barnato AE, McClellan MB, Kagay CR, et al. Trends in inpatient treatment intensity among Medicare beneficiaries at the end of life. Health Serv Res 2004;39: 363–75.
15. Santhirapala R, Moonesinghe R. Primum Non Nocere: is shared decision-making the answer? Perioper Med (Lond) 2016;5:16.
16. United States. President's commission for the study of ethical problems in medicine and biomedical and behavioral research. U S Code Annot U S 1982; Title 42 Sect. 300v as added 1978:Unknown.

17. Légaré F, Thompson-Leduc P. Twelve myths about shared decision making. Patient Educ Couns 2014;96(3):281–6.
18. Barry MJ, Edgman-Levitan S. Shared decision making—pinnacle of patient-centered care. N Engl J Med 2012;366(9):780–1.
19. Murthy S, Hepner DL, Cooper Z, et al. Leveraging the preoperative clinic to engage older patients in shared decision making about complex surgery: an illustrative case. A A Case Rep 2016;7(2):30–2.
20. Towle A, Godolphin W. Framework for teaching and learning informed shared decision making. BMJ 1999;319(7212):766–71.
21. Frongillo M, Feibelmann S, Belkora J, et al. Is there shared decision making when the provider makes a recommendation? Patient Educ Couns 2013;90(1):69–73.
22. Cooper Z, Hevelone N, Sarhan M, et al. Identifying patient characteristics associated with deficits in surgical decision making. J Patient Saf 2016. [Epub ahead of print].
23. Ankuda CK, Block SD, Cooper Z, et al. Measuring critical deficits in shared decision making before elective surgery. Patient Educ Couns 2014;94(3):328–33.
24. Urman RD, Lilley EJ, Changala M, et al. A pilot study to evaluate compliance with guidelines for preprocedural reconsideration of code status limitations. J Palliat Med 2018. [Epub ahead of print].
25. Fisher M, Ridley S. Uncertainty in end-of-life care and shared decision making. Crit Care Resusc 2012;14(1):81–7.
26. Yek JL, Lee AK, Tan JA, et al. Defining reasonable patient standards and preference for shared decision making among patients undergoing anesthesia in Singapore. BMC Med Ethics 2017;18(1):6.
27. Légaré F, Ratte S, Gravel K, et al. Barriers and facilitators to implementing shared decision-making in clinical practice: update of a systematic review of health professionals' perceptions. Patient Educ Couns 2008;73:526–35.
28. Santema TB, Stoffer EA, Kunneman M, et al. What are the decision making preferences of patients in vascular surgery? A mixed-methods study. BMJ Open 2017;7:e013272.
29. Gulbrandsen P, Clayman ML, Beach MC, et al. Shared decision-making as an existential journey: aiming for restored autonomous capacity. Patient Educ Couns 2016;99(9):1505–10.
30. Shay LA, Lafata JE. Where is the evidence? A systematic review of shared decision making and patient outcomes. Med Decis Making 2015;35(1):114–31.
31. Stubenrouch FE, Mus EMK, Lut JW, et al. The current level of shared decision-making in anesthesiology: an exploratory study. BMC Anesthesiol 2017;17(1):95.
32. Stacey D, Légaré F, Lewis K, et al. Decision aids to help people who are facing health treatment or screening decisions. Cochrane Database Syst Rev 2017;(4):CD001431.
33. Sepucha K, Atlas SJ, Chang Y, et al. Patient decision aids improve decision quality and patient experience and reduce surgical rates in routine orthopaedic care: a prospective cohort study. J Bone Joint Surg Am 2017;99(15):1253–60.
34. Volk RJ, Shokar NK, Leal VB, et al. Development and pilot testing of an online case-based approach to shared decision making skills training for clinicians. BMC Med Inform Decis Mak 2014;14:95.
35. Rahimi SA, Menear M, Robitaille H, et al. Are mobile health applications useful for supporting shared decision making in diagnostic and treatment decisions? BMC Med Inform Decis Mak 2014;14:95.

36. Elwyn G, Barr PJ, Grande SW, et al. Developing CollaboRATE: a fast and frugal patient-reported measure of shared decision making in clinical encounters. Patient Educ Couns 2013;93(1):102–7.
37. Kawamura Y, Takayashiki A, Ito M, et al. Stress factors associated with burnout among attending physicians: a cross-sectional study. J Clin Med Res 2018; 10(3):226–32.
38. Fahrenkopf AM, Sectish TC, Barger LK, et al. Rates of medication errors among depressed and burnt out residents: prospective cohort study. BMJ 2008; 336(7642):488–91.
39. Maslach C, Jackson S, Leiter M. Maslach burnout inventory. Palo Alto (CA): Consulting Psychologist Press; 1996.
40. Siedsma M, Emlet L. Physician burnout: can we make a difference together? Crit Care 2015;19:273.
41. Dobler CG, West CP, Montori VM. Can Shared decision making improve physician well-being and reduce burnout? Cureus 2017;9(8):e1615.
42. Beller JP, Scheinerman JA, Balsam LB, et al. Operative strategies and outcomes in type A aortic dissection after the enactment of a multidisciplinary aortic surgery team. Innovations 2015;10(6):410–5.
43. El Saghir NS, Keating NL, Carlson RW, et al. Tumor boards: optimizing the structure and improving efficiency of multidisciplinary management of patients with cancer worldwide. Am Soc Clin Oncol Educ Book 2014;e461–6.
44. Keating NL, Landrum MB, Lamont EB, et al. Tumor boards and the quality of cancer care. J Natl Cancer Inst 2013;105(2):113–21.
45. Glance LG, Osler TM, Neuman MD. Redesigning surgical decision making for high-risk patients. N Engl J Med 2014;370(15):1379–81.
46. Whiteman AR, Dhesi JK, Walker D. The high-risk surgical patient: a role for a multidisciplinary team approach? Br J Anaesth 2016;116(3):311–4.
47. Sroka R, Gabriel EM, Al-Hadidi D, et al. A novel anesthesiologist-led multidisciplinary model for evaluating high-risk surgical patients at a comprehensive cancer center. J Healthc Risk Manag 2018. [Epub ahead of print].

Preoperative Management of Medications

Zdravka Zafirova, MD[a],*, Karina G. Vázquez-Narváez, MD[b], Delia Borunda, MD[c]

KEYWORDS

- Perioperative medications • Perioperative serotonin syndrome
- Perioperative antihypertensive therapy • Perioperative stress dose steroids
- Perioperative anticoagulation

KEY POINTS

- The medication regimens of patients presenting for surgery need to be carefully evaluated to prevent perioperative complications.
- Some medications, such as cardiovascular, central nervous system, pulmonary, immuno-modulatory, and endocrine agents, are essential and should be continued without interruption during the perioperative period.
- Preoperative medications have a potential for interactions during anesthesia and surgery, and select agents may need to be adjusted, replaced, or held for a variable period of time before the surgery.
- Multidisciplinary approach to complex medication regimens is key to the comprehensive management of perioperative pharmacotherapy.

INTRODUCTION

Patients presenting for surgical and interventional procedures frequently use medications for various medical conditions. Sutherland and colleagues[1] showed that the average number of medications administered, stratified by age groups (<18, 18–64, and >64 years), is 0.4, 1.4, and 4.1. Furthermore, 59.7% of the adults aged 40 to 81 years in another study have been taking at least 1 medication. Polypharmacy (use of 5 or more drugs)- is increasing, especially in elderly, estimated to be between 11% and 40% in various population studies across the world.[2] The administration of multiple medications is a major risk factor for potentially inappropriate medication

Conflicts of Interest: All authors affirm that they have no conflicts of interest to disclose.
[a] Section of Critical Care, Department of Cardiovascular Surgery, Mount Sinai Hospital System, 1 Gustave L. Levy Place, Mail Box 1028, New York, NY 10029, USA; [b] Department of Anesthesiology and Perioperative Medicine, Instituto Nacional de Ciencias Médicas y Nutrición "Salvador Zubirán", Vaco de Quiroga #15, Col. Belisario Dominguez Sección XVI, Mexico City 14080, Mexico; [c] Department of Anesthesiology and Perioperative Medicine, Centro de Desarrollo de Destrezas Medicas, Instituto Nacional de Ciencias Médicas y Nutrición "Salvador Zubirán", Vaco de Quiroga #15, Col. Belisario Dominguez Sección XVI, Mexico City 14080, Mexico
* Corresponding author.
E-mail address: zzafirova@free.fr

Anesthesiology Clin 36 (2018) 663–675
https://doi.org/10.1016/j.anclin.2018.07.012
1932-2275/18/© 2018 Elsevier Inc. All rights reserved.

prescribing (PIP) and adverse drug events (ADEs).[3–5] Polypharmacy is linked to risk of drug withdrawal, complications, reduced survival, and increased use of health care resources in surgical and hospitalized medical patients.[6–8] During the preoperative assessment of surgical patients, a thorough documentation of all prescription and nonprescription pharmacotherapeutics must be done, including the indications, dose and frequency, and patient's compliance. The medication management should focus on the appropriateness of the drug regimen, identification of PIP and drug interactions, ADEs, and risk of withdrawal. Further optimization includes determination of medications that are to be continued or withheld, new agents to be initiated, the dose and timing adjustments, or substitution with an alternative regimen.

The specific instructions on the medication plan should be clearly explained to the patients, and supplied in writing, in the language in which they are fluent. Agreement between the perioperative clinicians is essential to avoid conflicting instructions. This agreement is best achieved via advanced communication among the teams involved, particularly when complex medical comorbidities require input from various specialists. Streamlining of the process of medication management via institutional guidelines on common medication regimens and designation of a point team to issue the instructions, such as the preoperative assessment clinic, ensures consistency and reliability. General medication management suggestions are outlined in **Tables 1–4**; however, an individualized approach by the perioperative clinician for each patient is required.

CENTRAL NERVOUS SYSTEM PHARMACOTHERAPY

Medications affecting the central nervous system (CNS) and peripheral nervous system are administered for wide range of comorbidities, including epilepsy, depression, schizoaffective disorders, dementia, Parkinson disease, attention-deficit/hyperactivity

Table 1
Antiplatelet and anticoagulant agents

Medication	Continue	Withhold	
Aspirin	Low dose on DOS: for stent, cardiac mechanical device, unless high BR	7–10 d: • High BR: may use bridging • Primary prophylaxis	
Clopidogrel/prasugrel/ ticagrelor	SAPT/DAPT: high TR (DES<6–12 mo, BMS<1 mo) and low BR	7–10 d (ticagrelor, 5 d): • Low TR • High TR/BR: may use bridging	
Warfarin	Very low BR/high TR	3–5 d • Bridge in high TR	
Novel Oral Anticoagulants		**CrCl ≥50 mL/min**	**CrCl <50 mL/min**
Dabigatran		>24–72 h	>72–120 h
Rivaroxaban		>24–48 h	>24–72 h
Apixaban		>24–48 h	>24–96 h
Edoxaban		>24–48 h	>24–48 h
Low-molecular weight heparin		12–24 h	

If regional anesthesia planned, additional adjustments need to be made.
Longer withholding time for higher bleeding risk procedures.
Abbreviations: BMS, bare metal stent; BR, bleeding risk; CrCl, creatinine clearance; DAPT, dual antiplatelet; DES, drug-eluting stent; DOS, day of surgery; SAPT, single antiplatelet; TR, thrombosis risk.

Table 2
Medications continued on day of surgery

Medication	Specific Considerations and Regimen Alterations
Antiepileptics	Interactions, ADEs
Anti-Parkinson and dementia	Interactions, ADEs; adjust in deep-brain stimulation procedures
Neuroleptics	Hold if concern for ADEs
TCAs, MAOIs	If discontinuation considered, slow taper over multiple days; ADEs
SSRIs/SNRIs/anxiolytics	
Anticholinesterases	Interactions with muscle relaxation
Antihypertensive, antianginal, antiarrhythmics, statins	Except ACEIs/ARBs
Diuretics	Monitor electrolytes; loop diuretics, hold unless heart or renal failure
Pulmonary inhalers, systemic therapy for reactive airway	
Systemic pulmonary vasodilators	Specialized consultation, vascular access
Immunosuppressants, antiallergics, corticosteroids	Stress dose steroids may be indicated
Cyclooxygenase-2 inhibitors	May hold if indicated
Thyroid, adrenal, pituitary modulators	Specialized consultation, transition to parenteral agents
Insulin pump	Basal rate only: may need to adjust rate or hold
Basal insulin (glargine, levemir)	Use usual or reduced dose, or hold, depending on glycemic control
Proton pump inhibitors, H2 blockers, nonparticulate antacids	
Oral contraceptives	If high thrombotic risk, hold days before and use alternative contraception
Ophthalmic drops	Effect on pupillary monitoring

Table 3
Medications withheld 12–48 hours before surgery

Medication	Specific Considerations and Regimen Alterations
ACEIs/ARBs	May continue in heart failure, refractory hypertension, aneurysm
Phosphodiestherase-5 inhibitors	Hold 48–72 h
Oral antihyperglycemics	Hold 12–24 h
Metformin	Hold 24–48 h
Short-acting insulin	Hold DOS
Intermediate-acting and long-acting insulin	Hold or dose adjustment night before or DOS, depending on glycemic control
Lithium	If need to continue, monitor for ADEs
Nonsteroidal antiinflammatory drugs	48–72 h
Vitamins, iron, topical creams	May continue some topical medications

Table 4
Medications withheld several days to a week before the surgery

Medication	Specific Considerations and Regimen Alterations
Antiplatelet, anticoagulants	See **Table 1**
Herbal, nonvitamin supplements, vitamin E	
Estrogen replacement; tamoxifen	Deep vein thrombosis risk; oncology consultation

syndrome, and posttraumatic stress disorder (PTSD), as well as for the management of anxiety, insomnia, migraines, acute and chronic pain, control of addiction, and prevention of substance withdrawal. Patients may take 1 or more medications for the specific disorder, and the same pharmacologic agent may be used for different indications. It is essential to determine the specific indications, disease control, dosing, and compliance. The potential for significant side effects (SEs) and interactions should be recognized. The withdrawal of these agents risks disease relapse, morbidity, and mortality.

Antiepileptic Medications

Various classes of established agents for the treatment of epilepsy are in use, as well as novel pharmaceuticals in development; clinicians should stay updated on their SEs and interactions to avoid complications. These medications are essential and should be continued in the perioperative period without interruption. Principal concerns with their use involve pharmacokinetic drug interactions among antiepileptics and with nonanticonvulsants: alterations of protein binding and increase in plasma levels of some antiepileptic drugs, specifically phenytoin, carbamazepine, and valproate; enzyme induction and metabolic rate increase, affected by drugs such as phenytoin, phenobarbital, carbamazepine, and topiramate, with reduction of levels of lamotrigine and lacosamide. Gabapentin, levetiracetam, and zonisamide have few major pharmacokinetic interactions.[9–11]

Psychiatric Agents

The pharmacologic drug classes used in psychiatric syndromes such as depression, psychotic syndromes, panic disorder, and PTSD include selective serotonin-uptake inhibitors (SSRIs), serotonin-norepinephrine reuptake inhibitors (SNRIs), tricyclic antidepressants (TCAs) and related cyclic agents, monoamine oxidase inhibitors (MAOIs), benzodiazepines, neuroleptic agents (NLAs), and lithium. Antidepressants are some of the most commonly prescribed medications in the United States and are used for anxiety, migraines, neuropathic pain, and other indications.[12]

SSRIs and SNRIs have good safety profiles without major cardiovascular, respiratory, or epileptogenic SEs. Investigators indicate association of SSRIs, particularly citalopram, fluoxetine, and sertraline, in higher doses, with QT prolongation, whereas others have questioned significant correlation or its clinical relevance.[13–15] SSRIs exert a variable inhibition on certain hepatic cytochrome P-450 enzymes, which should be considered with regard to drug interactions. Bleeding risk is another potential SE associated with SSRIs; the risk of increased surgical bleeding and transfusion rate has been indicated by studies in cardiac and noncardiac surgery.[16–19] However, the clinical significance and impact on mortality or reoperation rate continues to be debated in the literature. Furthermore, increase in mortality and 30-day readmissions rate from a retrospective study may reflect a higher-risk population, rather than causality.

The primary concern with SSRIs/SNRIs in the perioperative period, particularly the ones with short half-lives (paroxetine, venlafaxine, sertraline, citalopram, duloxetine, and escitalopram), is the risk of withdrawal syndromes with abrupt discontinuation, which should be avoided. Withdrawal symptoms include gastrointestinal, cardiovascular (tachycardia, palpitations), and neuropsychiatric (paresthesia, insomnia, agitation, confusion, and visual changes).[20] Given the risks of withdrawal and worsening of the primary disease for which they are prescribed, and the debated clinical significance of their SEs, SSRIs should generally be continued in the perioperative period.

Although TCAs have become less prevalent in the treatment of depression, because their SE profile is inferior to that of SSRIs/SNRIs, they remain in use as a second line in refractory depression. Furthermore, they have benefits in pain management, particularly in neuropathic pain syndromes, and seem to potentiate the analgesic effects of opiates.[12] The CNS and cardiovascular effects of TCA (delirium; tachycardia; dry mouth; blurred vision; delayed gastric, bowel, and bladder emptying) stem from their catecholamine-reuptake blocking and anticholinergic properties. CNS depression and reduction of the seizure threshold, and less frequently extrapyramidal symptoms, are also a concern.[21] Orthostatic hypotension, cardiodepression, arrhythmias, and conduction abnormalities are well recognized with TCAs; some of these effects are more significantly associated with supratherapeutic doses or in preexisting cardiac disease.[22,23] The hemodynamic activities of direct and indirect sympathomimetic agents in the setting of TCA therapy are variable and difficult to predict; in the initiation period of TCAs, exaggerated response to sympathomimetics may be anticipated and dose reduction necessary. Under chronic administration, the effectiveness of sympathomimetics may be reduced and higher doses and more potent agents may be required to restore hemodynamic balance.[24] TCAs have potential for significant ADEs in the perioperative period and consideration should be given to discontinuation well in advance of the surgery unless there is a strong clinical indication to continue. If they are continued, cardiovascular monitoring is essential and abnormal hemodynamics responses should be anticipated.

MAOIs are irreversible enzyme inhibitors with prolonged effects, major cardiovascular SEs, as well as interactions with drugs and dietary components, and the prescribing of nonselective MAOI-A/B antidepressants has waned.[12,25,26] Their use can be associated with CNS excitation or depression and significant orthostatic hypotension; there is a risk of hyperadrenergic crisis with use of indirect and direct sympathomimetics and in the setting of dietary ingestion of tyramine and other monoamines. In the past, preoperative discontinuation of MAOI was recommended 2 to 4 weeks before the surgery to avoid risk of cardiovascular collapse. Recent data indicate that MAOIs can be continued safely in the perioperative period for patients at high risk for depression relapse, as long as clinicians have a heightened awareness of the potential drug interactions and hemodynamic management impact.[27,28]

Serotonin syndrome (SS) is a potentially life-threatening state of enhanced serotonin activity, associated with single or combinations of medications with direct or indirect serotoninergic activity. The clinical presentations include altered mental status, hyperreflexia, rigidity, tremors, hyperthermia, and autonomic instability; the diagnosis and differentiation from other syndromes are challenging.[29,30] Drugs linked to SS are SSRIs, MAOIs, anti-Parkinson agents (selegiline), migraine drugs (triptans), lithium, opiate receptor agents (meperidine, fentanyl, sufentanil, methadone, tramadol), dextromethorphan, antiemetics (metoclopramide, 5-hydroxytryptamine [5-HT] 3 receptor antagonists), methylene blue, and linezolid. Furthermore, nonprescription substances (eg, St John's wort) and illicit drugs (LSD [lysergic acid diethylamide], MDMA [methylenedioxymethamphetamine]) have been implicated.[31–33] During the preoperative assessment, combinations of medications with potential for SS should be identified and withholding considered.

NLAs are in the categories of phenothiazines, thioxanthenes, dibenzodiazepines, butyrophenones, benzisoxalones, and diphenylbutylpiperidines, and second-generation antipsychotic drugs (SGAs), including risperidone, olanzapine, quetiapine, ziprasidone, aripiprazole, asenapine, lurasidone, and cariprazine. SEs of these medications may present a significant issue in the perioperative period; their incidence varies among different drugs and is generally lower for SGAs.[34] Cardiovascular effects are systemic hypotension caused by alpha-adrenergic blockade (risperidone, chlorpromazine), brainstem-medicated vasomotor reflex suppression, direct smooth-muscle relaxation, direct cardiac depression, and cardiac dysrhythmia (prolongation and risk of ventricular tachycardia [haloperidol, droperidol, thioridazine, pimozide]); chlorpromazine may have an antiarrhythmic effect caused by local anesthetic activity. Although the direct respiratory effects of these drugs are not significant, they may potentiate opioid-induced respiratory depression. Extrapyramidal effects manifest as tardive dyskinesia(involuntary movements of the orofacial, neck, trunk, and extremity muscle groups, potentially affecting breathing and swallowing) and acute dystonia with muscle rigidity, including laryngospasm, tremor, and akathisia. These medications can reduce the seizure threshold. Neuroleptic malignant syndrome (NMS) occurs in 0.02% to 3.23% of patients using NLA; carries a mortality risk of 5% to 50%; and contributing risk factors include polypharmacy, alcohol withdrawal, acute illness, dehydration, malnutrition, parenteral administration of antipsychotics, withdrawal of dopaminergic agonists such as are used in the treatment of Parkinson disease. SSRIs (paroxetine), amitriptyline, and lithium have been linked to NMS. Alteration of the dopaminergic pathway leads to hyperthermia, cardiovascular instability, arrhythmia, altered mental status, skeletal muscle hypertonicity, and renal and liver dysfunction; the treatment includes mechanical ventilation, hemodynamic support, and dantrolene and dopamine agonists (bromocriptine or amantadine). Differentiation from malignant hyperthermia, SS, and other syndromes can be challenging.[29,30,35–37] The endocrine impact of NLAs results from impaired release of corticotropin and insulin, leading to depressed corticosteroid secretion and glucose intolerance.

Lithium has a major role in the treatment of bipolar disorder; it can be continued in the perioperative period, taking into consideration the renal side effects, the exacerbation of SEs of other agents, and the impact of drugs on the lithium plasma concentration.

Pharmacotherapy for Parkinson Disease

Regimens include the dopamine precursor levodopa, synthetic dopamine agonists, along with peripheral decarboxylase inhibitors, and are associated with psychiatric and neurologic disturbances and cardiovascular manifestations such as orthostatic hypotension and arrhythmias. Anticholinergic agents and amantadine come with the associated SEs. The selective MAOI-B selegiline has lower likelihood of sympathetic potentiation; however, in higher doses it becomes less selective. Selegiline is linked to psychiatric reactions and occurrence of SS; selection of perioperative analgesic agents should be carefully reviewed. Anti-Parkinson therapy should be continued preoperatively because abrupt discontinuation can cause disease flare and NMS.[38,39]

Miscellaneous Central Nervous System Medications

Triptans are 5-HT receptor agonists for therapy for migraine; major concern is link with SS. These medications are continued in the preoperative period.[31]

Benzodiazepines and buspirone are used for anxiolysis and insomnia and generally have a low SE profile. They can be continued in the perioperative period; potentiation of the CNS depressant effects of other drugs should be considered.

CARDIOVASCULAR MEDICATIONS

Medications for management of cardiovascular disease (CVD) are among the most commonly prescribed classes and are most likely to be included in a multidrug regimen.

Antihypertensive Medications

Medications include alpha2-adrenergic agonists, beta-adrenergic agonists, angiotensin-converting enzyme inhibitors (ACEIs), angiotensin receptor blockers (ARBs), calcium-channel antagonists, direct vasodilators, and diuretics. Antihypertensive therapy reduces the incidence of major cardiovascular events (MACEs), especially in patients at increased CVD risk.[40–42] Antihypertensive regimens should not be interrupted preoperatively. Systematic initiation of alpha2-adrenergic or beta-adrenergic agonists in the immediate preoperative period cannot be recommended at present because of increased risk of stroke, adverse events, and all-cause mortality.[43,44] However, patients who use these agents as a long-term regimen should continue taking them to avoid withdrawal and increase in cardiovascular complications.[45–47] ACEIs and ARBs are associated with reduction in the incidence of MACEs and cerebrovascular events, particularly in ischemic heart disease, reduced ejection fraction, diabetes, or renal disease.[41,42,48] However, administration of ACEIs and ARBs until the day of surgery has been consistently linked to hypotension under anesthesia, which can be refractory to conventional therapy, particularly with general anesthesia (GA).[49–52] The clinical implications and outcome effects are still debated; some studies have shown an increased need for vasopressors, whereas others have contradicting results or have shown that optimization of fluids is sufficient for hemodynamic control. The decision to continue or withhold ACEIs and ARBs on the day of surgery depends on the particular clinical situation; a reasonable strategy is to withhold these agents for 24 or even 48 hours when GA is planned; in anticipated lengthy surgical procedures, involving significant blood loss risk, particularly spine or intracranial procedures, especially in prone position; in the setting of multiple antihypertensive medications, controlled hypertension, and use of potent loop diuretics; in the absence of significant heart failure; or increased risk for stroke.

Antiplatelet and Anticoagulation Medications

Antiplatelet treatment (APT) with single APT (SAPT) agent, dual APT (DAPT), or triple regimen includes aspirin; P_2Y_{12} inhibitors such as clopidogrel, prasugrel, and ticagrelor; as well as cilostazol and dipyridamole. The benefits of APT in reducing thrombotic risk and MACEs should be weighed against the impact on surgical bleeding. The indications for the APT and the bleeding risk of the specific procedure must be clarified in the preoperative visit.[53,54] Withholding APT used for primary prevention is reasonable, unless a minor surgery with insignificant bleeding risk is planned.[55,56] When APT is used in the setting of coronary revascularization, prior intervention on cardiac valve, and in the presence of coronary and vascular stents and cardiac support devices, a multidisciplinary approach to the decision to continue or hold therapy, and to use an alternative bridging agent, should be undertaken.[54,55]

Anticoagulant regimen, enteral or parenteral, in the perioperative period should be determined by the thromboembolic risk of the indicated comorbidity versus surgical bleeding risk. Oral anticoagulants, including warfarin, dabigatran, apixaban, and rivaroxaban, need to be held for most surgical and anesthetic procedures; the timing depends on the specific agent, the impact of the patient's pharmacokinetic function, and the availability of reversal. Depending on the indication for anticoagulation, bridging with parenteral agent may be indicated.

Other Cardiovascular Medications

Medications for symptomatic control of coronary ischemia, including nitroglycerin and isosorbide, should be continued, and their potential hemodynamic effects should be taken into account when planning the anesthetic and surgical plan.

Diuretics are routinely used in the management of systemic hypertension, heart failure, and pulmonary hypertension; in the setting of advanced chronic kidney disease, they help in the management of hypervolemia and electrolyte abnormalities, specifically hyperkalemia. Perioperative electrolyte monitoring is essential with diuretic use.

Thiazide diuretics administered for hypertension control can be continued on the day of surgery. Loop diuretics may be held, especially in surgery with expected significant fluid shifts; however, when they are administered for chronic heart failure (CHF) indications, consideration should be given to continuation, depending on the specific clinical situation. Although a paucity of trials specifically targeting loop diuretic withdrawal and outcomes in CHF exists, the evidence regarding the link between clinical congestion in CHF and poor outcomes is consistently shown.[57,58] Aldosterone antagonists may have utility not only as diuretics but in coronary artery disease and CHF and should be continued unless hyperkalemia risk exists.

Antiarrhythmia therapy in the perioperative period should be continued unless specific contraindications are identified, related to the anesthesia or surgical procedure; in such cases, alternative therapy should be considered.

Therapy for lipid disorders is typically continued in the perioperative period, with particular emphasis on continuation of HMG-CoA (3-hydroxy-3-methylglutaryl coenzyme A) reductase inhibitors, because of their added pleiotropic benefits.[59–61]

PULMONARY MEDICATIONS

The optimization of pulmonary comorbidities and reduction of perioperative pulmonary complications includes management of inhaled and systemic pulmonary medications. Inhaled beta agonists and anticholinergic bronchodilators and anti-inflammatory agents should not be interrupted in patients with reactive airway disease (RAD), including on the day of surgery. Initiation of perioperative inhaled therapy may be considered in specific situations. Additional inhaled short-acting bronchodilator dose before initiation of anesthesia and surgery is beneficial.

Systemic therapy includes enteral and parenteral medications for control of inflammation, steroids and montelukast, as well as agents targeting the pulmonary vasculature in pulmonary hypertension. Systemic regimens used for maintenance therapy should be continued. Evidence supporting initiation of prophylactic preoperative systemic steroid therapy in RAD is lacking; however, in the setting of acute exacerbation, treatment with short-term low-dose systemic steroids is reasonable.[62–64]

ENDOCRINE THERAPY

Modulators of hormonal function can be used as a replacement in hormonal deficiency or for their various therapeutic effects and include agents that affect the function of the anterior and posterior pituitary, thyroid and adrenal glands, the pancreas, and the reproductive organs. Many modulators of endocrine function are essential and should be continued throughout the perioperative period. Although generalized recommendations, particularly regarding the management of diabetes and thyroid dysfunction, can be used and are included in tables and other articles in this issue, an individualized approach in many situations is indispensable and may require the involvement of highly specialized health providers.

MODULATION OF IMMUNE FUNCTION AND INFLAMMATION

Inhaled and systemic glucocorticosteroid therapy is used for inflammatory and autoimmune disorders, as well as being part of immunosuppression in transplant recipients. Patients on chronic steroid therapy may develop adrenal suppression and, ultimately, secondary adrenal insufficiency with hemodynamic and metabolic manifestations. The risk for development of adrenal suppression is related to the potency of the agent, the dose and the duration of therapy; the signs and symptoms of adrenal insufficiency are influenced by the degree of suppression as well as the surgical stress. All patients should continue their chronic therapy regimens. The goal of the preoperative assessment is to identify the risk of adrenal insufficiency and the need for administration of a stress steroid regimen. Although the debate on the issue continues, with a paucity of good clinical data, the general consensus is that patients at low risk, taking glucocorticosteroid for 3 weeks or less, or a daily dose of prednisone less than or equal to 5 mg generally do not require additional steroid administration beyond their usual dose; patients at high risk include those with clinical manifestations of steroid administration and those taking greater than or equal to 20 mg/d for greater than or equal to 3 weeks and they are likely to require stress doses of steroids based on the determinations of surgical stress.[65–67] Patients at intermediate risk, taking steroids for greater than or equal to 3 weeks, at dosages 5 to 20 mg/d of prednisone, may require further clinical and biochemical evaluation, using the cosyntropin stimulation test, to determine their need for additional perioperative steroid administration.

SUMMARY

The perioperative evaluation of the pharmacotherapy for surgical patients should focus on assessment of drugs and indications; determination of the need to start, stop, modify, and substitute medications preoperatively; as well as a plan for postoperative management, including when to restart the agents, or to substitute, as well as a backup plan if the anticipated route of administration is not available, such as prolonged unavailability of enteral intake and limitations of parenteral access.

REFERENCES

1. Sutherland JJ, Daly TM, Liu X, et al. Co-prescription trends in a large cohort of subjects predict substantial drug-drug interactions. PLoS One 2015;10(3): e0118991.
2. Castioni J, Marques-Vidal P, Abolhassani N, et al. Prevalence and determinants of polypharmacy in Switzerland: data from the CoLaus study. BMC Health Serv Res 2017;17(1):840.
3. Jirón M, Pate V, Hanson LC, et al. Trends in prevalence and determinants of potentially inappropriate prescribing in the United States: 2007 to 2012. J Am Geriatr Soc 2016;64(4):788–97.
4. Ribeiro MR, Motta AA, Marcondes-Fonseca LA, et al. Increase of 10% in the rate of adverse drug reactions for each drug administered in hospitalized patients. Clinics (Sao Paulo) 2018;73:e185.

5. Johnell K, Klarin I. The relationship between number of drugs and potential drug-drug interactions in the elderly: a study of over 600,000 elderly patients from the Swedish Prescribed Drug Register. Drug Saf 2007;30(10):911–8.

6. McIsaac DI, Wong CA, Bryson GL, et al. Association of polypharmacy with survival, complications, and healthcare resource use after elective noncardiac surgery: a population-based cohort study. Anesthesiology 2018;128(6):1140–50.

7. Fried TR, O'Leary J, Towle V, et al. Health outcomes associated with polypharmacy in community-dwelling older adults: a systematic review. J Am Geriatr Soc 2014;62:2261–72.

8. Härstedt M, Rogmark C, Sutton R, et al. Polypharmacy and adverse outcomes after hip fracture surgery. J Orthop Surg Res 2016;11:151.

9. Perks A, Cheema S, Mohanraj R. Anaesthesia and epilepsy. Br J Anaesth 2012; 108(4):562–71.

10. Bialer M, Johannessen SI, Levy RH, et al. Progress report on new antiepileptic drugs: a summary of the thirteenth Eilat conference on new antiepileptic drugs and devices (EILAT XIII). Epilepsia 2017;58(2):181–221.

11. Stefanović S, Janković SM, Novaković M, et al. Pharmacodynamics and common drug-drug interactions of the third-generation antiepileptic drugs. Expert Opin Drug Metab Toxicol 2018;14(2):153–9.

12. Catalani B, Hamilton CS, Herron EW, et al. Psychiatric agents and implications for perioperative analgesia. Best Pract Res Clin Anaesthesiol 2014;28(2):167–81.

13. Jolly K, Gammage MD, Cheng KK, et al. Sudden death in patients receiving drugs tending to prolong the QT interval. Br J Clin Pharmacol 2009;68(5):743–51.

14. Alvarez PA, Pahissa J. QT alterations in psychopharmacology: proven candidates and suspects. Curr Drug Saf 2010;5(1):97–104.

15. Beach SR, Celano CM, Sugrue AM, et al. QT prolongation, torsades de pointes, and psychotropic medications: a 5-year update. Psychosomatics 2018;59(2): 105–22.

16. van Haelst IM, Egberts TC, Doodeman HJ, et al. Use of serotonergic antidepressants and bleeding risk in orthopedic patients. Anesthesiology 2010;112(3): 631–6.

17. Auerbach AD, Vittinghoff E, Maselli J, et al. Perioperative use of selective serotonin reuptake inhibitors and risks for adverse outcomes of surgery. JAMA Intern Med 2013;173(12):1075–81.

18. Singh I, Achuthan S, Chakrabarti A, et al. Influence of pre-operative use of serotonergic antidepressants (SADs) on the risk of bleeding in patients undergoing different surgical interventions: a meta-analysis. Pharmacoepidemiol Drug Saf 2015;24:237–45.

19. Sajan F, Conte JV, Tamargo RJ, et al. Association of selective serotonin reuptake inhibitors with transfusion in surgical patients. Anesth Analg 2016;123(1):21–8.

20. Bainum TB, Fike DS, Mechelay D, et al. Effect of abrupt discontinuation of antidepressants in critically ill hospitalized adults. Pharmacotherapy 2017;37(10): 1231–40.

21. Woolf AD, Erdman AR, Nelson LS, et al. Tricyclic antidepressant poisoning: an evidence-based consensus guideline for out-of-hospital management. Clin Toxicol (Phila) 2007;45(3):203–33.

22. Gheshlaghi F, Mehrizi MK, Yaraghi A, et al. ST-T segment changes in patients with tricyclic antidepressant poisoning. J Res Pharm Pract 2013;2(3):110–3.

23. Kerr GW, McGuffie AC, Wilkie S. Tricyclic antidepressant overdose: a review. Emerg Med J 2001;18(4):236–41.

24. Tran TP, Panacek EA, Rhee KJ, et al. Response to dopamine vs norepinephrine in tricyclic antidepressant-induced hypotension. Acad Emerg Med 1997;4(9): 864–8.
25. Shulman KI, Fischer HD, Herrmann N, et al. Current prescription patterns and safety profile of irreversible monoamine oxidase inhibitors: a population-based cohort study of older adults. J Clin Psychiatry 2009;70(12):1681–6.
26. Thomas SJ, Shin M, McInnis MG, et al. Combination therapy with monoamine oxidase inhibitors and other antidepressants or stimulants: strategies for the management of treatment-resistant depression. Pharmacotherapy 2015;35(4): 433–49.
27. Krings-Ernst I, Ulrich S, Adli M. Antidepressant treatment with MAO-inhibitors during general and regional anesthesia: a review and case report of spinal anesthesia for lower extremity surgery without discontinuation of tranylcypromine. Int J Clin Pharmacol Ther 2013;51(10):763–70.
28. van Haelst IM, van Klei WA, Doodeman HJ, et al, MAOI Study Group. Antidepressive treatment with monoamine oxidase inhibitors and the occurrence of intraoperative hemodynamic events: a retrospective observational cohort study. J Clin Psychiatry 2012;73(8):1103–9.
29. Katus LE, Frucht SJ. Management of serotonin syndrome and neuroleptic malignant syndrome. Curr Treat Options Neurol 2016;18(9):39.
30. Perry PJ, Wilborn CA. Serotonin syndrome vs neuroleptic malignant syndrome: a contrast of causes, diagnoses, and management. Ann Clin Psychiatry 2012; 24(2):155–62.
31. Orlova Y, Rizzoli P, Loder E. Association of coprescription of triptan antimigraine drugs and selective serotonin reuptake inhibitor or selective norepinephrine reuptake inhibitor antidepressants with serotonin syndrome. JAMA Neurol 2018;75(5): 566–72.
32. Uddin MF, Alweis R, Shah SR, et al. Controversies in serotonin syndrome diagnosis and management: a review. J Clin Diagn Res 2017;11(9):OE05–7.
33. Werneke U, Jamshidi F, Taylor DM, et al. Conundrums in neurology: diagnosing serotonin syndrome - a meta-analysis of cases. BMC Neurol 2016;16:97.
34. Werner FM, Coveñas R. Safety of antipsychotic drugs: focus on therapeutic and adverse effects. Expert Opin Drug Saf 2014;13(8):1031–42.
35. Sahin A, Cicek M, Gonenc Cekic O, et al. A retrospective analysis of cases with neuroleptic malignant syndrome and an evaluation of risk factors for mortality. Turk J Emerg Med 2017;17(4):141–5.
36. Oruch R, Pryme IF, Engelsen BA, et al. Neuroleptic malignant syndrome: an easily overlooked neurologic emergency. Neuropsychiatr Dis Treat 2017;13:161–75.
37. Velamoor R. Neuroleptic malignant syndrome: a neuro-psychiatric emergency: recognition, prevention, and management. Asian J Psychiatr 2017;29:106–9.
38. Akbar U, Kurkchubasche AG, Friedman JH. Perioperative management of Parkinson's disease. Expert Rev Neurother 2017;17(3):301–8.
39. Jacob JE, Wagner ML, Sage JI. Safety of selegiline with cold medications. Ann Pharmacother 2003;37(3):438–41.
40. Thomopoulos C, Parati G, Zanchetti A. Effects of blood pressure lowering on outcome incidence in hypertension: 3. effects in patients at different levels of cardiovascular risk–overview and meta-analyses of randomized trials. J Hypertens 2014;32:2305–14.
41. Thomopoulos C, Parati G, Zanchetti A. Effects of blood pressure lowering on outcome incidence in hypertension: 4. Effects of various classes of antihypertensive drugs–overview and meta-analyses. J Hypertens 2015;33:195.

42. Blood Pressure Lowering Treatment Trialists' Collaboration. Predicted cardiovascular risk can inform decisions to lower blood pressure with drugs: evidence from an individual patient data meta-analysis. Lancet 2014;384:591.

43. Wijeysundera DN, Duncan D, Nkonde-Price C, et al. Perioperative beta blockade in noncardiac surgery: a systematic review for the 2014 ACC/AHA guideline on perioperative cardiovascular evaluation and management of patients undergoing noncardiac surgery: a report of the American College of Cardiology/American Heart Association Task Force on Practice Guidelines. J Am Coll Cardiol 2014; 64:2406.

44. Devereaux PJ, Sessler DI, Leslie K, et al, POISE-2 Investigators. Clonidine in patients undergoing noncardiac surgery. N Engl J Med 2014;370:1504.

45. Bangalore S, Makani H, Radford M, et al. Clinical outcomes with β-blockers for myocardial infarction: a meta-analysis of randomized trials. Am J Med 2014; 127(10):939–53.

46. Li C, Sun Y, Shen X, et al. Relationship between β-blocker therapy at discharge and clinical outcomes in patients with acute coronary syndrome undergoing percutaneous coronary intervention. J Am Heart Assoc 2016;5:e004190.

47. Prins KW, Neill JM, Tyler JO, et al. Effects of beta-blocker withdrawal in acute decompensated heart failure: a systematic review and meta-analysis. JACC Heart Fail 2015;3:647–53.

48. Bertrand ME, Ferrari R, Remme WJ, et al. Perindopril and β-blocker for the prevention of cardiac events and mortality in stable coronary artery disease patients: a EUropean trial on Reduction Of cardiac events with Perindopril in stable coronary Artery disease (EUROPA) subanalysis. Am Heart J 2015;170:1092.

49. Zou Z, Yuan HB, Yang B, et al. Perioperative angiotensin-converting enzyme inhibitors or angiotensin II type 1 receptor blockers for preventing mortality and morbidity in adults. Cochrane Database Syst Rev 2016;(1):CD009210.

50. Rajgopal R, Rajan S, Sapru K, et al. Effect of pre-operative discontinuation of angiotensin-converting enzyme inhibitors or angiotensin II receptor antagonists on intra-operative arterial pressures after induction of general anesthesia. Anesth Essays Res 2014;8:32.

51. Twersky RS, Goel V, Narayan P, et al. The risk of hypertension after preoperative discontinuation of angiotensin-converting enzyme inhibitors or angiotensin receptor antagonists in ambulatory and same-day admission patients. Anesth Analg 2014;118(5):938–44.

52. Roshanov P, Rochwerg B, Patel A, et al. Withholding versus continuing angiotensin-converting enzyme inhibitors or angiotensin ii receptor blockers before noncardiac surgery: an analysis of the vascular events in noncardiac surgery patients cohort evaluation prospective cohort. Anesthesiology 2017;126:16.

53. Antithrombotic Trialists' Collaboration. Collaborative meta-analysis of randomized trials of antiplatelet therapy for prevention of death, myocardial infarction, and stroke in high risk patients. BMJ 2002;324:71.

54. Baigent C, Blackwell L, Collins R, et al. Aspirin in the primary and secondary prevention of vascular disease: collaborative meta-analysis of individual participant data from randomized trials. Lancet 2009;373:1849.

55. Bittl JA, Baber U, Bradley SM, et al. Duration of dual antiplatelet therapy: a systematic review for the 2016 ACC/AHA guideline focused update on duration of dual antiplatelet therapy in patients with coronary artery disease: a report of the American College of Cardiology/American Heart Association Task Force on Clinical Practice Guidelines. J Am Coll Cardiol 2016;68:1116.

56. Devereaux PJ, Mrkobrada M, Sessler DI, et al, POISE-2 Investigators. Aspirin in patients undergoing noncardiac surgery. N Engl J Med 2014;370:1494.
57. Hopper I, Samuel R, Hayward C, et al. Can medications be safely withdrawn in patients with stable chronic heart failure? Systematic review and meta-analysis. J Card Fail 2014;20:522–32.
58. Ambrosy AP, Pang PS, Khan S, et al. Clinical course and predictive value of congestion during hospitalization in patients admitted for worsening signs and symptoms of heart failure with reduced ejection fraction: findings from the EVEREST trial. Eur Heart J 2013;34:835–43.
59. Natsuaki M, Morimoto T, Furukawa Y, et al, CREDO-Kyoto PCI/CABG Registry Cohort-2 Investigators. Effect of statin therapy on cardiovascular outcomes after coronary revascularization in patients ≥80 years of age: observations from the CREDO-Kyoto registry cohort-2. Atherosclerosis 2014;237(2):821–8.
60. Fulcher J, O'Connell R, Voysey M, et al. Efficacy and safety of LDL-lowering therapy among men and women: meta-analysis of individual data from 174,000 participants in 27 randomised trials. Cholesterol Treatment Trialists' (CTT) Collaboration. Lancet 2015;385:1397–405.
61. Diamantis E, Kyriakos G, Quiles-Sanchez LV, et al. The anti-inflammatory effects of statins on coronary artery disease: an updated review of the literature. Curr Cardiol Rev 2017;13(3):209–16.
62. Vogelmeier CF, Criner GJ, Martinez FJ, et al. Global strategy for the diagnosis, management, and prevention of chronic obstructive lung disease 2017 report. GOLD executive summary. Am J Respir Crit Care Med 2017;195:557–82.
63. Dreger H, Schaumann B, Gromann T, et al. Fast-track pulmonary conditioning before urgent cardiac surgery in patients with insufficiently treated chronic obstructive pulmonary disease. J Cardiovasc Surg 2011;52:587–91.
64. Bölükbas S, Eberlein M, Eckhoff J, et al. Short-term effects of inhalative tiotropium/formoterol/budenoside versus tiotropium/formoterol in patients with newly diagnosed chronic obstructive pulmonary disease requiring surgery for lung cancer: a prospective randomized trial. Eur J Cardiothorac Surg 2011;39:995–1000.
65. Marik PE, Varon J. Requirement of perioperative stress doses of corticosteroids: a systematic review of the literature. Arch Surg 2008;143:1222–6.
66. Marik PE, Pastores SM, Annane D, et al. American College of Critical Care Medicine: recommendations for the diagnosis and management of corticosteroid insufficiency in critically ill adult patients: consensus statements from an international task force by the American College of Critical Care Medicine. Crit Care Med 2008;36:1937–49.
67. Liu MM, Reidy AB, Saatee S, et al. Perioperative steroid management: approaches based on current evidence. Anesthesiology 2017;127:166–72.

Perioperative Surgical Home Models

Thomas R. Vetter, MD, MPH[a,b],*

KEYWORDS

- Surgical home • Perioperative assessment • Perioperative optimization
- Value-based health care • Perioperative population health management

KEY POINTS

- The comprehensive perioperative management afforded by various perioperative surgical home models can play a pivotal role in delivering this higher quality and lower cost patient care, thereby achieving greater health care value.
- The perioperative surgical home can be considered a programmatic umbrella, under which several related entities can be positioned.
- Any variant of a perioperative surgical home model should contribute to its organization being a rapid-learning health system.
- There are several specific ethical opportunities that can be afforded by a bona fide perioperative surgical home model.

INTRODUCTION

According to the latest available data from the Centers for Disease Control and Prevention and its National Center for Health Statistics, 51 million inpatient surgical procedures were performed in the United States in 2010.[1] The combined effects of expanded health insurance coverage, sustained economic development and growth, continued diagnostic and therapeutic technological advances, and an ever-aging population (the so-called Silver Tsunami) are expected to result in an even greater demand for health care goods and services, including for surgery, anesthesiology, and perioperative medicine.[2–5]

Disclosures: The author has no relationship with a commercial company that has a direct financial interest in the subject matter or materials discussed in this article, or with a company making a competing product.
[a] Department of Surgery and Perioperative Care, Dell Medical School at the University of Texas at Austin, Health Discovery Building, Room 6.812, 1701 Trinity Street, Austin, TX 78712-1875, USA; [b] Department of Population Health, Dell Medical School at the University of Texas at Austin, Health Discovery Building, Room 6.812, 1701 Trinity Street, Austin, TX 78712-1875, USA
* Corresponding author. Department of Population Health, Dell Medical School at the University of Texas at Austin, Health Discovery Building, Room 6.812, 1701 Trinity Street, Austin, TX 78712-1875.
E-mail address: thomas.vetter@austin.utexas.edu

Anesthesiology Clin 36 (2018) 677–687
https://doi.org/10.1016/j.anclin.2018.07.015
1932-2275/18/© 2018 Elsevier Inc. All rights reserved.

However, continued widely variable and often fragmented diagnostic and treatment plans, undertaken by different practitioners, will

1. Expose surgical patients to lapses in evidence-based and well-defined standards of care
2. Increase the risk of mishaps and complications
3. Result in unnecessary, more costly, and potentially detrimental interventions
4. Ultimately, adversely affect the patient health care experience.[3,6–10]

The perioperative surgical home (PSH) model per se was initially developed and implemented in an effort to help remedy existing suboptimal and overly costly perioperative care in the United States.[10–14] At its conception, Vetter and colleagues[15] noted that there would very likely be multiple future variations of the surgical home concept that may work effectively, depending on institutional infrastructure, available resources, and internal and external organizational forces that were yet to be identified. Now, nearly a decade on, it is fitting to review the tenets of the PSH and to examine its continued evolution, opportunity, utility, and impact.

THE PERIOPERATIVE SURGICAL HOME

The PSH remains essentially an intentionally patient-centered approach to surgical care, with a strong emphasis on shared decision-making, rigorous process standardization, and use of evidence-based clinical care pathways, as well as robust coordination and integration of processes across the preoperative, intraoperative, postoperative, and postdischarge phases of care.[10–13]

This physician-led, yet highly interdisciplinary and collaborative, team-based model of care (**Fig. 1**) is intended to improve clinical outcomes, enhance patient and provider satisfaction, and reduce overall cost, thereby delivering greater health care value[10–13] and achieving the newly recognized quadruple aim of health care.[16–19]

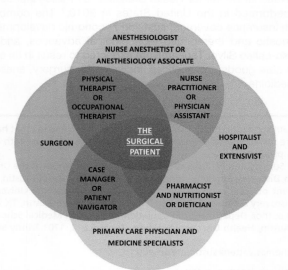

Fig. 1. Interdisciplinary web of key perioperative stakeholders and players. (*Courtesy of* T.R. Vetter, MD, MPH, Austin, TX.)

Patients and Their Transitions of Care Are Paramount

Undergoing a major surgical procedure is among the most psychologically and physiologically stressful events in an individual's life. Even an independently functioning, well-informed, and proactive person can become a dependent, confused, and passive patient who is bewildered by the very foreign and often ironically hostile health care environment.[15] Nevertheless, 2 very appropriate questions often considered, if not effectively openly posed, by surgical patients are

1. What outcomes matter most to me?
2. What can I do to improve these outcomes that matter most important to me?

These 2 questions speak directly to the fundamental PSH tenets of patient engagement and patient empowerment.[15]

Therefore, any PSH model of care should consistently inform and guide patients, their family members, and other caregivers through the complexities of the perioperative continuum, from making the decision for surgery through the extended postacute care and postoperative rehabilitation phase care. Based on shared decision-making, elective and semiurgent surgical procedures are appropriately and judiciously delayed, or comprehensive long-term medical management is pursued in lieu of surgery (**Fig. 2**).[10–13]

Furthermore, building on the seminal work of Coleman and colleagues,[20,21] and the leading recommendations of the Institute for Healthcare Improvement,[22–24] a preemptive approach to postacute care discharge planning should ideally be undertaken by

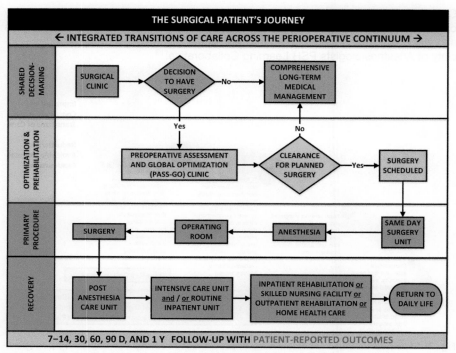

Fig. 2. The multiple phases of a surgical patient's perioperative journey. (*Courtesy of* T.R. Vetter, MD, MPH, Austin, TX.)

any PSH team. Rather than waiting until the postoperative, acute care hospital discharge is imminent but the available disposition options are limited or access is constrained or delayed, the likely needed type of postacute care is identified preoperatively and a plan is set and kept in motion (**Fig. 3**).

A novel perioperative transitions across levels of care (TLC) service can be implemented to improve coordination and outcomes across the entire surgical episode of care.[25] This TLC service expands on existing, conventional, internal medicine-based inpatient comanagement services by promoting greater collaboration, communication, and teamwork among the surgeon, anesthesiologist, hospitalist, intensivist, and other key members of the health care team, particularly during transitions across the 4 phases and within all the elements of perioperative care.[25] This service is especially apropos for more complex, higher risk surgical patients who need extra TLC (tender loving care).

Recent evidence suggests that such improvement in health care teamwork can result in significant gains in efficiency of care and patient safety as measured by complication and mortality rates. Interventions to improve teamwork in health care will likely lead to the next major advance in patient outcomes.[26]

Specifically, a 2016 systematic review observed that discharge planning programs, patient education interventions, primary care follow-up, and home health care visits all reduced hospital readmissions after high-risk surgeries, leading the investigators to posit that improving discharge planning, patient education, and follow-up communication may reduce hospital readmissions.[27]

THE PERIOPERATIVE SURGICAL HOME AS A PROGRAMMATIC UMBRELLA

Components or elements of a PSH model or an entire PSH model have reportedly been trialed and implemented by a large number of organizations in the United States and elsewhere, both independently[28–36] and under the auspices of the American Society of Anesthesiologists PSH Learning Collaborative.[13]

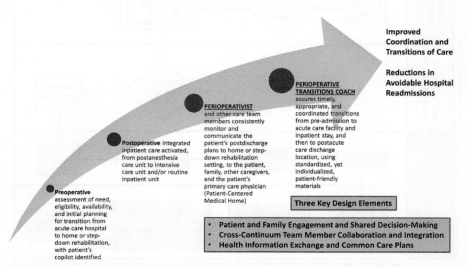

Fig. 3. Modified Institute for Healthcare Improvement roadmap for improving perioperative transitions in care during and after hospitalization, and reducing avoidable hospital readmissions. (*Courtesy of* T.R. Vetter, MD, MPH, Austin, TX.)

Nevertheless, the PSH model has also generated confusion, controversy, and even political conflict related to the challenges of expanding anesthesiologists' traditional services outside the immediate operating room setting,[37,38] leadership of the PSH,[39,40] and even the name itself.[41] As observed by Mariano and colleagues,[42] unfortunate resulting tensions among surgeons, anesthesiologists, and internal medicine hospitalists locally, and among their respective professional societies nationally, have likely hampered the acceptance of the PSH as an optimal model of care.

Mariano and colleagues[42] have suggested that this confusion, controversy, and push-back have resulted largely from misinterpretation of the PSH. The PSH is viewed by many of its stakeholders as a single, all-or-none, and hence massive undertaking. It would seem prudent to step back from this global concept and demonstrate how variations of the PSH can work across the spectrum of institutional practices.[42]

One tactical and operational strategy is to consider the PSH as a programmatic umbrella (**Fig. 4**) under which several related entities can be positioned, thereby mitigating duplicated institutional efforts and competition for ubiquitous finite organizational resources.

THE ROLE OF A PERIOPERATIVE SURGICAL HOME WITHIN A RAPID-LEARNING HEALTH SYSTEM

Health care systems and practicing clinicians collectively continue to face widespread challenges, including implementing meaningful use of electronic medical or health records; adapting to payment reforms and resulting operational austerity measures; and caring for an increasing number of insured, yet chronically ill and aging, patients. They are also expected to adopt new scientific discoveries and technologies, yet curb escalating costs.[43,44]

Reorganizing health care delivery to meet these challenges and expectations requires a fundamental transformation in how health care systems generate and apply knowledge. The rapid-learning health system is a proposed strategy to foster such transformation.[43–45] A rapid-learning system uses enhanced health information technology and health database infrastructure to access and apply evidence in real-time,

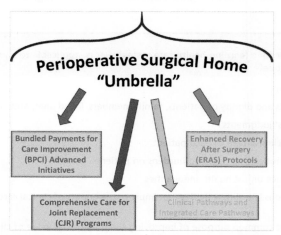

Fig. 4. The PSH as a programmatic umbrella, under which several closely related entities can be strategically and operationally positioned. (*Data from* Refs.[22–24]; and *Courtesy of* T.R. Vetter, MD, MPH, Austin, TX.)

while simultaneously drawing knowledge from its real-world care delivery to promote innovation and health system change.[43,46,47] This has been aptly described as rapid-cycle, bidirectional learning, in which evidence informs practice and practice informs evidence.[43] Any variant of a PSH should capitalize on the opportunity to contribute to its organization being a rapid-learning health system.

THE ETHICAL OPPORTUNITIES WITH A PERIOPERATIVE SURGICAL HOME

Thought leaders have proposed that there is a moral imperative for an organization to become a learning health system. An ethics framework for such learning heath care systems and their clinicians has been proposed to assess the ethical utility of their activities (**Box 1**).[48,49] As posited by Goeddel and colleagues,[50] there are in turn at least 5 specific ethical opportunities that can and should be afforded by a bona fide PSH model (**Fig. 5**):

- Serve as a disruptive innovation
- Enhance patient-centered care
- Embrace shared decision-making
- Increase health literacy
- Reduce futile surgery.

Although all 5 of these ethical opportunities clearly first present themselves in the preoperative phase, they continue throughout the surgical continuum.

THE RISING PROMINENCE OF VALUE-BASED CARE AND POPULATION HEALTH MANAGEMENT

In the United States and other Western countries, there is an ongoing transition from traditional volume-based toward value-based health care payment models.[51-55] Delivering value-based health care requires effectively managing not only the long-term but also the short-term health of patient populations, especially high-risk patents and during disproportionately costly acute care episodes such as surgery.[5,54-59] Managing the short-term health of the surgical population certainly begins in the preoperative

---

Box 1
Ethics framework for a learning health care system that is, applicable to a perioperative surgical home model

Ethical obligation

Respect the rights and dignity of patients, family members, loved ones, and patient surrogates

Respect clinicians' judgments

Provide optimal clinical care to each patient

Avoid imposing nonclinical risks and burdens on patients

Address and reduce unjust health inequalities

Conduct continuous learning activities that improve the quality of clinical care and health care systems

Contribute to the common purpose of improving the quality and value of clinical care health care systems

Data from Refs.[48-50]

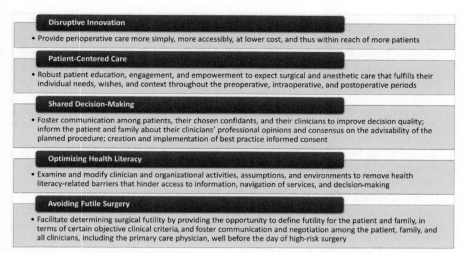

Fig. 5. Ethical opportunities with a PSH. (*Courtesy of* T.R. Vetter, MD, MPH, Austin, TX.)

phase but continues throughout the intraoperative, postoperative, and postdischarge phases of care.[5,12,55,59]

This rising prominence of value-based health care and population health management supports the continued need and role for evolving PSH models, which rely extensively on continuously evolving evidence-based best practice, as well as telemedicine and telehealth, including mobile technologies and connectivity. However, to successfully deliver greater valued-based care and to effectively contribute to sustained and meaningful perioperative population health management, the scope of existing, primarily preoperative, assessment and its associated services and clinician skills must expand.[12,55,60]

SUMMARY

There will almost assuredly be a continued increased need for and volume of not only medical but also surgical and perioperative care in coming decade.[2,61] There will be attendant demands from key stakeholders for a maximum return on their investment; namely, greater realized value for this surgical and perioperative care.[61] This movement toward value-based payment models, driven by governmental policies, federal statutes, and market forces, is propelling the importance of effectively managing the health of populations to the forefront in the United States and other developed countries.[55] This article has thus focused on various PSH models as continued opportunities and mechanisms for delivering greater value-based, comprehensive perioperative assessment and global optimization of the surgical patient.

Comprehensive perioperative management will play a pivotal role in delivering this higher quality and lower cost care to surgical patients. The aging population is especially increasing demand for high-quality surgical care. Of note, the Coalition for Quality in Geriatric Surgery includes 58 diverse stakeholder organizations committed to improving geriatric surgery.[62] Although anesthesiologists have played and will continue to play a seminal role in any PSH model,[42] they would be well-advised to acknowledge and to embrace the equally vital role of surgeons, hospitalists, and geriatricians.[63,64]

REFERENCES

1. Centers for Disease Control and Prevention, National Center for Health Statistics. National hospital discharge survey: 2010. FastStats. Atlanta (GA): Centers for Disease Control and Prevention; 2017. Available at: https://www.cdc.gov/nchs/data/nhds/4procedures/2010pro4_numberprocedureage.pdf. Accessed February 21, 2018.
2. Sisko AM, Keehan SP, Cuckler GA, et al. National health expenditure projections, 2013-23: faster growth expected with expanded coverage and improving economy. Health Aff (Millwood) 2014;33(10):1841–50.
3. Grocott MPW, Pearse RM. Perioperative medicine: the future of anaesthesia? Br J Anaesth 2012;108(5):723–6.
4. Vetter TR, Pittet JF. The perioperative surgical home: a panacea or Pandora's box for the specialty of anesthesiology? Anesth Analg 2015;120(5):968–73.
5. Aronson S, Sangvai D, McClellan MB. Why a proactive perioperative medicine policy is crucial for a sustainable population health strategy. Anesth Analg 2018;126(2):710–2.
6. Phipps D, Meakin GH, Beatty PC, et al. Human factors in anaesthetic practice: insights from a task analysis. Br J Anaesth 2008;100(3):333–43.
7. Schimpff SC. Improving operating room and perioperative safety: background and specific recommendations. Surg Innov 2007;14(2):127–35.
8. Cormier JN, Cromwell KD, Pollock RE. Value-based health care: a surgical oncologist's perspective. Surg Oncol Clin N Am 2012;21(3):497–506, x.
9. Tsai TC, Orav EJ, Jha AK. Care fragmentation in the postdischarge period: surgical readmissions, distance of travel, and postoperative mortality. JAMA Surg 2015;150(1):59–64.
10. Vetter TR, Goeddel LA, Boudreaux AM, et al. The perioperative surgical home: how can it make the case so everyone wins? BMC Anesthesiol 2013;13:6.
11. Kain ZN, Vakharia S, Garson L, et al. The perioperative surgical home as a future perioperative practice model. Anesth Analg 2014;118(5):1126–30.
12. Vetter TR, Boudreaux AM, Jones KA, et al. The perioperative surgical home: how anesthesiology can collaboratively achieve and leverage the triple aim in health care. Anesth Analg 2014;118(5):1131–6.
13. Schweitzer M, Vetter TR. The perioperative surgical home: more than smoke and mirrors? Anesth Analg 2016;123(3):524–8.
14. Wanderer JP, Rathmell JP. A brief history of the perioperative surgical home. Anesthesiology 2015;123(1):A23.
15. Vetter TR, Ivankova NV, Goeddel LA, et al. An analysis of methodologies that can be used to validate if a perioperative surgical home improves the patient-centeredness, evidence-based practice, quality, safety, and value of patient care. Anesthesiology 2013;119(6):1261–74.
16. Bodenheimer T, Sinsky C. From triple to quadruple aim: care of the patient requires care of the provider. Ann Fam Med 2014;12(6):573–6.
17. Epperson WJ, Childs SF, Wilhoit G. Provider burnout and patient engagement: the quadruple and quintuple aims. J Med Pract Manage 2016;31(6):359–63.
18. Gergen Barnett KA. In pursuit of the fourth aim in health care: the joy of practice. Med Clin North Am 2017;101(5):1031–40.
19. Sikka R, Morath JM, Leape L. The quadruple aim: care, health, cost and meaning in work. BMJ Qual Saf 2015;24(10):608–10.
20. Coleman EA, Parry C, Chalmers S, et al. The care transitions intervention: results of a randomized controlled trial. Arch Intern Med 2006;166(17):1822–8.

21. Coleman EA, Smith JD, Frank JC, et al. Preparing patients and caregivers to participate in care delivered across settings: the care transitions intervention. J Am Geriatr Soc 2004;52(11):1817–25.
22. Sevin C, Evdokimoff M, Sobolewski S, et al. How-to guide: improving transitions from the hospital to home health care to reduce avoidable rehospitalizations. Cambridge (MA): Institute for Healthcare Improvement; 2013. Available at: www.ihi.org. Accessed March 4, 2018.
23. Herndon LBC, Bradke P, Rutherford P. How-to guide: improving transitions from the hospital to skilled nursing facilities to reduce avoidable rehospitalizations. Cambridge (MA): Institute for Healthcare Improvement; 2013. Available at: www.ihi.org. Accessed March 4, 2018.
24. Rutherford P, Nielsen GA, Taylor J, et al. How-to guide: improving transitions from the hospital to community settings to reduce avoidable rehospitalizations. Cambridge (MA): Institute for Healthcare Improvement; 2013. Available at: www.ihi.org. Accessed March 4, 2018.
25. Vetter TR, Uhler LM, Bozic KJ. Value-based Healthcare: a novel transitional care service strives to improve patient experience and outcomes. Clin Orthop Relat Res 2017;475(11):2638–42.
26. Weller J, Boyd M, Cumin D. Teams, tribes and patient safety: overcoming barriers to effective teamwork in healthcare. Postgrad Med J 2014;90(1061):149–54.
27. Jones CE, Hollis RH, Wahl TS, et al. Transitional care interventions and hospital readmissions in surgical populations: a systematic review. Am J Surg 2016; 212(2):327–35.
28. Kash BA, Zhang Y, Cline KM, et al. The perioperative surgical home (PSH): a comprehensive review of US and non-US studies shows predominantly positive quality and cost outcomes. Milbank Q 2014;92(4):796–821.
29. Vetter TR, Barman J, Hunter JM Jr, et al. The effect of implementation of preoperative and postoperative care elements of a perioperative surgical home model on outcomes in patients undergoing hip arthroplasty or knee arthroplasty. Anesth Analg 2017;124(5):1450–8.
30. Chaurasia A, Garson L, Kain ZL, et al. Outcomes of a joint replacement surgical home model clinical pathway. Biomed Res Int 2014;2014:296302.
31. Cyriac J, Garson L, Schwarzkopf R, et al. Total joint replacement perioperative surgical home program: 2-year follow-up. Anesth Analg 2016;123(1):51–62.
32. Garson L, Schwarzkopf R, Vakharia S, et al. Implementation of a total joint replacement-focused perioperative surgical home: a management case report. Anesth Analg 2014;118(5):1081–9.
33. Qiu C, Cannesson M, Morkos A, et al. Practice and outcomes of the perioperative surgical home in a California integrated delivery system. Anesth Analg 2016; 123(3):597–606.
34. Qiu C, Rinehart J, Nguyen VT, et al. An ambulatory surgery perioperative surgical home in Kaiser Permanente settings: practice and outcomes. Anesth Analg 2017; 124(3):768–74.
35. Raphael DR, Cannesson M, Schwarzkopf R, et al. Total joint perioperative surgical home: an observational financial review. Perioper Med (Lond) 2014;3:6.
36. Aronson S, Westover J, Guinn N, et al. A perioperative medicine model for population health: an integrated approach for an evolving clinical science. Anesth Analg 2018;126(2):682–90.
37. Butterworth JF 4th, Green J. The anesthesiologist-directed perioperative surgical home: a great idea that will succeed only if it is embraced by hospital administrators and surgeons. Anesth Analg 2014;118(5):896–7.

38. Hooper VD. Who staffs the perioperative surgical home? Anesth Analg 2013; 116(4):754–5.

39. Powell AC, Thearle MS, Cusick M, et al. Early results of a surgeon-led, perioperative surgical home. J Surg Res 2017;211:154–62.

40. Soybel DI, Knuf K. The perioperative surgical home: cui bono? JAMA Surg 2016; 151(11):1003–4.

41. Schonberger RB. Rebranding the perioperative surgical home: lessons from the Duke experience. J Cardiothorac Vasc Anesth 2016;30(4):1064–6.

42. Mariano ER, Vetter TR, Kain ZN. The perioperative surgical home is not just a name. Anesth Analg 2017;125(5):1443–5.

43. Greene SM, Reid RJ, Larson EB. Implementing the learning health system: from concept to action. Ann Intern Med 2012;157(3):207–10.

44. Smith M, Halvorson G, Kaplan G. What's needed is a health care system that learns: recommendations from an IOM report. JAMA 2012;308(16):1637–8.

45. Etheredge LM. A rapid-learning health system. Health Aff (Millwood) 2007;26(2): w107–18.

46. Krumholz HM. Big data and new knowledge in medicine: the thinking, training, and tools needed for a learning health system. Health Aff (Millwood) 2014; 33(7):1163–70.

47. Krumholz HM, Terry SF, Waldstreicher J. Data acquisition, curation, and use for a continuously learning health system. JAMA 2016;316(16):1669–70.

48. Faden RR, Kass NE, Goodman SN, et al. An ethics framework for a learning health care system: a departure from traditional research ethics and clinical ethics. Hastings Cent Rep 2013;Spec No:S16–27.

49. Grady C, Wendler D. Making the transition to a learning health care system. Commentary. Hastings Cent Rep 2013;Spec No:S32–3.

50. Goeddel LA, Porterfield JR Jr, Hall JD, et al. Ethical opportunities with the perioperative surgical home: disruptive innovation, patient-centered care, shared decision making, health literacy, and futility of care. Anesth Analg 2015;120(5): 1158–62.

51. Thaker NG, Feeley TW. Creating the healthcare transformation from volume to value. In: Phillips RA, editor. America's healthcare transformation: strategies and innovations. New Brunswick (NJ): Rutgers University Press; 2016. p. 295–318.

52. Gordon JE, Leiman JM, Deland EL, et al. Delivering value: provider efforts to improve the quality and reduce the cost of health care. Annu Rev Med 2014; 65:447–58.

53. Stadhouders N, Koolman X, Tanke M, et al. Policy options to contain healthcare costs: a review and classification. Health Policy 2016;120(5):486–94.

54. Shah NN, Vetter TR. Comprehensive preoperative assessment and global optimization. Anesthesiol Clin 2018;36(2):259–80.

55. Boudreaux AM, Vetter TR. A primer on population health management and its perioperative application. Anesth Analg 2016;123(1):63–70.

56. Peterson TA, Bernstein SJ, Spahlinger DA. Population health: a new paradigm for medicine. Am J Med Sci 2016;351(1):26–32.

57. Steenkamer BM, Drewes HW, Heijink R, et al. Defining population health management: a scoping review of the literature. Popul Health Manag 2017;20(1):74–85.

58. Andrieni JD. Population health management: the lynchpin of emerging healthcare delivery models. In: Phillips RA, editor. America's healthcare transformation: strategies and innovations. New Brunswick (NJ): Rutgers University Press; 2016. p. 113–27.

59. Peden CJ, Mythen MG, Vetter TR. Population health management and perioperative medicine: the expanding role of the anesthesiologist. Anesth Analg 2018; 126(2):397–9.
60. Alem N, Kain Z. Evolving healthcare delivery paradigms and the optimization of 'value' in anesthesiology. Curr Opin Anaesthesiol 2017;30(2):223–9.
61. Vetter TR, Jones KA. Perioperative surgical home: perspective II. Anesthesiol Clin 2015;33(4):771–84.
62. Berian JR, Rosenthal RA, Baker TL, et al. Hospital standards to promote optimal surgical care of the older adult: a report from the coalition for quality in geriatric surgery. Ann Surg 2018;267(2):280–90.
63. Mohanty S, Rosenthal RA, Russell MM, et al. Optimal perioperative management of the geriatric patient: a best practices guideline from the American College of Surgeons NSQIP and the American Geriatrics Society. J Am Coll Surg 2016; 222(5):930–47.
64. Thompson RE, Pfeifer K, Grant PJ, et al. Hospital medicine and perioperative care: a framework for high-quality, high-value collaborative care. J Hosp Med 2017;12(4):277–82.

Preoperative Evaluation of the Pediatric Patient

Allison Basel, MD[a,b], Dusica Bajic, MD, PhD[b,c,*]

KEYWORDS

- Pediatric • Preoperative evaluation • Premature • Congenital heart disease
- Respiratory infection • Preoperative anxiety

KEY POINTS

- Infants and children are a unique population requiring special consideration during the preoperative period.
- Former premature infants up to 48 to 50 weeks postgestational age are at an increased risk for postoperative apnea and bradycardia, requiring close postoperative monitoring.
- Infants and children with congenital cardiac disease need thorough evaluation of their current anatomy and previous surgeries to evaluate their need for further cardiac evaluation and endocarditis prophylaxis.
- Infants and children with recent upper or lower respiratory infections are at risk of respiratory complications with administration of anesthesia.
- Both patient and parental anxiety should be anticipated and addressed before the day of surgery to increase the likelihood of a smooth operative course.

INTRODUCTION

This article is intended to assist the general anesthesiologist in preparing pediatric patients for the procedure or intervention. The preoperative workup discussed mainly focuses on infants and toddler-aged children. Neonatal and premature infant preoperative evaluation is outside the scope of this article and require additional discussion and depth of conversation. In general, most preoperative evaluation of adults can be applied to children. A thorough history and physical is needed, laboratory work is done if indicated, and specialty referral when deemed necessary.[1] However, there are special considerations with pediatric patients that make them unique and warrant

Disclosure Statement: There are no conflicts of interest to disclose.
[a] Department of Anesthesia, Critical Care, and Pain Medicine, Beth Israel Deaconess Medical Center, 330 Brookline Avenue, Boston, MA 02215, USA; [b] Department of Anesthesiology, Critical Care and Pain Medicine, Boston Children's Hospital, 300 Longwood Avenue, Boston, MA 02115, USA; [c] Department of Anaesthesia, Harvard Medical School, 25 Shattuck Street, Boston, MA 02115, USA
* Corresponding author. Department of Anesthesiology, Critical Care and Pain Medicine, Boston Children's Hospital, 300 Longwood Avenue, Bader 3, Boston, MA 02115.
E-mail address: dusica.bajic@childrens.harvard.edu

Anesthesiology Clin 36 (2018) 689–700
https://doi.org/10.1016/j.anclin.2018.07.016
1932-2275/18/© 2018 Elsevier Inc. All rights reserved.

anesthesiology.theclinics.com

further evaluation and attention. They also have a unique physiology that must be considered. Children naturally have less cardiorespiratory reserve and may be easily prone to cyanosis, bradycardia, and cardiac arrest. Specifically, the estimated anesthesia-related cardiac arrest in noncardiac cases is 1 per 10,000 to 15,000.[2–4] Outcomes for pediatric patients undergoing anesthesia have improved over the years as a result of advances in monitoring and equipment, safer and more easily titratable anesthetic agents, and possibly the practice of subspecialization.[4] However, knowledge of frequently encountered possible complications during administration of pediatric anesthesia should direct detailed preoperative evaluation, ultimately serving as a foundation for earlier detection and possible prevention of potential perioperative problems, leading to better outcomes. The article covers the subjects of gestational age, respiratory and cardiovascular concerns, fasting guidelines, and management of preoperative anxiety, all unique for pediatric population, as well as the current hot topic of the potential neurotoxic effects of anesthetics on the developing brain.

PREOPERATIVE EVALUATION
History, Physical, and Laboratory Examinations

Although the standard adult history and physical exam can be adapted to preoperative evaluation of children, there are some topics that require further emphasis in children. Preexisting pediatrician's notes can be a valuable resource when evaluating a child in the preoperative period because parents may not remember all the medical details. Specifically, birth history is an important factor that can potentially be overlooked in an adult. It is particularly important to find out if the child was born prematurely because sequela of prematurity can affect anesthesia management and anticipated complications.[5,6] It is also prudent to investigate the patient's neurologic development, airway anomalies, surgical history, previous intubations, and general medical health (heart, lung, endocrine, renal disorders). A child with a genetic or dysmorphic syndrome should be thoroughly evaluated because anomalies in the cervical spine (eg, Down syndrome) or craniofacial dysmorphia can significantly affect anesthetic management.[7,8] Psychological issues should be addressed because they can alter how smoothly the operative course runs.[1] Children with psychological conditions may require intervention of a child life specialist to make a successful transition to the operating room.

Certain aspects of the family history are key. Specifically, a history of (1) malignant hyperthermia (MH), (2) pseudocholinesterase deficiency, (3) postoperative nausea and vomiting, (4) congenital myopathies, and (5) bleeding disorders should be explored.[1] It is extremely important that children at risk of MH be identified preoperatively. At-risk children include those with a family or personal history of MH or congenital myopathies, such as central core disease.[9,10] Children account for 52.1% of all MH reactions.[9] If an at-risk child is encountered, anesthetic management with total intravenous anesthesia should be strongly considered because it minimizes the chance of being exposed to a volatile anesthetic trigger. Succinylcholine should also be avoided because it can also be a trigger. It is essential that all anesthetizing facilities, especially ambulatory surgery centers, are prepared for the eventuality of an acute life-threatening MH event.[11] If MH is suspected intraoperatively, all volatile anesthetics should be stopped immediately and intravenous dantrolene should be given.[12] Detailed information on the management of MH can be found on *The Malignant Hyperthermia Association of the United States* Web site (https://www.mhaus.org/). To learn more about the history of MH in pediatric population, refer to article by King and colleagues.[13]

No laboratory work is indicated for healthy children undergoing a procedure with minimal blood loss anticipated. A hematocrit test may be ordered if a great amount of blood loss is expected and may be required for infants at some institutions.[1] Bleeding time, prothrombin time and partial thromboplastin time, and platelet count have not proven to be reliable predictors of bleeding risk; therefore, they are not routinely recommended.[14–16] Routine pregnancy testing is controversial because some parents may decline the test and history alone can be unreliable in predicting the need for the test. It is recommended that, at the minimum, the test be discussed with the patient and family, although institutional guidelines may vary. The test should especially be offered to patients if it would affect their management. At the current time, there is a knowledge gap regarding the risks of anesthesia in early pregnancy.[17]

Although allergies are a part of every preoperative evaluation, special attention should be given to a known or possible latex allergy. Although the incidence of latex allergy throughout the general population has been estimated between 1% and 6%, for certain pediatric populations (eg, spinal bifida and bladder exstrophy) its incidence has been reported as high as 73%.[18,19] Specifically, those with an increased risk include pediatric patients with spina bifida, myelodysplasia, urinary tract malformations,[20–22] as well as multiple previous surgeries.[23] It has been recommended that high-risk patients with a history of multiple surgeries be also screened preoperatively for a latex allergy with not only questioning but also skin prick or radioallergosorbent testing.[23] Studies show that latex-allergic children can be safely anesthetized if exposure to latex in the medical environment is avoided, and that administration of prophylactic medications to decrease the allergic response is unnecessary.[24] Although many clinical institutions are latex-free, it is still prudent to become familiar with the common symptoms of latex allergy. For more detailed information on latex allergy; recognition of symptoms; and operative latex-free setup, precautions, and treatment, refer to the *American Latex Allergy Association* Web site (http://latexallergyresources.org/).

Former Premature Infant

Premature infants are born less than 37-weeks gestational age. The former premature infant is at an increased risk for postoperative apnea, periodic breathing, and bradycardia up to 24 hours after surgery when compared with term infants.[25] Therefore, it is generally advisable to admit these patients for 24 hours postanesthesia monitoring. This should be arranged during the preoperative assessment period. Postoperative apnea and bradycardia are associated with immaturity of the brainstem, leading to ineffective central and peripheral chemoreceptors that do not respond properly to hypoxia and hypercarbia stimuli.[26] There are some interventions that have been used to minimize postoperative apnea, including

1. The administration of perioperative caffeine
2. The use of spinal anesthesia as opposed to general anesthesia
3. Delaying surgery until 48 to 50 weeks postconception.[27]

These infants should also have their hematocrit checked because hematocrit values less than 30% in this group are associated with a higher incidence of postoperative apnea.[28] Another concern in this population is bronchopulmonary dysplasia, a chronic lung disease that premature infants may suffer from.[29] This can cause an exaggerated risk of bronchospasm and oxygen desaturation in the perioperative period within the first year of life. Affected children are also more susceptible to pulmonary vasoconstriction in response to the variety of possible assaults during anesthesia, such as hypothermia, pain, and acidosis.[30]

Congenital Heart Disease

Congenital heart disease is a common problem encountered in pediatric anesthesia and often needs special consideration during the preoperative period. Intracardiac murmurs, shunts, and the need for antibiotic prophylaxis should to be evaluated because all these can affect the anesthetic management and possible perioperative complications.

It is vital that innocent versus pathologic nature of the heart murmurs be distinguished. At minimum, evaluation for a murmur should include a thorough medial history and a physical evaluation, as well as electrocardiogram testing. Generally speaking, if a child is acyanotic, has normal first and second heart sounds, is growing well, and has good exercise tolerance, the murmur will most likely not cause significant consequences during anesthesia. If there is a question of a significant structural heart defect, an echocardiogram and evaluation by a pediatric cardiologist should be done. Intracardiac shunts (eg, ventricular septal defect) need to be identified in the preoperative period because anesthesia agents can affect the functioning of these shunts. Understanding the basic physiology of shunts is essential for anticipation of potential perioperative circulatory problems. With a decrease in pulmonary vascular resistance, pulmonary overcirculation can occur in the presence of the left-to-right shunts leading to failure due to pulmonary overcirculation. On the other hand, pulmonary vascular resistance can also increase due to various assaults possible during anesthesia, such as hypoxia, hypercarbia, hypotension, and hypothermia. This decrease can actually cause a left-to-right shunt to reverse (to a right-to-left shunt) producing serious consequences (ie, hypoxemia). Children who have intracardiac shunts are at risk for paradoxic embolism and, therefore, should be identified preoperatively despite that stroke is less common in children than adults.[31] The need for antibiotic prophylaxis to prevent bacterial endocarditis should be evaluated in the preoperative period. Surgical procedures at risk for bacteremia, such as dental procedures, require prophylaxis in patients with certain shunts or other congenital heart defects. Those with prosthetic heart valves and/or history of endocarditis also require prophylaxis (**Box 1**). The antibiotic prophylactic regiment should be followed as outlined by the *American Heart Association* recommendations.[32–34]

In a child with known complex congenital heart disease (eg, single ventricle), the current anatomy should be evaluated, noting any previous corrective or palliative surgeries.[35] Even with surgical evaluation, there can still be residual defects capable of causing physiologic compromise. Children with congenital heart disease who present

---

Box 1
Endocarditis prophylaxis

Dental procedures only (no longer gastrointestinal or genitourinary)

- Prosthetic heart valves

- Previous endocarditis

- Heart transplant with abnormal heart valve function

- Complex congenital heart defects
  - Cyanotic, not fully repaired
  - Fully repaired for first 6 months after repair
  - Repaired with residual defects

Dental procedures but not gastrointestinal or genitourinary should be considered for endocarditis prophylaxis in pediatric patients with listed cardiac conditions.
Reprinted with permission www.heart.org. ©2018 American Heart Association, Inc.

for noncardiac surgery are at increased risk of perioperative morbidity. Those high-risk children require transfer to a specialist center because full pediatric intensive care and cardiology services may be required. Involvement of the pediatric cardiac anesthesia team may be warranted for many cases. Children with low-risk for perioperative morbidity may undergo surgery at the local hospital. More detailed information about providing noncardiac anesthesia care for cardiac pediatric patient should be sought elsewhere.[36–38]

Respiratory Infection

Children can have multiple respiratory infections each year, making this condition very common in the preoperative course. The average child gets 3 to 9 upper respiratory infections per year, with each lasting between 7 to 10 days.[39] Although respiratory infections are common, they pose a considerable threat to the perioperative course. An active respiratory infection increases the risk of perioperative respiratory complications from 2-fold to 7-fold.[40] These complications include laryngospasm, bronchospasm, atelectasis, postextubation croup, and postoperative pneumonia.[41] There is a correlation between the child's age and the risk of pulmonary complications due to a respiratory infection, with children younger than 5 years being at a significantly increased risk compared with children older than 5 years.[42] There are no definitive rules for canceling a procedure based on the presence of a respiratory tract infection. However, generally speaking, signs of active lower respiratory infection, such as wheezing, productive cough, chest radiograph findings, as well as presence of systemic illness (presence of fever), should warrant canceling an elective procedure.[43] Although complications are most severe during an active respiratory infection, the take-home message for the anesthesia providers is that the airway reactivity can remain for up to 6 weeks postinfection.[42] Given this information, it is advisable to delay an elective procedure 4 to 6 weeks if deemed necessary.[42,43] One can proceed with planned surgery if minor symptoms of upper respiratory infection are present, such as clear rhinorrhea and upper airway congestion.[42] If the procedure needs to move forward despite presence of the upper respiratory infection symptoms, there are perioperative considerations. Endotracheal intubation increases the risk of respiratory complications 11-fold in children with respiratory infectious symptoms.[40] Using a mask airway instead of tracheal intubation may minimize the risk if appropriate.[44]

Asthma

Asthma is a common childhood respiratory disorder that results in a hyperreactive airway. Laryngoscopy and tracheal intubation are both potent airway stimulators. It is extremely important the preoperative history include specific details pertaining to the child's asthma. It is necessary to understand the severity of the illness, current symptoms, age of onset, current medications, prior hospitalizations, the date of the last attack, and prior need of mechanical ventilation.[45] As a rule, medical therapy should be optimized before surgery to minimize incidence of perioperative respiratory complications.[46] Even in children whose asthma is well-controlled, medical therapy should be escalated before surgery to prevent or minimize bronchospasm.[47] The therapy should be escalated according to their baseline needs. For example, in a child who takes a beta-agonist on an as-needed basis, a scheduled beta-agonist should begin 3 to 5 days before surgery.[48] If the child is actively wheezing or has had a recent asthma attack, strong consideration should be given to delaying the procedure.[49] All medications should be continued up to and on the morning of surgery, including oral steroids.

Obstructive Sleep Apnea

Obstructive sleep apnea syndrome is a sleep disorder characterized by partial upper airway obstruction and/or temporary complete obstruction. It can be central (neurologic; <5%) or obstructive (>95%) in origin, and possibly mixed in nature of presentation. It is a relatively prevalent condition in children, affecting 1% to 5% of children 2 to 8 years of age and is caused by a variety of different pathophysiologic abnormalities.[50] More common obstructive apnea results from a physical airway obstruction, whereas central apnea is the result of a lack of airflow, as well as respiratory effort.[50,51] Polysomnography is the gold standard of diagnosis and should be reviewed during the preoperative period if available.[52] Although this condition is also found in adults, there are some important differences to note in the pediatric population. In children, obstructive sleep apnea affects both sexes equally and is associated with all body types, as opposed to largely being linked to obesity in adults. In children, this condition is treated surgically, compared with more noninvasive techniques in adults, such as continuous positive airway pressure. Although these differences exist, children can suffer the same serious sequelae as adults, including cor pulmonale, pulmonary hypertension, cognitive difficulties, learning disabilities, and behavioral issues.[53] In the preoperative period, these children may require additional testing to evaluate their cardiovascular status, especially if there are signs of right ventricular dysfunction, systemic hypertension, or multiple episodes of desaturation less than 70%.[54] Furthermore, children with obstructive sleep apnea are usually more susceptible to the respiratory depressant effects of opioids,[55] which is an important fact to consider when managing postoperative pain. This has been linked to a possible increase in central opioid receptors due to chronic hypoxemia.[56] In one study, children with oxygenation less than 85% required only 50% of the postoperative morphine dose for analgesia.[53] Children with obstructive sleep apnea may also require a higher level of monitoring in the postoperative period. The intensive care or step-down unit may be required for those with severe obstructive sleep apnea, body mass index greater than 40, or very young children.[57] This requirement should be arranged in the preoperative period.

Fasting Guidelines

Fasting guidelines are designed to minimize gastric volume and, it is hoped, to reduce the risk of pulmonary aspiration; however, recent data suggest gastric fluid volume is more of a surrogate marker than a risk factor for pulmonary aspiration.[58] The following fasting guidelines are generally agreed on, but institutional guidelines may vary. Clear liquids can be given up to 2 hours before surgery and breast milk up to 4 hours before surgery. Formula, nonhuman milk, and a light meal can be given up to 6 hours before surgery and solids up to 8 hours before surgery. These guidelines allow for a smoother preoperative course and a more comfortable child.[59] The preoperative *nil per os* (nothing by mouth) instructions should be explicitly explained to the parent because they are frequently misunderstood (**Box 2**).

Patient or Parental Preoperative Anxiety

Presenting for surgery can be an overwhelming and frightening idea for both children and their parents. It is the job of the anesthesiologist to calm these fears in the preoperative period to allow for a smooth perioperative course. Factors associated with higher preoperative anxiety include younger age, the child's first surgery, problems with prior health care encounters, length of procedure, and anxious parents.[60,61] The anesthesia course should be explained in terms that are appropriate for the age

---

Box 2
Pediatric nil per os (nothing by mouth) guidelines

- 8 hours prior: heavy, fatty meal
- 6 hours prior: light meal, formula, nonhuman milk
- 4 hours prior: human milk
- 2 hours prior: clear liquids

These are fasting guidelines before surgical procedure for pediatric patients.
Adapted from Ferrari L. Introduction and definitions. In Ferrari L, editor. Anesthesia and Pain Management for the Pediatrician. Baltimore: The Johns Hopkins University Press; 1999. p. 1–10.

---

of the child, taking into consideration their level of development. For example, preschool aged children are concrete thinkers and will take literally what you say to them. Adolescents may not adequately express either their fears or questions directly. It is important to clearly explain the anesthesia course and indirectly calm these fears without the adolescent having to explicitly state them.[45] Parents are often most concerned with the anesthesia aspect of the surgical procedure. In the preoperative period, parents should be educated about the anesthesia course and common complications. Major adverse events include laryngospasm, bronchospasm, drug reactions, pneumonia, hypoxemia, and dental trauma. Laryngospasm (1.7% of cases) is the most common complication. Some minor risks include oral trauma, sore throat, nausea, vomiting, cough, and hoarseness (**Table 1**).[62] It is often helpful to give parents perspective when discussing risks. For example, the risk of an adverse event in a healthy child undergoing an uncomplicated surgery is 1 in 200,000.[63]

There is much controversy over parents' presence at induction. Some possible benefits of the practice include decreased need for preoperative sedation, avoiding separation anxiety when going to the operating room, increasing child compliance with induction, and increasing parental satisfaction. However, there are potential drawbacks to the practice, including disrupting or crowding the operating room, potential adverse reaction by the parents, and slowing the induction process. Although there are potential benefits to the process, randomized controlled trials suggest the practice is not beneficial.[64–66] When comparing parental presence to traditional preoperative sedation with oral midazolam, patients who have received midazolam were less anxious and more amenable during induction. The reaction of the parent should also be considered because an anxious parent accompanying the child to the operating room may cause the patient to be more anxious.

Table 1
Pediatric complications of anesthesia

Minor	Major
• Oral trauma	• Laryngospasm
• Sore throat	• Bronchospasm
• Nausea and vomiting	• Drug reactions
• Cough	• Pneumonia
• Hoarseness	• Hypoxemia

Summary of some minor and major common pediatric complications of anesthesia administration.
Adapted from Ferrari LR. Introduction and definitions. In: Ferrari LR, editor. Anesthesia and pain management for the pediatrician. Baltimore (MD): Johns Hopkins University Press; 1999; with permission.

Effects of Anesthesia on the Developing Brain

The effects of anesthesia on the developing brain are an area of much interest that has been a subject of concern and considerable research interest. This topic has been the focus of 3 public hearings by the US Food and Drug Administration (FDA) since 2007, including an FDA Science Board meeting in November 2014. These served to better inform the public and practitioners about the most recent findings, and to foster a discussion between parents and physicians about the potential risks posed when using anesthesia in young children.[67,68] Although in vitro and animal research studies from roundworms to nonhuman primates support evidence of neurotoxicity in the presence of anesthetic agents,[69] the impact of surgery on anesthetic-induced brain injury in the developing brain has not yet been adequately addressed. A retrospective study done at the Mayo Clinic showed children who received more than 2 anesthetics before age 4 were at an increased risk for developing learning disabilities.[70] In another retrospective study, greater behavioral problems were seen in children who had anesthesia before 24 months compared with those who had not received anesthesia.[71] However, the overall literature consensus is that clinical data, comprising largely of retrospective cohort database analyses, are inconclusive, in part due to confounding variables inherent in these observational epidemiologic approaches.[69] In contrast, a twin study showed no discrepancies in learning capability between twins: one who had received anesthesia before age 3 years and one who had not received anesthesia.[72,73] This places even greater emphasis on prospective approaches to this problem, such as the ongoing General Anesthesia and Awake-Regional Anesthesia in Infancy (General Anesthesia compared to Spinal Anesthesia; GAS) trial[74–77] and the Pediatric Anesthesia Neurodevelopment Assessment (PANDA) study.[78,79] The resulting data do not show any long-term sequelae from early anesthesia exposure in otherwise healthy infants. It is advisable to present the parent with the current data but to note that more extensive human studies need to be done to fully understand the short-term and long-term consequences of anesthesia administration in pediatric patients.

SUMMARY

Preoperative planning for infants and children encompasses many of the same steps as adults; however, there are important differences to be noted. In addition to the traditional history and physical examination, attention should be paid to the child's overall development and the presence of any syndromes. A careful personal or family history of MH should be elicited, as well as risk factors for latex allergy. Due to their immature physiology and development, these age groups are more susceptible to certain conditions that can dramatically affect anesthesia management. Notably, any recent or current respiratory infection can have drastic effects perioperatively, leading to higher anesthetic complications. It is also prudent to investigate a history of former prematurity, congenital heart disease, and asthma. An especially unique concern for this age group is parental, as well as patient, anxiety. There are several techniques used to calm these anxieties and each plan should be tailored to the individual family. By taking these special considerations into account, the preoperative evaluation of the pediatric patient can be accomplished, allowing a successfully operative course.

REFERENCES

1. Section on A, Pain M. The pediatrician's role in the evaluation and preparation of pediatric patients undergoing anesthesia. Pediatrics 2014;134(3):634–41.

2. Bharti N, Batra YK, Kaur H. Paediatric perioperative cardiac arrest and its mortality: database of a 60-month period from a tertiary care paediatric centre. Eur J Anaesthesiol 2009;26(6):490–5.
3. Ramamoorthy C, Haberkern CM, Bhananker SM, et al. Anesthesia-related cardiac arrest in children with heart disease: data from the Pediatric Perioperative Cardiac Arrest (POCA) registry. Anesth Analg 2010;110(5):1376–82.
4. Lee C, Mason L. Complications in paediatric anaesthesia. Curr Opin Anaesthesiol 2006;19(3):262–7.
5. Welborn LG, Greenspun JC. Anesthesia and apnea. Perioperative considerations in the former preterm infant. Pediatr Clin North Am 1994;41(1):181–98.
6. Conran AM, Kahana M. Anesthetic considerations in neonatal neurosurgical patients. Neurosurg Clin N Am 1998;9(1):181–5.
7. Baker S, Parico L. Pathologic paediatric conditions associated with a compromised airway. Int J Paediatr Dent 2010;20(2):102–11.
8. Lewanda AF, Matisoff A, Revenis M, et al. Preoperative evaluation and comprehensive risk assessment for children with Down syndrome. Paediatr Anaesth 2016;26(4):356–62.
9. Bamaga AK, Riazi S, Amburgey K, et al. Neuromuscular conditions associated with malignant hyperthermia in paediatric patients: a 25-year retrospective study. Neuromuscul Disord 2016;26(3):201–6.
10. Brandom BW, Muldoon SM. Unexpected MH deaths without exposure to inhalation anesthetics in pediatric patients. Paediatr Anaesth 2013;23(9):851–4.
11. Litman RS, Joshi GP. Malignant hyperthermia in the ambulatory surgery center: how should we prepare? Anesthesiology 2014;120(6):1306–8.
12. Pardo MC, Miller RD. Inhaled anesthetics. In: Pardo MC, Miller RD, editors. Basics of anesthesia. Philadelphia: Elselvier; 2018. p. 101.
13. King MR, Firth PG, Yaster M, et al. Malignant hyperthermia in the early days of pediatric anesthesia: an interview with anesthesiology pioneer, Dr John F. Ryan. Paediatr Anaesth 2015;25(9):871–6.
14. Burk CD, Miller L, Handler SD, et al. Preoperative history and coagulation screening in children undergoing tonsillectomy. Pediatrics 1992;89(4 Pt 2):691–5.
15. Suchman AL, Mushlin AI. How well does the activated partial thromboplastin time predict postoperative hemorrhage? JAMA 1986;256(6):750–3.
16. Rodgers RP, Levin J. A critical reappraisal of the bleeding time. Semin Thromb Hemost 1990;16(1):1–20.
17. Committee on Standards and Practice Parameters, Apfelbaum JL, Connis RT, et al. Practice advisory for preanesthesia evaluation: an updated report by the American Society of Anesthesiologists Task Force on preanesthesia evaluation. Anesthesiology 2012;116(3):522–38.
18. Levy DA, Charpin D, Pecquet C, et al. Allergy to latex. Allergy 1992;47(6):579–87.
19. Holzman RS. Latex allergy: an emerging operating room problem. Anesth Analg 1993;76(3):635–41.
20. Meeropol E, Frost J, Pugh L, et al. Latex allergy in children with myelodysplasia: a survey of Shriners hospitals. J Pediatr Orthop 1993;13(1):1–4.
21. Kelly KJ, Pearson ML, Kurup VP, et al. A cluster of anaphylactic reactions in children with spina bifida during general anesthesia: epidemiologic features, risk factors, and latex hypersensitivity. J Allergy Clin Immunol 1994;94(1):53–61.
22. Adler S, Stehr M. High latex allergy risk in children with urologic abnormalities. Aktuelle Urol 2004;35(5):361–2 [in German].
23. Porri F, Pradal M, Lemière C, et al. Association between latex sensitization and repeated latex exposure in children. Anesthesiology 1997;86(3):599–602.

24. Holzman RS. Clinical management of latex-allergic children. Anesth Analg 1997; 85(3):529–33.
25. Welborn LG, Rice LJ, Hannallah RS, et al. Postoperative apnea in former preterm infants: prospective comparison of spinal and general anesthesia. Anesthesiology 1990;72(5):838–42.
26. Kurth CD, Spitzer AR, Broennle AM, et al. Postoperative apnea in preterm infants. Anesthesiology 1987;66(4):483–8.
27. Welborn LG, Hannallah RS, Fink R, et al. High-dose caffeine suppresses postoperative apnea in former preterm infants. Anesthesiology 1989;71(3):347–9.
28. Welborn LG, Hannallah RS, Luban NL, et al. Anemia and postoperative apnea in former preterm infants. Anesthesiology 1991;74(6):1003–6.
29. Bancalari E, Claure N, Sosenko IR. Bronchopulmonary dysplasia: changes in pathogenesis, epidemiology and definition. Semin Neonatol 2003;8(1):63–71.
30. Maxwell LG. Age-associated issues in preoperative evaluation, testing, and planning: pediatrics. Anesthesiol Clin North America 2004;22(1):27–43.
31. Dowling MM, Ikemba CM. Intracardiac shunting and stroke in children: a systematic review. J Child Neurol 2011;26(1):72–82.
32. Wilson W, Taubert KA, Gewitz M, et al. Prevention of infective endocarditis: guidelines from the American Heart Association: a guideline from the American Heart Association Rheumatic Fever, Endocarditis and Kawasaki Disease Committee, Council on Cardiovascular Disease in the Young, and the Council on Clinical Cardiology, Council on Cardiovascular Surgery and Anesthesia, and the Quality of Care and Outcomes Research Interdisciplinary Working Group. J Am Dent Assoc 2008;139(Suppl):3S–24S.
33. Sakai Bizmark R, Chang RR, Tsugawa Y, et al. Impact of AHA's 2007 guideline change on incidence of infective endocarditis in infants and children. Am Heart J 2017;189:110–9.
34. American Heart Association (AHA). Infective endocarditis. Available at: http://www.heart.org/HEARTORG/Conditions/CongenitalHeartDefects/TheImpactofCongenitalHeartDefects/Infective-Endocarditis_UCM_307108_Article.jsp#.Wz-dqqjwaUk. Accessed August 22, 2018.
35. Pardo MC, Miller RD. Congenital heart disease. In: Pardo MC, Miller RD, editors. Basics of anesthesia. Philadelphia: Elselvier; 2018. p. 454.
36. Junghare SW, Desurkar V. Congenital heart diseases and anaesthesia. Indian J Anaesth 2017;61(9):744–52.
37. Burrows FA. Anaesthetic management of the child with congenital heart disease for non-cardiac surgery. Can J Anaesth 1992;39(5 Pt 2):R60–70.
38. White MC, Peyton JM. Anaesthetic management of children with congenital heart disease for non-cardiac surgery. Cont Educat Anaesth Crit Care & Pain 2012; 12(1):17–22.
39. Van der Walt J. Anaesthesia in children with viral respiratory tract infections. Paediatr Anaesth 1995;5(4):257–62.
40. Parnis SJ, Barker DS, Van Der Walt JH. Clinical predictors of anaesthetic complications in children with respiratory tract infections. Paediatr Anaesth 2001;11(1): 29–40.
41. Martin LD. Anesthetic implications of an upper respiratory infection in children. Pediatr Clin North Am 1994;41(1):121–30.
42. Cohen MM, Cameron CB. Should you cancel the operation when a child has an upper respiratory tract infection? Anesth Analg 1991;72(3):282–8.
43. Jacoby DB, Hirshman CA. General anesthesia in patients with viral respiratory infections: an unsound sleep? Anesthesiology 1991;74(6):969–72.

44. Tait AR, Pandit UA, Voepel-Lewis T, et al. Use of the laryngeal mask airway in children with upper respiratory tract infections: a comparison with endotracheal intubation. Anesth Analg 1998;86(4):706–11.
45. Ferrari LR. Do children need a preoperative assessment that is different from adults? Int Anesthesiol Clin 2002;40(2):167–86.
46. Pien LC, Grammer LC, Patterson R. Minimal complications in a surgical population with severe asthma receiving prophylactic corticosteroids. J Allergy Clin Immunol 1988;82(4):696–700.
47. Woods BD, Sladen RN. Perioperative considerations for the patient with asthma and bronchospasm. Br J Anaesth 2009;103(Suppl 1):i57–65.
48. Franceschini F, De Benedictis FM, Peroni DG, et al. Anesthesia in children with asthma and rhinitis. Int J Immunopathol Pharmacol 2011;24(3 Suppl):S83–90.
49. Rajesh MC. Anaesthesia for children with bronchial asthma and respiratory infections. Indian J Anaesth 2015;59(9):584–8.
50. Li Z, Celestin J, Lockey RF. Pediatric sleep apnea syndrome: an update. J Allergy Clin Immunol Pract 2016;4(5):852–61.
51. Moreira GA, Pradella-Hallinan M. Sleepiness in children: an update. Sleep Med Clin 2017;12(3):407–13.
52. Rosen CL. Obstructive sleep apnea syndrome (OSAS) in children: diagnostic challenges. Sleep 1996;19(10 Suppl):S274–7.
53. Collins CE, Everett LL. Challenges in pediatric ambulatory anesthesia: kids are different. Anesthesiol Clin 2010;28(2):315–28.
54. Schwengel DA, Sterni LM, Tunkel DE, et al. Perioperative management of children with obstructive sleep apnea. Anesth Analg 2009;109(1):60–75.
55. Brown KA, Laferrière A, Lakheeram I, et al. Recurrent hypoxemia in children is associated with increased analgesic sensitivity to opiates. Anesthesiology 2006;105(4):665–9.
56. Brown KA, Laferriere A, Moss IR. Recurrent hypoxemia in young children with obstructive sleep apnea is associated with reduced opioid requirement for analgesia. Anesthesiology 2004;100(4):806–10 [discussion: 5A].
57. Leong AC, Davis JP. Morbidity after adenotonsillectomy for paediatric obstructive sleep apnoea syndrome: waking up to a pragmatic approach. J Laryngol Otol 2007;121(9):809–17.
58. Schreiner MS. Gastric fluid volume: is it really a risk factor for pulmonary aspiration? Anesth Analg 1998;87(4):754–6.
59. Hanna AH, Mason LJ. Challenges in paediatric ambulatory anesthesia. Curr Opin Anaesthesiol 2012;25(3):315–20.
60. Litman RS, Berger AA, Chhibber A. An evaluation of preoperative anxiety in a population of parents of infants and children undergoing ambulatory surgery. Paediatr Anaesth 1996;6(6):443–7.
61. Chahal N, Manlhiot C, Colapinto K, et al. Association between parental anxiety and compliance with preoperative requirements for pediatric outpatient surgery. J Pediatr Health Care 2009;23(6):372–7.
62. Ferrari LR. Introduction and definitions. In: Ferrari LR, editor. Anesthesia and pain management for the pediatrician. Baltimore (MD): Johns Hopkins University Press; 1999. p. 1–10.
63. Eichhorn JH. Effect of monitoring standards on anesthesia outcome. Int Anesthesiol Clin 1993;31(3):181–96.
64. McCann ME, Kain ZN. The management of preoperative anxiety in children: an update. Anesth Analg 2001;93(1):98–105.

65. Kain ZN, Mayes LC, Wang SM, et al. Parental presence and a sedative premedicant for children undergoing surgery: a hierarchical study. Anesthesiology 2000; 92(4):939–46.
66. Kain ZN, Mayes LC, Caramico LA, et al. Parental presence during induction of anesthesia. A randomized controlled trial. Anesthesiology 1996;84(5):1060–7.
67. Olutoye OA, Baker BW, Belfort MA, et al. Food and Drug Administration warning on anesthesia and brain development: implications for obstetric and fetal surgery. Am J Obstet Gynecol 2018;218(1):98–102.
68. Andropoulos DB, Greene MF. Anesthesia and developing brains - implications of the FDA warning. N Engl J Med 2017;376(10):905–7.
69. Sanders RD, Hassell J, Davidson AJ, et al. Impact of anaesthetics and surgery on neurodevelopment: an update. Br J Anaesth 2013;110(Suppl 1):i53–72.
70. Wilder RT, Flick RP, Sprung J, et al. Early exposure to anesthesia and learning disabilities in a population-based birth cohort. Anesthesiology 2009;110(4): 796–804.
71. Kalkman CJ, Peelen L, Moons KG, et al. Behavior and development in children and age at the time of first anesthetic exposure. Anesthesiology 2009;110(4): 805–12.
72. Bartels M, Althoff RR, Boomsma DI. Anesthesia and cognitive performance in children: no evidence for a causal relationship. Twin Res Hum Genet 2009; 12(3):246–53.
73. Flick RP, Wilder RT, Sprung J, et al. Anesthesia and cognitive performance in children: no evidence for a causal relationship. Are the conclusions justified by the data? Response to Bartels et al., 2009. Twin Res Hum Genet 2009;12(6):611–2 [discussion: 613–4].
74. McCann ME, Withington DE, Arnup SJ, et al. Differences in blood pressure in infants after general anesthesia compared to awake regional anesthesia (GAS Study-a prospective randomized trial). Anesth Analg 2017;125(3):837–45.
75. Davidson AJ, Morton NS, Arnup SJ, et al. Apnea after awake regional and general anesthesia in infants: the general anesthesia compared to spinal anesthesia study–comparing apnea and neurodevelopmental outcomes, a randomized controlled trial. Anesthesiology 2015;123(1):38–54.
76. Davidson AJ, Disma N, de Graaff JC, et al. Neurodevelopmental outcome at 2 years of age after general anaesthesia and awake-regional anaesthesia in infancy (GAS): an international multicentre, randomised controlled trial. Lancet 2016;387(10015):239–50.
77. McCann ME, de Graaff J. Current thinking regarding potential neurotoxicity of general anesthesia in infants. Curr Opin Urol 2017;27(1):27–33.
78. Sun LS, Li G, Miller TL, et al. Association between a single general anesthesia exposure before age 36 months and neurocognitive outcomes in later childhood. JAMA 2016;315(21):2312–20.
79. Sun LS, Li G, Dimaggio C, et al. Anesthesia and neurodevelopment in children: time for an answer? Anesthesiology 2008;109(5):757–61.

Optimizing Preoperative Anemia to Improve Patient Outcomes

Brittany N. Burton, MHS[a], Alison M. A'Court, MD[b],
Ethan Y. Brovman, MD[c],
Michael J. Scott, MD, ChB, FRCP, FRCA, FFICM[d,e],
Richard D. Urman, MD, MBA[f], Rodney A. Gabriel, MD, MAS[g,h,*]

KEYWORDS

- Anemia • Hemoglobin • Outcomes • Transfusion

KEY POINTS

- Several studies have shown that preoperative anemia leads to increased morbidity and mortality following major surgery.
- The varying degrees of perioperative practice patterns and the health-related impact of preoperative anemia highlight the urgent need to identify new strategies to optimize preoperative anemia.
- Multiple published protocols recommend testing patients for hemoglobin at least 1 month before surgery, to allow intervention and treatment to take effect before surgery. This initial testing can be done at the preoperative clinic visit.
- Although professional society guidelines exist for the perioperative management of blood products, including transfusion triggers and cancellation guidance, less clear guidance exists on the perioperative optimization of patient red blood cell volume to improve clinical outcomes.

Disclosures: None.
[a] School of Medicine, University of California, San Diego, 9500 Gilman Dr, La Jolla, CA 92093, USA; [b] Department of Anesthesiology, Preoperative Care Clinic, University of California, San Diego, 9500 Gilman Dr, La Jolla, CA 92093, USA; [c] Department of Anesthesiology, Perioperative and Pain Medicine, Cardiothoracic Anesthesia, Harvard Medical School, Brigham & Women's Hospital, 75 Francis St, Boston, MA 02115, USA; [d] Department of Anesthesiology, Virginia Commonwealth University Health System, 1200 East Broad Street, PO Box 980695, Richmond, VA 23298, USA; [e] Department of Anesthesiology, Perelman School of Medicine, University of Pennsylvania, 3400 Spruce St, Philadelphia, PA 19104, USA; [f] Department of Anesthesiology, Perioperative and Pain Medicine, Harvard Medical School, Brigham & Women's Hospital, 75 Francis St, Boston, MA 02115, USA; [g] Division of Regional Anesthesia and Acute Pain, Department of Anesthesiology, University of California, San Diego, 9500 Gilman Dr, La Jolla, CA 92093, USA; [h] Department of Medicine, Division of Biomedical Informatics, University of California, San Diego, 9500 Gilman Dr, La Jolla, CA 92093, USA
* Corresponding author. Department of Anesthesiology, University of California, San Diego, 9500 Gilman Drive, MC 0881, La Jolla, CA 92093-0881.
E-mail address: ragabriel@ucsd.edu

Anesthesiology Clin 36 (2018) 701–713
https://doi.org/10.1016/j.anclin.2018.07.017
1932-2275/18/© 2018 Elsevier Inc. All rights reserved.

anesthesiology.theclinics.com

INTRODUCTION

Anemia is a decrease in red blood cell mass, which leads to a reduction in oxygen delivery to tissues. The 2003 to 2012 National Health and Nutrition Examination Surveys (NHANES) estimated that an average of 5.6% of the United States population met the World Health Organization (WHO) criteria for anemia and 1.5% met the criteria for moderate to severe anemia during the study period.[1] In practice, a low hematocrit or hemoglobin concentration is widely used to screen and estimate the degree of anemia. The WHO defines anemia as a hemoglobin concentration less than 13 g/dL in men and less than 12 g/dL in women.[2] The WHO and the National Cancer Institute published revised cutoffs for the evaluation of anemia secondary to complications of cancer, in which anemia is defined as a hemoglobin concentration of less than 14 g/dL and less than 12 g/dL for men and women, respectively.[2]

Iron deficiency is the most common cause of anemia and can be caused by chronic blood loss, poor intake/absorption of iron from the gastrointestinal tract, or a functional state of iron deficiency induced by chronic disease. There are several other causes, such as anemia of chronic disease (eg, cancer, tuberculosis, human immunodeficiency virus), vitamin deficiencies (eg, folate and vitamin B_{12}), blood loss secondary to traumatic injury, chronic renal failure, and hemoglobinopathies. The WHO estimates that 50% of anemia cases are secondary to iron deficiency anemia,[2] However, this estimate is based largely on the geographic region and the population under study. Symptoms of anemia range from weakness and fatigue to angina and reduced cognitive performance. Anemia is the most common preoperative hematologic diagnosis and the reduced oxygen carrying capacity of the blood plays a critical role in causing perioperative morbidity and mortality. Estimates of anemia prevalence in the surgical population have been found to range from 25% to as high as 75% in orthopedic and colorectal surgeries, respectively.[3]

The increasing burden of chronic diseases (eg, heart disease, renal disease, cancer) coupled with an aging population pose unique challenges in optimizing preoperative anemia. Randomized controlled trials have established a hemoglobin concentration of less than 7 g/dL for transfusion, and, although transfusions are used perioperatively in the management of anemia, they are associated with inherent complications. Complications include acute/delayed hemolytic reactions, anaphylactic reactions, and transfusion associated with graft-versus-host disease.[4] Irrespective of degree of preoperative anemia, patients receiving perioperative transfusions were more likely to experience inpatient mortality.[5] As such, anemia and consequent blood transfusion pose a significant threat to postoperative rehabilitation and increases the risk of poor outcomes.

In a Web-based survey of preoperative anemia management practice patterns among liver surgeons and anesthesiologists, Bennet and colleagues[6] found that anesthesiologists (47%) relied heavily on hemoglobin concentration, whereas liver surgeons (33%) relied on hemodynamics when determining intraoperative transfusion. In their evaluation of 97,443 patients who underwent cardiac and noncardiac surgery, Sim and colleagues[7] showed that anemia predicted 1-year mortality. The varying degrees of perioperative practice patterns and the health-related impact of preoperative anemia highlight the urgent need to identify new strategies to optimize preoperative anemia. With this, an understanding of preoperative anemia and postoperative outcomes in various surgical settings is crucial. This article:

1. Reviews the relevant literature and highlights consequences of preoperative anemia in the surgical setting
2. Suggests strategies for screening and optimizing anemia in the preoperative setting

PREOPERATIVE ANEMIA AND POSTOPERATIVE OUTCOMES

The literature on preoperative anemia and postoperative outcomes is discussed here, based on surgical specialty, including cardiac surgery, general surgery, thoracic surgery, spine surgery, orthopedic (eg, joint arthroplasty), and vascular surgery.

Cardiac Surgery

Cardiac surgery patients with anemia commonly present with several comorbidities.[8,9] Studies have identified anemia as an independent predictor of postoperative morbidity and mortality in this surgical population.[10–13] Studies have also shown that anemia is associated with increased risk of postoperative renal dysfunction, for which patients may require renal replacement therapy.[11,14,15] In their evaluation of anemic patients with chronic kidney disease, Shavit and colleagues[16] showed that, for every 1 g/dL decrease in hemoglobin concentration, the odds of mortality, sepsis, postoperative hemodialysis, and cerebrovascular accident significantly increased.

The prevalence of anemia was 26% in a retrospective study that identified 10,589 patients who underwent elective cardiac operations. After adjusting for red blood cell transfusion, anemia remained a risk factor of renal failure, inpatient death, arrhythmias, and longer hospital and intensive care unit (ICU) length of stay.[17] Ranucci and colleagues[18] showed in a retrospective propensity-matched analysis of 401 severely anemic patients undergoing cardiac surgery that anemic patients had significantly higher rates of cerebrovascular accident, major postoperative morbidity, and operative mortality. Moreover, the severity of preoperative anemia and intraoperative blood transfusion both independently led to decreased long-term survival.[19] Hallward and colleagues[20] assessed the relationship between hemoglobin concentration and blood transfusion requirements, hospital length of stay, reoperation, and mortality. For every 1 g/dL increase in hemoglobin, there was a relative 11% decrease in red blood cell units transfused, an 8% decrease in number of platelets transfused, and a 3% decrease in fresh frozen plasma transfused. In addition, lower hemoglobin concentration has been shown to be associated with increased postoperative hospital and ICU length of stay. In a matched case-control study of 1170 cardiac surgery patients, Padmanabhan and colleagues[21] showed that anemic patients were significantly more likely to require postoperative airway support and had higher rates of surgical site infection and postoperative atrial fibrillation. Researchers have evaluated the impact of treating preoperative anemia with strategies other than transfusion. Cladellas and colleagues[22] showed that administration of recombinant human erythropoietin decreases postoperative mortality, blood transfusions, and hospitalization. Based on the existing data, prospective studies are needed to evaluate new strategies to optimally manage perioperative anemia in patients undergoing cardiac surgery.

General Surgery

Preoperative anemia is the most common hematologic disorder in many malignancies and its prevalence ranges from 30% to 90%.[23] In their single-institution retrospective evaluation of 2163 gastric surgery patients, Liu and colleagues[23] showed that preoperative anemia was associated with overall lower survival and an increased rate of perioperative transfusions and postoperative complications. Anemia has been identified as a marker of disease severity in inflammatory bowel disease (IBD), and the prevalence of colectomy for IBD is roughly 30% worldwide.[24] Michailidou and Nfonsam[24] showed that preoperative anemia predicted morbidity and increased hospital length of stay in patients with IBD following colorectal surgery. Preoperative anemia is also an independent risk factor of postoperative venous thromboembolism in patients with IBD following colectomy.[25] After adjustment, preoperative anemia is associated with increases risk of morbidity following hepatectomy.[26] Similarly, Lucas and colleagues[27] showed that hepatopancreatobiliary surgery patients with preoperative hematocrit less than 36% were significantly more likely to require postoperative transfusion. Furthermore, in patients undergoing resection of colorectal liver metastases, correction of preoperative anemia with allogenic red blood cell transfusion was independently associated with lower recurrence-free survival.[28] Despite the well-understood pathology and ease of diagnosis, perioperative anemia continues to be a challenging issue. Physicians should continue efforts to develop guidelines for perioperative management of anemia.

Thoracic Surgery

Postoperative complications directly influence postoperative mortality following thoracic surgery. Using the American College of Surgeons (ACS) National Surgical Quality Improvement Program (NSQIP), Jean and colleagues[29] evaluated 6434 lung resection patients and showed that the odds of 30-day mortality were 53% higher in patients with preoperative anemia compared with those without. Likewise, in their retrospective analysis of 125 patients with non–small cell lung cancer, Yovino and colleagues[30] found that preoperative hemoglobin level less than 12 g/dL predicted worse relapse-free and overall survival. Berardi and colleagues[31] found that perioperative anemia predicted postoperative mortality and this relationship remained after correction of anemia with red blood cell transfusion. In contrast, Melis and colleagues[32] showed that preoperative anemia was not associated with poor outcomes in patients undergoing esophagectomy, but preoperative anemia was independently associated with increased rate of perioperative blood transfusions, and such transfusions were associated with higher risk of overall complications and surgical site infections.

Spine Surgery

Over the last decade, the prevalence of spine surgeries has dramatically increased. With an increasing elderly population, there is also an increase in perioperative comorbidities that consequently increase the risk of postoperative morbidity and mortality.[33] Patients with anemia are significantly more likely to have several preoperative risk factors of poor outcomes, including diabetes mellitus, American Society of Anesthesiologists physical status classification greater than or equal to 3, and dependent functional status.[34] In patients undergoing posterior cervical fusion, preoperative anemia was associated with roughly a 3-fold increase in any complications, pulmonary complications, perioperative transfusions, reoperation, readmission, and extended hospital length of stay (ie, >5 days).[34] Similarly, in a retrospective study using data from ACS NSQIP, 3500 patients undergoing anterior cervical discectomy and fusion were included in the final analysis. Preoperative anemia was a prognostic indicator of any complication, pulmonary complications, intraoperative blood transfusions, reoperation, and hospital length of stay greater than 5 days.[35] Moreover, low preoperative hematocrit (ie, <40%) was shown to be associated with hospital stay greater than 5 days in patients receiving lumbar spinal procedures.[36] In adult patients undergoing elective spine surgeries, anemic patients had an increased risk of perioperative blood transfusion, which was associated with morbidity and mortality.[33] Preoperative hematocrit was also identified as an independent risk factor of postoperative 30-day reintubation in a cohort of 8648 cervical spine surgery patients.[33]

Orthopedic Surgery

In patients undergoing total hip and knee arthroplasty, preoperative anemia was associated with postoperative complications, extended hospital length of stay, and increased rates of allogenic red blood cell transfusions.[37] Similarly, after total knee arthroplasty in noncardiac patients, preoperative anemia was shown to be associated with higher odds of transfusions and pulmonary and renal postoperative complications.[38] After controlling for potential confounders, preoperative hematocrit less than 38% was associated with short-term inpatient complications following total shoulder arthroplasty.[39] Perioperative red blood cell transfusion is also associated with significantly higher rates of myocardial infarction, pneumonia, sepsis, venous thromboembolism, and cerebrovascular accident in patients undergoing shoulder arthroplasty.[40] Dix and colleagues[41] evaluated 39 patients who underwent hindfoot and ankle arthrodesis and found that preoperative anemia was associated with surgery-specific complications (ie, delayed union, nonunion, and malunion), postoperative infection, and longer hospital stay.

Elderly anemic patients are at increased risk of postoperative adverse events secondary to the aging process and the comorbidity burden associated with perioperative anemia. Furthermore, anemia is common in orthopedic surgery. A systematic literature review of perioperative anemia in hip or knee arthroplasty showed that preoperative anemia was prevalent in 24% to 44% of the patients and postoperative anemia occurred in 51% of patients.[42] Furthermore, that review showed that anemic patients had significantly higher rates of red blood cell transfusion, postoperative infection, and mortality, as well as poor postoperative recovery and increased hospital length of stay.[42] In their assessment of postoperative outcomes after total hip and knee arthroplasty in patients more than 85 years old, Pittert and colleagues[43] found that preoperative anemia was associated with 90-day readmission. In Medicare patients, Bozic and colleagues[44] showed that several comorbidities along with preoperative anemia were associated with an increased risk of periprosthetic joint infections and postoperative 90-day mortality following total hip arthroplasty.

Vascular Surgery

Anemic patients undergoing vascular surgery are at higher risk of several postoperative adverse events. Bodewes and colleagues[45] evaluated 5081 patients with chronic limb-threatening ischemia undergoing infrainguinal bypass surgery and showed that anemic patients tended to be older with higher comorbidity burden. Severe preoperative anemia was associated with increased odds of short-term mortality, major amputation, adverse postoperative cardiovascular events, and reoperation. The relationship between preoperative anemia and mortality remains significant for patients following carotid endarterectomy.[46] It is well established that blood transfusions are common among patients receiving vascular surgery. Obi and colleagues[47] investigated the impact of perioperative transfusions on 30-day morbidity and mortality in 2964 patients undergoing peripheral arterial disease procedures and aneurysm repair and found a 25% transfusion rate with preoperative anemia predicting perioperative transfusions. With advancements in technology, there is an increasing prevalence of elderly patients undergoing vascular surgery. Peripheral arterial disease is estimated to occur at a rate of 29% in this population. Using the ACS NSQIP database to evaluate 31,857 patients 65 years of age or older, Gupta and colleagues[48] found an inverse relationship between postoperative mortality and preoperative hematocrit following elective vascular procedures. Moreover, there is a lower perioperative hematocrit following open surgery versus endovascular repair of ruptured abdominal aortic aneurysm.[49]

ANEMIA SCREENING IN THE PREOPERATIVE ASSESSMENT CLINIC

Patient blood management is defined by the Society for the Advancement of Blood Management as the timely application of evidence-based medical and surgical concepts designed to maintain hemoglobin concentration, optimize hemostasis, and minimize blood loss to improve patient outcome. The 3 pillars include the optimization of red blood cell mass, reduction of blood loss and bleeding, and optimization of the patient's physiologic tolerance of anemia (**Fig. 1**).[50]

In the setting of the preoperative clinic, integrating the principles of patient blood management focuses on the first pillar: optimization of red blood cell mass to reduce perioperative transfusions. The preoperative clinic identifies patients with anemia before major elective surgery (**Fig. 2**). Once these patients are identified, the anemia can be evaluated and treated per protocols before surgery. These protocols vary by institution, but common approaches to these protocols are discussed later. Correcting anemia before surgery reduces the risk of perioperative transfusion in joint arthroplasty patients, with a relative risk of 0.48 in a meta-analysis.[51] It is reasonable to consider that patient outcomes should be improved by avoiding the known risks of severe anemia and transfusion as well as by treating underlying diseases. In addition, reductions in perioperative transfusion can result in reduced costs to the blood bank and health care system.[52] The Duke Perioperative Enhancement Team implemented a thorough financial modeling of a perioperative anemia screening program that showed a positive net value of more than $2.5 million over 5 years.[53]

Time Frame: When to Screen

Treatment of anemia in the preoperative period has a stronger level of evidence in improving anemia and transfusion-related outcomes than in the immediate perioperative period or the postoperative period.[52] Accordingly, multiple published protocols recommend testing patients for hemoglobin at least 1 month before surgery, to allow intervention and treatment to take effect before surgery.[54,55] This initial testing can be done at the preoperative clinic visit with a point-of-care test for a real-time result, or by ordering a complete blood count (CBC) as part of the preoperative laboratory tests.

Surgery Types: Who to Test/Screen

The decision regarding which patients to screen varies by institution. Screening all patients for hemoglobin is one approach, but several institutions make the decision to screen all patients presenting for specific surgeries with higher blood loss (>500 mL) or higher transfusion rates (>10%).[55] Most commonly, this includes major orthopedic (eg, total joint) and spine surgeries.[53] A third approach is to screen all patients for whom surgical orders include a crossmatch order.

What to Do with Identified Anemic Patients

The WHO criteria for anemia are hemoglobin level less than 13 g/dL in men and less than 12 g/dL in women.[56] Despite the gender differences in the WHO definition of anemia, some algorithms choose a hemoglobin level of 13 g/dL as the screening criteria

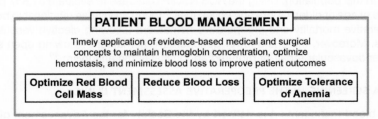

Fig. 1. Patient blood management goals.

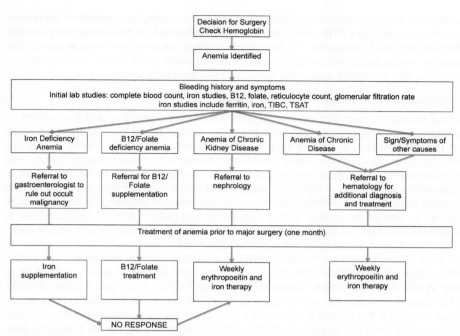

Fig. 2. Proposed evaluation and treatment algorithm for preoperative anemia. TIBC, total iron-binding capacity; TSAT, transferrin saturation.

for both genders. The reasoning is that female patients have a lower circulating blood volume, therefore a given amount of surgical blood loss would have a larger impact on perioperative anemia.[52] Once the syndrome of anemia is identified by these initial criteria, the triage of initial assessment and referral is summarized in **Fig. 2**. In parallel to referral for follow-up, the patient can also start treatment in the preoperative clinic for preoperative correction of the anemia before surgery.

TREATMENT OF ANEMIA FOR PREOPERATIVE OPTIMIZATION

Although professional society guidelines exist for the perioperative management of blood products, including transfusion triggers and cancellation guidance, less clear guidance exists on the perioperative optimization of patient red blood cell volume to improve clinical outcomes.[57–60] Preoperative anemia is clearly associated with worsened outcomes postoperatively. A holistic approach to perioperative blood management focuses on preoperative optimization of red blood cell mass, minimization and mitigation of intraoperative blood loss, and goal-directed management of postoperative anemia.[61] This article focuses on preoperative management and therefore the optimization of red blood cell mass. Treatment strategies can be broadly broken down into correction of reversible causes of anemia, enhanced red blood cell production, and preoperative transfusion.

Assessment of Anemia

Recommendations from the European Society of Anaesthesiology recommend that hemoglobin concentrations be measured 4 to 8 weeks before surgery, particularly if the patient is at risk for perioperative bleeding.[62] The goal of early identification is to allow time for preoperative interventions to result in meaningful increases in the hemoglobin concentration. At this time, no recommendation can be made regarding a target hemoglobin level preoperatively. Although increasing severity of anemia is associated with worsened postoperative outcomes, a clear causal link between preoperative optimization and improved outcomes has not been definitively shown.

Identification of Reversible Causes of Anemia

Once anemia is identified on preoperative laboratory screening and the patient is scheduled to undergo a surgery with moderate to high blood loss, further evaluation of potential reversible causes of anemia is warranted. Initial laboratory evaluation should focus on common, easily reversible causes, with assessment of serum iron and transferrin levels, total iron binding capacity, and ferritin levels to identify potential iron deficiency anemia. A CBC with assessment of the mean corpuscular volume can identify macrocytosis and should prompt assessment of vitamin B_{12} and folic acid levels, as well as prompting further assessment of patient alcohol consumption. A measure of systemic inflammation, such as the C-reactive protein or erythrocyte sedimentation rate, is often useful in the interpretation of iron studies. In addition, a marker of renal function, such as the serum creatinine level, should be assessed. This evaluation allows determination of the major, most common causes of anemia, as shown in **Fig. 2**: iron deficiency, other nutritional deficiency, anemia of chronic disease, anemia of chronic kidney disease, or the category of other less common hematologic or oncologic causes. If this testing is done and treatment is started in the preoperative clinic, patients still need to be referred for follow-up of the underlying cause of anemia. Iron deficiency anemia is the most common cause of anemia in preoperative patients, accounting for approximately 33% of cases.[2] If iron deficiency anemia is identified as the cause, referral may be made to a gastroenterologist to rule out occult malignancy, and the primary care provider should be notified. If glomerular filtration rate is less than 60 mL/min, a referral is made to nephrology. If folate or B_{12} levels are low, referral is made to primary care or nutrition for treatment. If these are all normal, the diagnosis of anemia of chronic disease is considered. If the anemia is severe (hemoglobin level <8 g/dL), other components of the CBC are abnormal, or history and physical suggest other causes of anemia, referral is made to primary care or hematology.

Management of Iron Deficiency Anemia

Iron deficiency anemia is a common cause of preoperative anemia and is readily corrected with administration of exogenous iron. Both oral and intravenous (IV) formulations of iron exist. Oral iron is an easily accessible, low-cost method of iron repletion that has been shown to decrease the likelihood of perioperative blood transfusion.[63] However, oral iron administration is limited by several factors, including patient adherence because of induced gastrointestinal upset, poor bioavailability, and the need for prolonged oral administration to restore adequate iron stores.

IV iron formulations have shown equivalent efficacy to enteral iron in the treatment of iron deficiency anemia, with fewer adverse effects and decreased time to efficacy. IV iron may be preferred in situations in which oral iron is not practical, such as when the time to surgery is less than 6 to 8 weeks, or the required intake is impossible because of patient adherence. IV iron has been shown to decrease the need for perioperative blood transfusion and improve hospital stay in several studies.[64,65]

Enhanced Red Blood Cell Production

In patients with adequate iron stores and without evidence of other macronutrient deficiencies, preoperative anemia is often assumed to be caused by impaired erythropoiesis. Use of recombinant human erythropoietin has been shown in several meta-analyses to effectively increase the preoperative hemoglobin level and reduce the need for perioperative blood transfusions.[66,67] The precise dosing, route of administration, frequency, and duration of treatment remain unknown. The most frequent dosing regimen is once-weekly erythropoietin injections, and usually results in an increase in hemoglobin level of between 0.5 g/dL and 1 g/dL per week. Clinicians considering implementation of erythropoietin treatment in the preoperative clinic should be aware of the contraindications to erythropoietin treatment, which include uncontrolled hypertension; severe or recent coronary, cerebral, or peripheral disease; and uncontrolled seizure disorder.[68] Erythropoietin is avoided in patients with cancer not on myelosuppressive chemotherapy because of increased risk of recurrence and progression in several cancers. In addition, although the adverse effects of erythropoietin administration have been well described in multiple other populations, the specific risks of preoperative administration are unclear.[69–71] Specifically, whether erythropoietin increases the rates of perioperative thrombotic events, including venous thromboembolism and myocardial infarction, in patients receiving erythropoietin is uncertain.[66,72]

Preoperative Blood Transfusion

Routine preoperative blood transfusion is not routinely recommended except in situations of symptomatic anemia in which transfusion is recommended by guidelines, or in cases of hemoglobinopathies such as sickle cell anemia.[73] The optimal method of transfusion for patients with sickle cell disease remains unknown. Consultation with a hematologist is recommended in these situations.[74]

SUMMARY

Anemia is a common preoperative finding in surgical populations. With only subtle clinical symptoms except when anemia becomes severe, a systematic approach to the screening and clinical assessment of anemia is needed when performing a preoperative assessment. Given the association between the severity of anemia and increased complication rates, mortality, and hospital length of stay, it is important to identify and optimize these patients. The risk factors associated with transfusion of blood products during the perioperative period mean that preoperative treatment of anemia is a key strategy for improving postsurgical outcomes.

REFERENCES

1. Le CH. The prevalence of anemia and moderate-severe anemia in the US population (NHANES 2003-2012). PLoS One 2016;11(11):e0166635.
2. Benoist BD, McLean E, Egll I, et al. Worldwide prevalence of anaemia 1993-2005: WHO global database on anaemia. Worldwide prevalence of anaemia 1993-2005. WHO Global Database on Anaemia; 2008.
3. Kansagra AJ, Stefan MS. Preoperative anemia: evaluation and treatment. Anesthesiol Clin 2016;34(1):127–41.
4. Hendrickson JE, Hillyer CD. Noninfectious serious hazards of transfusion. Anesth Analg 2009;108(3):759–69.
5. Gabriel RA, Clark AI, Nguyen AP, et al. The association of preoperative hematocrit and transfusion with mortality in patients undergoing elective non-cardiac surgery. World J Surg 2018;42(7):1939–48.
6. Bennett S, Ayoub A, Tran A, et al. Current practices in perioperative blood management for patients undergoing liver resection: a survey of surgeons and anesthesiologists. Transfusion 2018;58(3):781–7.

7. Sim YE, Wee HE, Ang AL, et al. Prevalence of preoperative anemia, abnormal mean corpuscular volume and red cell distribution width among surgical patients in Singapore, and their influence on one year mortality. PLoS One 2017;12(8): e0182543.

8. Matsuda S, Fukui T, Shimizu J, et al. Associations between preoperative anemia and outcomes after off-pump coronary artery bypass grafting. Ann Thorac Surg 2013;95(3):854–60.

9. Mirhosseini SJ, Sayegh SA. Effect of preoperative anemia on short term clinical outcomes in diabetic patients after elective off-pump CABG surgery. Acta Med Iran 2012;50(9):615–8.

10. Miceli A, Romeo F, Glauber M, et al. Preoperative anemia increases mortality and postoperative morbidity after cardiac surgery. J Cardiothorac Surg 2014;9:137.

11. Oprea AD, Del Rio JM, Cooter M, et al. Pre- and postoperative anemia, acute kidney injury, and mortality after coronary artery bypass grafting surgery: a retrospective observational study. Can J Anaesth 2018;65(1):46–59.

12. Deepak B, Balaji A, Pramod A, et al. The prevalence and impact of preoperative anemia in patients undergoing cardiac surgery for rheumatic heart disease. J Cardiothorac Vasc Anesth 2016;30(4):896–900.

13. Zhang L, Hiebert B, Zarychanski R, et al, Cardiovascular Health Research in Manitoba Investigator Group. Preoperative anemia does not increase the risks of early surgical revascularization after myocardial infarction. Ann Thorac Surg 2013;95(2):542–7.

14. Paparella D, Guida P, Mazzei V, et al. Hemoglobin and renal replacement therapy after cardiopulmonary bypass surgery: a predictive score from the Cardiac Surgery Registry of Puglia. Int J Cardiol 2014;176(3):866–73.

15. De Santo L, Romano G, Della Corte A, et al. Preoperative anemia in patients undergoing coronary artery bypass grafting predicts acute kidney injury. J Thorac Cardiovasc Surg 2009;138(4):965–70.

16. Shavit L, Hitti S, Silberman S, et al. Preoperative hemoglobin and outcomes in patients with CKD undergoing cardiac surgery. Clin J Am Soc Nephrol 2014;9(9): 1536–44.

17. Dai L, Mick SL, McCrae KR, et al. Preoperative anemia in cardiac operation: does hemoglobin tell the whole story? Ann Thorac Surg 2018;105(1):100–7.

18. Ranucci M, Di Dedda U, Castelvecchio S, et al. Impact of preoperative anemia on outcome in adult cardiac surgery: a propensity-matched analysis. Ann Thorac Surg 2012;94(4):1134–41.

19. von Heymann C, Kaufner L, Sander M, et al. Does the severity of preoperative anemia or blood transfusion have a stronger impact on long-term survival after cardiac surgery? J Thorac Cardiovasc Surg 2016;152(5):1412–20.

20. Hallward G, Balani N, McCorkell S, et al. The relationship between preoperative hemoglobin concentration, use of hospital resources, and outcomes in cardiac surgery. J Cardiothorac Vasc Anesth 2016;30(4):901–8.

21. Padmanabhan H, Aktuerk D, Brookes MJ, et al. Anemia in cardiac surgery: next target for mortality and morbidity improvement? Asian Cardiovasc Thorac Ann 2016;24(1):12–7.

22. Cladellas M, Farre N, Comin-Colet J, et al. Effects of preoperative intravenous erythropoietin plus iron on outcome in anemic patients after cardiac valve replacement. Am J Cardiol 2012;110(7):1021–6.

23. Liu X, Qiu H, Huang Y, et al. Impact of preoperative anemia on outcomes in patients undergoing curative resection for gastric cancer: a single-institution retrospective analysis of 2163 Chinese patients. Cancer Med 2018;7(2):360–9.

24. Michailidou M, Nfonsam VN. Preoperative anemia and outcomes in patients undergoing surgery for inflammatory bowel disease. Am J Surg 2018;215(1):78–81.
25. Henke PK, Arya S, Pannucci C, et al. Procedure-specific venous thromboembolism prophylaxis: a paradigm from colectomy surgery. Surgery 2012;152(4): 528–34 [discussion: 534–6].
26. Tohme S, Varley PR, Landsittel DP, et al. Preoperative anemia and postoperative outcomes after hepatectomy. HPB (Oxford) 2016;18(3):255–61.
27. Lucas DJ, Schexneider KI, Weiss M, et al. Trends and risk factors for transfusion in hepatopancreatobiliary surgery. J Gastrointest Surg 2014;18(4):719–28.
28. Schiergens TS, Rentsch M, Kasparek MS, et al. Impact of perioperative allogeneic red blood cell transfusion on recurrence and overall survival after resection of colorectal liver metastases. Dis Colon Rectum 2015;58(1):74–82.
29. Jean RA, DeLuzio MR, Kraev AI, et al. Analyzing risk factors for morbidity and mortality after lung resection for lung cancer using the NSQIP database. J Am Coll Surg 2016;222(6):992–1000.e1.
30. Yovino S, Kwok Y, Krasna M, et al. An association between preoperative anemia and decreased survival in early-stage non-small-cell lung cancer patients treated with surgery alone. Int J Radiat Oncol Biol Phys 2005;62(5):1438–43.
31. Berardi R, Brunelli A, Tamburrano T, et al. Perioperative anemia and blood transfusions as prognostic factors in patients undergoing resection for non-small cell lung cancers. Lung Cancer 2005;49(3):371–6.
32. Melis M, McLoughlin JM, Dean EM, et al. Correlations between neoadjuvant treatment, anemia, and perioperative complications in patients undergoing esophagectomy for cancer. J Surg Res 2009;153(1):114–20.
33. Seicean A, Seicean S, Alan N, et al. Preoperative anemia and perioperative outcomes in patients who undergo elective spine surgery. Spine (Phila Pa 1976) 2013;38(15):1331–41.
34. Phan K, Dunn AE, Kim JS, et al. Impact of preoperative anemia on outcomes in adults undergoing elective posterior cervical fusion. Global Spine J 2017;7(8): 787–93.
35. Phan K, Wang N, Kim JS, et al. Effect of preoperative anemia on the outcomes of anterior cervical discectomy and fusion. Global Spine J 2017;7(5):441–7.
36. Guan J, Karsy M, Schmidt MH, et al. Impact of preoperative hematocrit level on length of stay after surgery on the lumbar spine. Global Spine J 2015;5(5):391–5.
37. Pujol-Nicolas A, Morrison R, Casson C, et al. Preoperative screening and intervention for mild anemia with low iron stores in elective hip and knee arthroplasty. Transfusion 2017;57(12):3049–57.
38. Chamieh JS, Tamim HM, Masrouha KZ, et al. The association of anemia and its severity with cardiac outcomes and mortality after total knee arthroplasty in noncardiac patients. J Arthroplasty 2016;31(4):766–70.
39. Anthony CA, Westermann RW, Gao Y, et al. What are risk factors for 30-day morbidity and transfusion in total shoulder arthroplasty? A review of 1922 cases. Clin Orthop Relat Res 2015;473(6):2099–105.
40. Grier AJ, Bala A, Penrose CT, et al. Analysis of complication rates following perioperative transfusion in shoulder arthroplasty. J Shoulder Elbow Surg 2017;26(7):1203–9.
41. Dix B, Grant-McDonald L, Catanzariti A, et al. Preoperative anemia in hindfoot and ankle arthrodesis. Foot Ankle Spec 2017;10(2):109–15.
42. Spahn DR. Anemia and patient blood management in hip and knee surgery: a systematic review of the literature. Anesthesiology 2010;113(2):482–95.
43. Pitter FT, Jorgensen CC, Lindberg-Larsen M, et al, Lundbeck Foundation Center for Fast-track Hip and Knee Replacement Collaborative Group. Postoperative

morbidity and discharge destinations after fast-track hip and knee arthroplasty in patients older than 85 years. Anesth Analg 2016;122(6):1807–15.

44. Bozic KJ, Lau E, Kurtz S, et al. Patient-related risk factors for periprosthetic joint infection and postoperative mortality following total hip arthroplasty in Medicare patients. J Bone Joint Surg Am 2012;94(9):794–800.

45. Bodewes TCF, Pothof AB, Darling JD, et al. Preoperative anemia associated with adverse outcomes after infrainguinal bypass surgery in patients with chronic limb-threatening ischemia. J Vasc Surg 2017;66(6):1775–85.e2.

46. Pothof AB, Bodewes TCF, O'Donnell TFX, et al. Preoperative anemia is associated with mortality after carotid endarterectomy in symptomatic patients. J Vasc Surg 2018;67(1):183–90.e1.

47. Obi AT, Park YJ, Bove P, et al. The association of perioperative transfusion with 30-day morbidity and mortality in patients undergoing major vascular surgery. J Vasc Surg 2015;61(4):1000–9.e1.

48. Gupta PK, Sundaram A, Mactaggart JN, et al. Preoperative anemia is an independent predictor of postoperative mortality and adverse cardiac events in elderly patients undergoing elective vascular operations. Ann Surg 2013; 258(6):1096–102.

49. Davenport DL, O'Keeffe SD, Minion DJ, et al. Thirty-day NSQIP database outcomes of open versus endoluminal repair of ruptured abdominal aortic aneurysms. J Vasc Surg 2010;51(2):305–9.e1.

50. Society for the Advancement of Blood Management (SABM). Administrative and clinical standards for patient blood management programs 4th edition. 2017. Available at: https://www.sabm.org/publications. Accessed February 28, 2018.

51. Alsaleh K, Alotaibi GS, Almodaimegh HS, et al. The use of preoperative erythropoiesis-stimulating agents (ESAs) in patients who underwent knee or hip arthroplasty: a meta-analysis of randomized clinical trials. J Arthroplasty 2013; 28(9):1463–72.

52. Desai N, Schofield N, Richards T. Perioperative patient blood management to improve outcomes. Anesth Analg 2017. [Epub ahead of print]. https://doi.org/10.1213/ANE.0000000000002549.

53. Guinn NR, Guercio JR, Hopkins TJ, et al. How do we develop and implement a preoperative anemia clinic designed to improve perioperative outcomes and reduce cost? Transfusion 2016;56(2):297–303.

54. Goodnough LT, Maniatis A, Earnshaw P, et al. Detection, evaluation, and management of preoperative anaemia in the elective orthopaedic surgical patient: NATA guidelines. Br J Anaesth 2011;106(1):13–22.

55. Goodnough LT, Shander A. Patient blood management. Anesthesiology 2012; 116(6):1367–76.

56. Nutritional anaemias. Report of a WHO scientific group. World Health Organ Tech Rep Ser 1968;405:5–37.

57. American Society of Anesthesiologists Task Force on Perioperative Blood Management. Practice guidelines for perioperative blood management: an updated report by the American Society of Anesthesiologists Task Force on Perioperative Blood Management*. Anesthesiology 2015;122(2):241–75.

58. Fleisher LA, Fleischmann KE, Auerbach AD, et al. 2014 ACC/AHA guideline on perioperative cardiovascular evaluation and management of patients undergoing noncardiac surgery: executive summary: a report of the American College of Cardiology/American Heart Association Task Force on Practice Guidelines. Developed in collaboration with the American College of Surgeons, American Society of Anesthesiologists, American Society of Echocardiography, American

Society of Nuclear Cardiology, Heart Rhythm Society, Society for Cardiovascular Angiography and Interventions, Society of Cardiovascular Anesthesiologists, and Society of Vascular Medicine endorsed by the Society of Hospital Medicine. J Nucl Cardiol 2015;22(1):162–215.

59. Society of Thoracic Surgeons Blood Conservation Guideline Task Force, Ferraris VA, Ferraris SP, Saha SP, et al. Perioperative blood transfusion and blood conservation in cardiac surgery: the Society of Thoracic Surgeons and The Society of Cardiovascular Anesthesiologists clinical practice guideline. Ann Thorac Surg 2007;83(5 Suppl):S27–86.

60. Carson JL, Stanworth SJ, Roubinian N, et al. Transfusion thresholds and other strategies for guiding allogeneic red blood cell transfusion. Cochrane Database Syst Rev 2016;10:CD002042.

61. National Clinical Guideline Centre (UK). Blood transfusion. London: National Institute for Health and Care Excellence (UK); 2015.

62. Kozek-Langenecker SA, Ahmed AB, Afshari A, et al. Management of severe perioperative bleeding: guidelines from the European Society of Anaesthesiology: first update 2016. Eur J Anaesthesiol 2017;34(6):332–95.

63. Clevenger B, Gurusamy K, Klein AA, et al. Systematic review and meta-analysis of iron therapy in anaemic adults without chronic kidney disease: updated and abridged Cochrane Review. Eur J Heart Fail 2016;18(7):774–85.

64. Munoz M, Gomez-Ramirez S, Cuenca J, et al. Very-short-term perioperative intravenous iron administration and postoperative outcome in major orthopedic surgery: a pooled analysis of observational data from 2547 patients. Transfusion 2014;54(2):289–99.

65. Froessler B, Palm P, Weber I, et al. The important role for intravenous iron in perioperative patient blood management in major abdominal surgery: a randomized controlled trial. Ann Surg 2016;264(1):41–6.

66. Lin DM, Lin ES, Tran MH. Efficacy and safety of erythropoietin and intravenous iron in perioperative blood management: a systematic review. Transfus Med Rev 2013;27(4):221–34.

67. Weltert L, Rondinelli B, Bello R, et al. A single dose of erythropoietin reduces perioperative transfusions in cardiac surgery: results of a prospective single-blind randomized controlled trial. Transfusion 2015;55(7):1644–54.

68. Prescriber's Digital Reference. Epoetin alfa-drug summary. 2018. Available at: http://www.pdr.net/drug-summary/Procrit-epoetin-alfa-280.2692. Accessed March 8, 2018.

69. Swedberg K, Young JB, Anand IS, et al. Treatment of anemia with darbepoetin alfa in systolic heart failure. N Engl J Med 2013;368(13):1210–9.

70. Macdougall IC, Provenzano R, Sharma A, et al. Peginesatide for anemia in patients with chronic kidney disease not receiving dialysis. N Engl J Med 2013; 368(4):320–32.

71. Solomon SD, Uno H, Lewis EF, et al. Erythropoietic response and outcomes in kidney disease and type 2 diabetes. N Engl J Med 2010;363(12):1146–55.

72. Duce L, Cooter ML, McCartney SL, et al. Outcomes in patients undergoing cardiac surgery who decline transfusion and received erythropoietin compared to patients who did not: a matched cohort study. Anesth Analg 2018;127(2):490–5.

73. Carson JL, Grossman BJ, Kleinman S, et al. Red blood cell transfusion: a clinical practice guideline from the AABB*. Ann Intern Med 2012;157(1):49–58.

74. Estcourt LJ, Fortin PM, Trivella M, et al. Preoperative blood transfusion for sickle cell disease. Cochrane Database Syst Rev 2016;(4):CD003149.